Sixth Edition

Textbook of Biochemistry for Dental Students

Including Practical Exercises

Other Books by the Same Author

- *Textbook of Biochemistry, 4th ed*
- *Biochemistry for BSc Nursing Students, 4th ed*
- *Food and Nutrition: Medical, Nursing and Allied Sciences, 2nd ed*
- *MCQs in Biochemistry*
- *Essentials of Pharmaceutical Biochemistry, 2nd ed*
- *Essentials of Biochemistry for BSc Nursing Students*

Sixth Edition

Textbook of Biochemistry for Dental Students

Including Practical Exercises

Harbans Lal PhD FIAO FACBI FSOBSI
Former Senior Professor and Head
Department of Biochemistry
Maharaja Agrasen Medical College, Agroha (Hisar)
Former Senior Professor
Department of Biochemistry
Pt BD Sharma Postgraduate Institute of Medical Sciences
Rohtak (Haryana)
Ex-WHO Fellow

CBSPD

CBS Publishers & Distributors Pvt Ltd
New Delhi • Bengaluru • Chennai • Kochi • Kolkata • Lucknow • Mumbai
Hyderabad • Jharkhand • Nagpur • Patna • Pune • Uttarakhand

Sixth Edition

Textbook of
Biochemistry
for Dental Students
Including Practical Exercises

ISBN: 978-93-5466-863-0

Sixth Edition: 2025
First Edition: 1997
Reprint: 1999
Second Edition: 2000
Reprint: 2000, 2003, 2004
Third Edition: 2006
Reprint: 2006, 2008
Fourth Edition: 2010
Reprint: 2011, 2012, 2013, 2014, 2015, 2016
Fifth Edition: 2019

Published by **Satish Kumar Jain** and produced by **Varun Jain** for

CBS Publishers & Distributors Pvt Ltd

4819/XI Prahlad Street, 24 Ansari Road, Daryaganj, New Delhi 110 002, India
Ph: 011-23266838, 23289259   Website: www.cbspd.com
e-mail: delhi@cbspd.com

Corporate Office: 204 FIE, Industrial Area, Patparganj, Delhi 110 092, India
Ph: 011-49344934   Fax: 011-49344935   e-mail: publishing@cbspd.com; publicity@cbspd.com

Branches

- **Bengaluru:** Seema House 2975, 17th Cross, K.R. Road, Banasankari 2nd Stage, Bengaluru 560 070, Karnataka, India
  Ph: +91-80-26771678/79   Fax: +91-80-26771680   e-mail: bangalore@cbspd.com
- **Chennai:** 18/8B, Subbaraya Street, Shenoy Nagar, Chennai 600 030, Tamil Nadu, India
  Ph: +91-44-42032115, 26681266   e-mail: chennai@cbspd.com
- **Kochi:** 42/1325, 1326, Power House Road, Opposite KSEB, Power House, Ernakulum 682018, Kochi, Kerala, India
  Ph: +91-484-4059061–65   Fax: +91-484-4059065   e-mail: kochi@cbspd.com
- **Kolkata:** 147, Hind Ceramics Compound, 1st Floor, Nilgunj Road, Belghoria, Kolkata 700056, West Bengal, India
  Ph: +91-33-25330055/56   e-mail: kolkata@cbspd.com
- **Lucknow:** Basement, Khushuma Complex, 7 Meerabai Marg (behind Jawahar Bhawan), Lucknow 226001, UP, India
  Ph: +91-522-4000032   e-mail: tiwari.lucknow@cbspd.com
- **Mumbai:** PWD Shed, Gala No. 25/26, Ramchandra Bhatt Marg, Next JJ Hospital, Gate No. 2, Opp. Union Bank of India, Noorbaug, Mumbai 400009, Maharashtra, India
  Ph: +91-22-66661880/89   e-mail: mumbai@cbspd.com

Representatives

- **Hyderabad** 0-9885175004
- **Jharkhand** 0-9811541605
- **Nagpur** 0-8692091830
- **Patna** 0-9334159340
- **Pune** 0-9664372571
- **Uttarakhand** 0-9716462459

Printed at: Sri Prints and Sales, Delhi, India

Preface to the Sixth Edition

It gives me immense pleasure to present the sixth edition of the *Textbook of Biochemistry for Dental Students*. The book has been thoroughly revised and updated. Like the previous editions, the new edition intends to convey the knowledge of time-old principles, which has been supplemented with modern developments in biochemistry. The figures and diagrams have been updated and simplified. Information regarding Recommended Daily Allowances for Indians has been updated as per Indian Council of Medical Research-National Institute of Nutrition Expert Group 2020. The subject matter has been written in a simple, precise and lucid manner which will not only help the dental students to grasp the basics of the subject but also prepare them for future integration with the clinical subjects in their journey to become knowledgeable dental graduates. My endeavour always has been to keep the subject matter simple, relevant and easy to understand for the students.

I express my sincere thanks and acknowledgements to the Director, National Institute of Nutrition (ICMR), Hyderabad, for the use RDA for Indians as per recommendations of the ICMR-NIN Group 2020. I am also thankful to Mr Satish Kumar Jain, CMD and the entire team from CBS Publishers & Distributors Pvt. Ltd., New Delhi, for bringing out this edition of the book in a very short time.

Keeping aside some shortcomings that may have crept in, it is expected that the book will be welcomed by the teachers and the students of the various dental colleges not only in India but also other countries worldwide. Comments and constructive criticism, of course, will ensure further improvement of the book.

Harbans Lal

July 2024

hl.biopgimsr@gmail.com

Preface to the First Edition

In the past few years, a number of textbooks in biochemistry have been published primarily for students of medicine, but none for students of dentistry. This textbook *A textbook of Biochemistry for Dental Students* has been written to meet the needs of dental students. While compiling this book of author has consulted several syllabi so as to cover all the topics prescribed for the BDS students of various universities. However, though concise, this textbook provides sufficient up-to-date material for learners of biochemistry even in Pharmacy, Nursing and other allied disciplines at the undergraduate level. The quantum of knowledge that is to be imparted to the students, in this period of ever-growing interdisciplinary speciality, has been presented in a simple and easily understandable language. Wherever necessary, the text has been illustrated with the help of self-explanatory reactions, diagrams, and tables. Some important questions have also been given at the end of each chapter for the benefit of students.

The text consists of 14 chapters and begins with an introduction to the subject. After a note on the cell and functions of the various organelles, is a chapter covering some aspects of enzymes. In the next 3 chapters the chemistry of carbohydrates, lipids, amino acids and proteins has been discussed. Various metabolic pathways have been given with an emphasis on those reactions that have particular relevance for health. Bone and teeth metabolism has also been included, briefly. Following this, is a description of nutrients considered regulatory in nature, namely, the minerals and trace elements, and vitamins. A chapter has also been written about nucleic acids to give an idea regarding the brief chemistry and functions of the macromolecules which form the chemical basis of heredity and are involved in the process of protein synthesis. After a focus on nutrition, there is mention about the regulatory molecules (hormones) which act as messengers for the various metabolic processes which occur within the cell. To cover the practicals, gastric juice and bile, have been given.

I wish to express my gratitude of my colleague, Dr SK Aggarwal, Associate Professor of Biochemistry for numerous helpful suggestions and comments. I also wish to express my appreciation to my daughter Anubha and son Ashish who rendered consistent help in the completion of this book. I am also thankful to my wife Veena for her patience. The enthusiastic cooperation received from Mr SK Jain and the staff members of CBS Publishers & Distributors, New Delhi, is acknowledged.

Suggestions and comments for its improvement are welcome.

Harbans Lal

May, 1997
Rohtak (Haryana)

Contents

Unit VII: Metabolic Regulation

Unit VIII: Structural Components and Blood Proteins

Unit IX: Medical Biochemistry

Unit X: Practicals

Unit I

Chemistry of Bio-organic Molecules

1. Carbohydrates
2. Lipids
3. Proteins
4. Nucleic Acids
5. High-energy Compounds
6. Enzymes

Chapter 1

Carbohydrates

Carbohydrates, also called saccharides (Greek, Sakcharon: sugar), are the most abundant biological molecules containing C, H, and O, which are combined in the ratio of 2:1, i.e. as $(CH_2O)_n$, where n is 3 or more. They may be defined as the aldehyde or ketone derivatives of higher polyhydroxy-alcohols, or their anhydrides.

BIOLOGICAL IMPORTANCE OF CARBOHYDRATES

- Carbohydrates provide significant fraction of energy in the diet.
- They also act as the storage form of energy in the body.
- Carbohydrates also serve as component of a cell membrane that mediates intracellular communication.
- They also serve as structural component of many organisms, including cell wall of bacteria, exoskeleton of insects as well as the fibrous cellulose portion of the plants.

CLASSIFICATION OF CARBOHYDRATES

Depending upon the number of the monomeric units present in the molecule, carbohydrates are classified as monosaccharides, disaccharides and polysaccharides (Fig. 1.1).

1. MONOSACCHARIDES

Monosaccharides are the simple sugars which can join in several ways to form disaccharides and polysaccharides. These are the aldehyde or ketone derivatives of the straight chain polyhydroxy-alcohols which contain 3 or more carbons.

Monosaccharides are **divided into different groups** either according to the chemical nature of the carbonyl group, or according to the number of the carbon atoms (Table 1.1).

Table 1.1: Classification of monosaccharides

Monosaccharides	*Number of carbons*	*Aldoses*	*Ketoses*
Trioses	3	Glyceraldehyde	Dihydroxyacetone
Tetroses	4	Erythrose	Erythrulose
Pentoses	5	Ribose	Ribulose
Hexoses	6	Glucose	Fructose

According to the chemical nature of the carbonyl group

According to the chemical nature of the carbonyl group, monosaccharides are divided into two groups as aldoses and ketoses:

- **Aldoses:** A sugar is an aldose when it has an **aldehyde** (–CHO) **group** on carbon-l, e.g. **glucose**.
- **Ketoses:** The sugar is a ketose when it has a **ketone** (–CO) **group** at carbon-2, e.g. **fructose**.

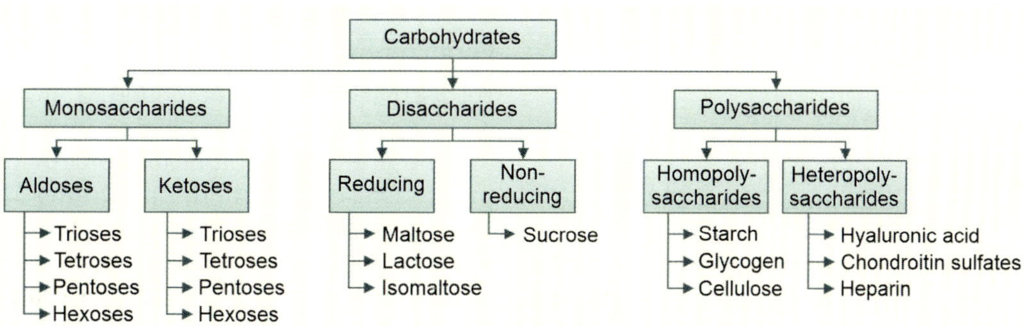

Fig. 1.1: Classification of carbohydrates

Some of the ketoses are named by inserting '**-ul**' before the suffix '**-ose**' with the name of the corresponding aldose, e.g. **erythrulose**. It is a ketose corresponding to erythrose, which is an aldose.

According to the number of the carbon atoms

According to the number of the carbon atoms monosaccharides are designated as trioses, tetroses, pentoses, hexoses, etc.:

- **Trioses:** Trioses are the smallest monosaccharides having **three carbon atoms**, e.g. **glyceraldehyde** (an aldo-triose) and dihydroxyacetone (a keto-triose). Both, of these are of physiological significance as their phosphate esters, which are referred to as glyceraldehyde-3-phosphate and dihydroxyacetone phosphate. They occur as intermediates of glycolysis.
- **Tetroses:** Tetroses have **four carbon atoms**, e.g. **erythrose** (an aldo-tetrose) and erythrulose (a keto-tetrose). Erythrose, as erythrose-4-phosphate, occurs as an intermediate in the hexose monophosphate (HMP) shunt.
- **Pentoses:** Pentoses contain **five carbon atoms**, e.g. **ribose** (an aldo-pentose) and **xylulose** (a keto-pentose). Both of them are found as intermediates of the HMP shunt. Ribose is also a constituent of the nucleotides present in RNAs.
- **Hexoses:** Hexoses contain **six carbon atoms**, e.g. **glucose** (an aldo-hexose) and fructose (a keto-hexose). Glucose, commonly known as dextrose, is used as a source of energy in the body. Galactose is a constituent of milk sugar lactose. Fructose is a constituent of the common sugar called sucrose.

Some monosaccharides of biological importance are exhibited in Fig. 1.2.

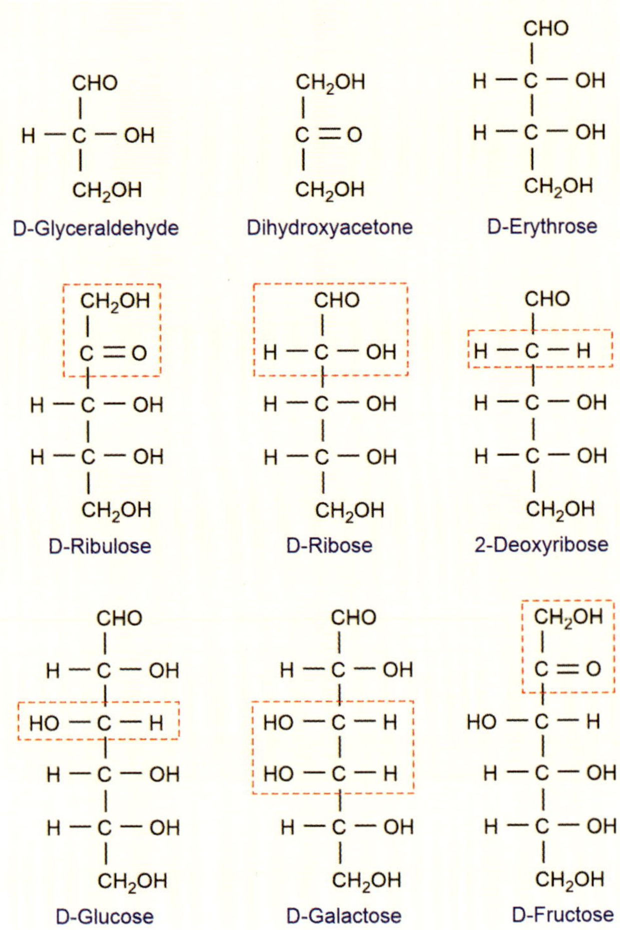

Fig. 1.2: Some monosaccharides of biological importance

PROPERTIES OF MONOSACCHARIDES

Carbohydrates exhibit different types of isomerism, such as stereoisomerism, optical isomerism, etc.

Stereoisomerism

Carbon-containing compounds commonly exist as stereoisomers, the molecules with the same chemical bonds but different stereochemistry, i.e. different configurations (the fixed spatial arrangement of atoms). This configuration is conferred by the presence of either:

- **Double bond** around which there is no freedom of rotation, or
- **Chiral centers** around which substituent groups are arranged in a specific sequence.

Asymmetric carbon: Asymmetric carbon refers to the carbon having four different atoms or groups attached to it. It is also referred to as **asymmetric center** or **chiral center** (Fig. 1.3).

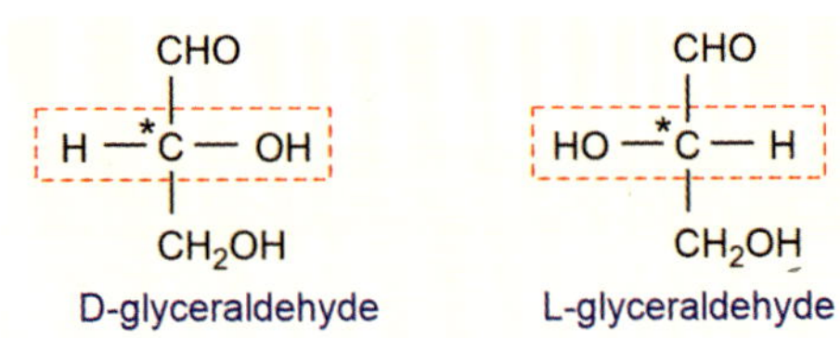

Fig. 1.3: Asymmetric carbon atom (*C)

All the monosaccharides except dihydroxyacetone, contain one or more asymmetric carbon atoms.

A molecule with one chiral center can have two stereoisomers. When two or more chiral carbons, suppose **'n'** are present, there can be **2^n** stereoisomers.

Enantiomers

As discussed above, a compound having one asymmetric carbon atom may occur in two forms, both of which are the non-super-imposable mirror images of each other. These are called enantiomers. For example, **D-glyceraldehyde** and **L-glyceraldehyde**.

- D- or L-form of a monosaccharide, in turn, is determined with respect to its spatial relationship with glyceraldehyde, which is referred to as the parent compound of carbohydrate family.

- In the Fischer projection, glyceraldehyde molecule with –OH group around the asymmetric center (i.e., the α-carbon atom or the carbon atom adjacent to the carbon atom with the terminal primary alcoholic group) on the right-hand side, when –CHO group is at the top, is designated as **D-glyceraldehyde**.
- Its non-superimposable mirror image, which has –OH group around the asymmetric center on the left-hand side is designated as **L-glyceraldehyde**.
- Any successive addition of a carbon atom, in the form of –CHOH (secondary alcoholic group), to the parent compound (D-glyceraldehyde), gives rise to the family of D-sugars. Thus, D-sugars have same absolute configuration at the asymmetric center, farthest from their carbonyl group, as does D-glyceraldehyde (e.g. –OH at fifth carbon of D-glucose is on the right hand, similar to the –OH at the second carbon of D-glyceraldehyde).
- Since each new carbon atom (as a secondary alcoholic group) is added as an asymmetric center, the number of isomers increase with the increasing number of carbon atoms. The number of isomers so formed, thus, depends upon the number of the asymmetric carbon atoms. For example, as we know that the number of the asymmetric carbon atoms in a glucose molecule are four (i.e. n = 4), hence glucose has 2^4 (16) stereoisomers.

Optical Isomerism

Enantiomers have nearly identical chemical properties but differ in a characteristic physical property, i.e. their interaction with the plane-polarized light.

- In separate solutions, two enantiomers rotate the plane of the polarized light in the opposite direction.
- An isomer which rotates the plane of the polarized light to the right is designated as **dextrorotatory (d** or +).
- On the other hand, another isomer which rotates the plane of the polarized light to the left is designated as **levorotatory (l** or –).
- A chiral molecule with D-configuration can be either dextrorotatory [D (+)] or levorotatory [D (–)], indicating its structural relationship to D- or L-glyceraldehyde but exhibiting different types of optical rotations.
- An equimolar solution of the two enantiomers shows no optical rotation and is called a **racemic mixture (dl-mixture)**.

Epimerism

Sugars that differ in configuration of its –H and –OH groups around only one of the optically active carbon atoms are called **epimers**. For example:

- D-Mannose differs in configuration around the second carbon atom (C2) with respect to D-glucose.
- D-galactose has a different configuration than D-glucose around the fourth carbon atom (C4).
- **D-Mannose** and **D-galactose**, therefore, are the **epimers of D-glucose** (Fig. 1.4).

Formation of the Ring Structure

Generally, monosaccharides have a ring conformation.

- Cyclization of D-glucose forms a six-membered ring, which has a hemiacetal bond between the aldehyde carbonyl group of carbon-1 and the hydroxyl group of carbon-5. The ring structure, so formed, is analogous to the structure of **pyran**, which is a six-membered ring that has five carbon atoms and one oxygen atom (Fig. 1.5).

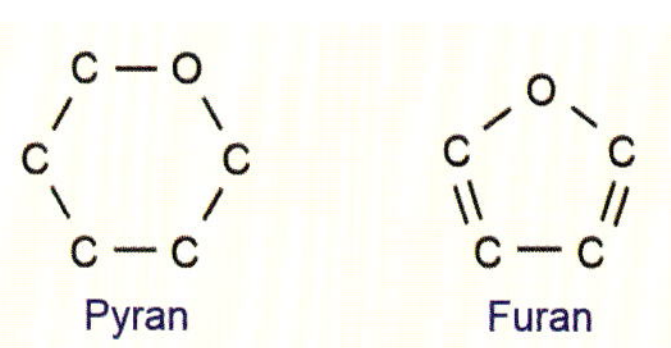

Fig. 1.5: Pyran and furan rings

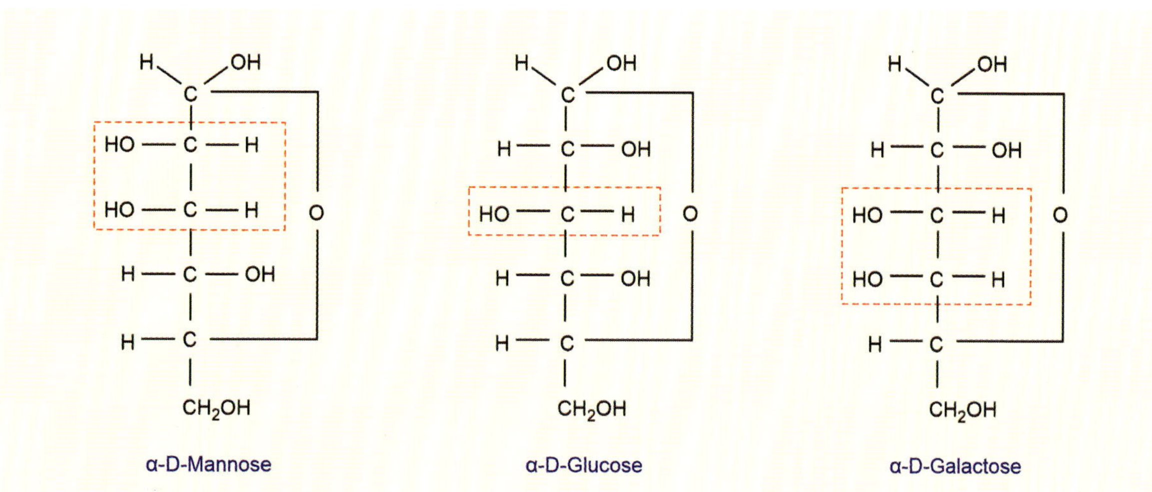

Fig. 1.4: Epimers of glucose

- Monosaccharides having a pyran ring are designated as pyranoses. Accordingly, glucose is referred to as **glucopyranose**.
- On the other hand, cyclization of D-fructose forms a five-membered ring, which has a hemiketal bond between the carbonyl group of carbon-2 and the alcoholic group of carbon-5. The ring structure, so formed, is analogous to the structure of **furan**, which is a five-membered ring that has four carbon atoms and one oxygen atom (Fig. 1.5).
- Monosaccharides having furan rings are designated as furanoses. Accordingly, fructose is referred to as **fructo-furanose**.
- The smallest monosaccharide having a furan ring is ribose.
- Ring structures of monosaccharides were proposed by Haworth and, thus, are also called **Haworth structures**.
- When a monosaccharide cyclizes, its carbonyl carbon, called anomeric carbon, also becomes asymmetric and exhibits two configurations, which are referred to as α and β **anomers**.

Anomerism

Isomeric forms of the monosaccharides that differ only in their configuration at the anomeric carbon, i.e. the first carbon (C1) in an aldose (e.g. glucopyranose) or the second carbon (C2) in a ketose (e.g. fructofuranose) are called **anomers**.

- An **α-anomer** has –OH group (at the anomeric carbon) below the plane.
- The other anomer, which has –OH group at the anomeric carbon above the plane is designated as **β-anomer** (Fig. 1.6).
- Two anomers of D-glucose, i.e. α-D-glucopyranose and β-D-gluco-pyranose have different physical and chemical properties, including optical rotation.
- They are, however, freely interconvertible in an aqueous solution.

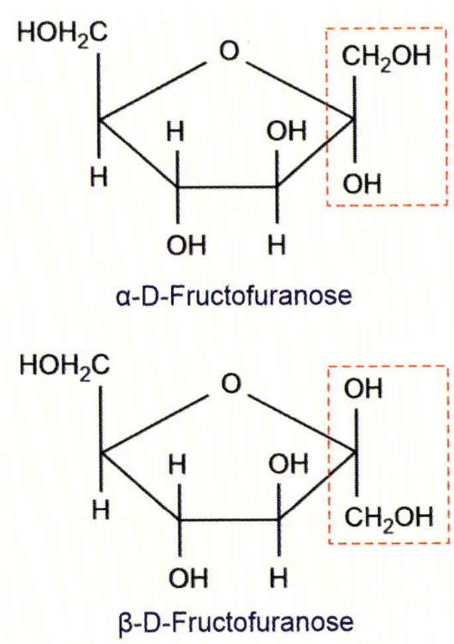

Fig. 1.6: α- and β-anomers of fructose

- During equilibrium, optical rotation of D-glucose also changes with time and reaches a constant value of 52.5°.
- At equilibrium, D-glucose is a mixture of β-anomer and α-anomer in a ratio of nearly 2:1.

SUGAR DERIVATIVES

Several derivatives of monosaccharides such as acids, alcohols, amines and methyl-glycosides are known to occur.

Acids

Monosaccharides have reducing (oxidation–reduction) properties. They act as reducing agents because they have a free aldehyde or ketone group. Due to the presence of this group, they reduce some other compound and, in turn, get oxidized.

- Monosaccharides can be oxidized by relatively, mild oxidizing agents such as ferric (Fe^{3+}) or cupric (Cu^{2+}) ions. This property forms the basis of the Fehling's reaction, a qualitative test used to show the presence of a reducing sugar.
- Oxidation of the carbonyl (aldehyde) carbon of an aldose (C1) to the carboxyl group produces **aldonic acid**, such as **D-gluconic acid**, which is formed by the oxidation of D-glucose.
- Oxidation of the carbon at C6 forms **uronic acid**, such as **D-glucuronic acid**, which is formed from glucose (Fig. 1.7).
- Oxidation of both the carbon atoms (i.e. C1 as well as C6) forms **saccharic acid** or **aldaric acid**.

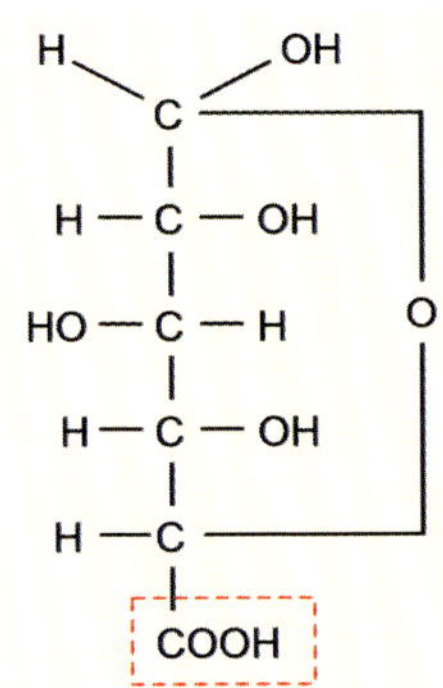

Fig. 1.7: D-Glucuronic acid

Alcohols

Sugars reduce under mild conditions and produce cyclic polyhydroxy alcohols called **alditols**, e.g. **ribitol** (a component of FMN and FAD) and **xylitol** (a sweetener used in the formation of gums and candies).

Amines

Amines, such as **glucosamine** and **galactosamine**, are formed when the —OH group at carbon-2 is substituted by the $-NH_2$ group.

- Some of the amines also **occur** as their **acetylated derivatives**.
- Several derivatives of these amines are **found in glycosaminoglycans**, such as in hyaluronic acid, chondroitin sulfates, erythromycin, etc.
- N-acetyl-neuraminic acid and its derivatives are called **sialic acids**. They are important constituents of glycoproteins and glycolipids.

Methyl-glycosides

A glycoside is a molecule that is formed by the condensation reaction, between a sugar and the hydroxyl group of some other compound, which may be another sugar (glycone) or some non-sugar molecule (aglycone).

- Glycosides can be linked by O- (an O-glycoside), N- (a glycosylamine), S- (a thio-glycoside), or C- (a C-glycoside) glycosidic bond.
- If the carbohydrate portion is glucose, the resulting glycoside is a **glucoside**; if galactose, it is referred to as a **galactoside**, etc.
- Carbon atom number-1 of a monosaccharide can also react with an alcohol, such as methanol and form **methyl-glycosides**. Methyl-glycosides are **found in glycosaminoglycans**.
- Molecules containing N-glycosidic bonds are known as **glycosyl-amines**.

2. DISACCHARIDES

Disaccharides consist of **two similar or dissimilar monosaccharides**, which are linked together by a glycosidic bond. Maltose, lactose, and sucrose are the disaccharides, which have biological importance.

Maltose

Maltose consists of **two glucose** (α-D-glucopyranose) **units**, which are linked together by α-1, 4-glycosidic linkage.

- In maltose, **C1** of a glucose molecule is linked to **C4** of the other molecule of glucose.
- Since –OH group at C4 of a glucose molecule is linked to the –OH group at C1 (the anomeric carbon) of the other glucose molecule, there remains the free –OH group at the anomeric carbon (C1) of the first glucose molecule. Thus, maltose is a **reducing disaccharide** (Fig. 1.8).

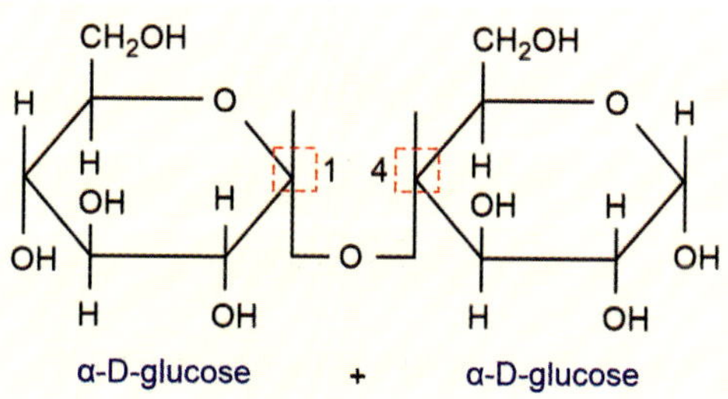

Fig. 1.8: Maltose

- Maltose is obtained as a **hydrolyzed product of polysaccharides**, such as starch and glycogen.
- Maltose is **hydrolyzed to two glucose units by** the enzyme **maltase**, in the intestinal lumen.

Lactose

Lactose consists of **galactose** (β-D-galacto-pyranose) and **glucose** (β-D-glucopyranose), which are linked together by α-1,4-glycosidic linkage.

- In lactose, glycoside bond links C1 of galactose to C4 of glucose.
- There is a free –OH group at the anomeric carbon (C1) of β-D-glucose. Thus, lactose is a **reducing disaccharide** (Fig. 1.9).
- Lactose **occurs** naturally **in milk**; hence lactose is also called **milk sugar**.
- In females, lactose is **synthesized during lactation** and is **secreted in milk**.
- During late pregnancy and lactation, lactose may be excreted in urine. This is referred to as **physiological lactosuria**.
- Lactose is **hydrolyzed by** the intestinal enzyme, called **lactase** (β-D-galactosidase) to **glucose and galactose**.

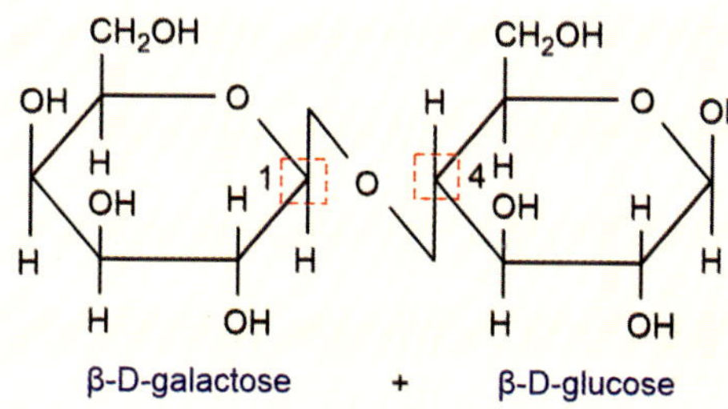

Fig. 1.9: Lactose

Sucrose

Sucrose consists of **glucose** (α-D-glucopyranose) and **fructose** (β-D-fructo-furanose), which are linked by the β-1,2-glycosidic linkage (Fig. 1.10).

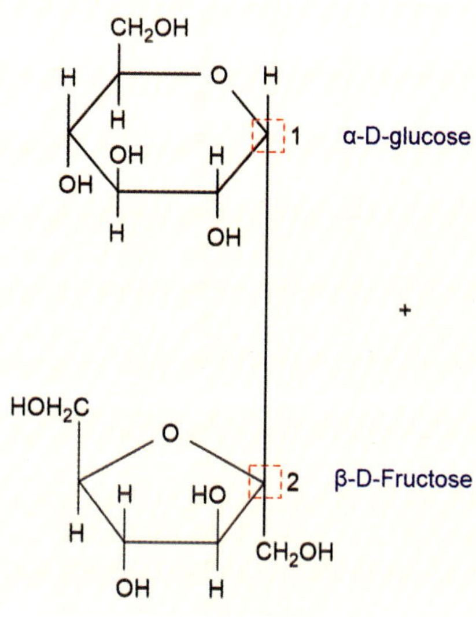

Fig. 1.10: Sucrose

- As carbonyl groups of both the monosaccharides, i.e. C1 of glucose and C2 of fructose, participate in the synthesis of the glycosidic bond and there is no free carbonyl carbon on any of its monosaccharides, thus, sucrose is a **nonreducing sugar**.
- Sucrose is also known as **table sugar, cane sugar** or **invert sugar**.
- It is the most abundant disaccharide **found in plants**.
- Sucrose is **hydrolyzed to glucose** and **fructose** by the intestinal enzyme, called **sucrase**, also referred to as **invertase**.

3. POLYSACCHARIDES

Polysaccharides are the carbohydrates which are built by the linking several monosaccharide units.

When three to ten monosaccharide units are linked by the O-glycosidic bonds, e.g. **malto-triose, raffinose,** etc. these **are** referred to as **oligosaccharides**. Most of the oligosaccharides are not digested in human. Oligosaccharides are, usually, attached to proteins, at the sequences that form surface loops or turns. Some oligosaccharides also play structural roles. A single protein may contain several N- or O-linked oligosaccharide chains. High extent of O-linked oligosaccharides occurs in mucin. Glycosylation may affect structure, stability, or activity of a protein.

Polymers of **large number of monosaccharides,** usually more than ten, are **called polysaccharides** or **glycans**.

Polysaccharides are **sparingly soluble in cold water,** but **form a colloidal solution in hot water**. They are **neither sweet in taste nor have reducing properties**.

Polysaccharides are further classified into two groups as homopolysaccharides and heteropolysaccharides.

A. Homopolysaccharides

Homopolysaccharides, also called **homoglycans**, are polymers, which have **identical monosaccharide units**.

Homopolysaccharides of biological significance include:

- Homopolymers of glucose, i.e. starch, glycogen and cellulose, and
- Homopolymer of fructose, called inulin.

i. Starch: Starch is stored as a **reservoir of food,** commonly **found in cereals** and **tubers of plants**.

- Starch **consists of two polysaccharide subunits,** referred to as α-amylose and amylopectin.
- **α-Amylose** is a **linear polymer of glucose**. Glucose molecules are linked together by α-(1→4) glycosidic bonds.
- **Amylopectin** is a **branched molecule** having, both α-(1→4) (straight chain) and α-(1→6) (branch points). Branching occurs after every 24 to 30 glucose residues (Fig. 1.11).

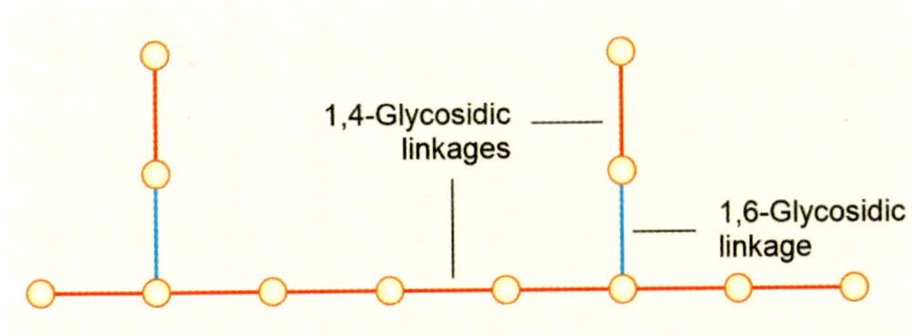

Fig. 1.11: Starch

- Starch is a **main source of carbohydrate in the human diet**.
- **Amylase**, found **in saliva and pancreatic juice,** randomly **hydrolyses α-(1→4) glycosidic bonds of amylose** (starch) and degrades starch **to** give a mixture of **maltose, malto-triose** and **dextrins**.

ii. Glycogen: Glycogen is a **polysaccharide found in animals**; hence, it is also **called animal starch**.

- Although, glycogen is found in all the cells in animals, it is **most prevalent in skeletal muscle and liver**.
- In the liver, glycogen is **degraded by the enzyme phosphorylase** and **serves as a readily available source of glucose**, especially, during initial 18–24 hours of fasting.
- Structure of glycogen is similar to amylopectin having both, a linear chain consisting of α-(1→4) glycosidic bonds and the branch points consisting of α-(1→6) glycosidic bonds. However, compared to amylopectin, in glycogen, branching occurs more frequently, i.e. after every 10–12 glucose residues. Thus, glycogen is **highly branched**, having a tree-like structure (Fig. 1.12).
- In the **liver glycogen is used as a** readily available **source of glucose during starvation**.

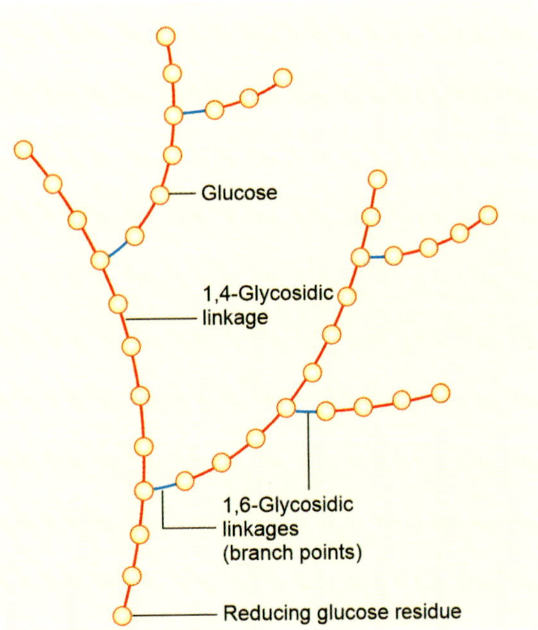

Fig. 1.12: Glycogen

Differences between starch and glycogen are shown in Table 1.2.

Table 1.2: Differences between starch and glycogen

Starch	*Glycogen*
It is a plant reserve food, mainly stored in grains	It is an animal reserve food, mainly stored in the liver and muscle
It is less branched. Branching occurs after every 24 to 30 glucose units	It is highly branched. Branching occurs after every 10 to 12 glucose units
It consists of two subunits, called amylose and amylopectin	No such structural subunits are found
It is sparingly soluble in cold water and forms a paste in hot water	It forms an opalescent solution in water
It gives violet color with iodine	It gives brown to red color with iodine

iii. Cellulose: Cellulose is found in plants. It is a **linear polymer of β-D-glucose**, and, thus, has β-(1→4) glycosidic bonds.

Though cellulose cannot be utilized by human beings, it forms a considerable part of the vegetarian food and adds to the bulk of the feces.

iv. Inulin: Inulin is found in plants such as in the bulbs of dahlia, onion and garlic.

- It is also not utilized by human beings.
- However, it is of biological significance as it is used for determining glomerular filtration rate (GFR).

v. Dextrans: Dextrans are produced by various microorganisms that are grown in sucrose media.

- Dextrans have high molecular weight.
- These are the highly branched homopolymers of glucose, having 1–6, 1–4 and 1–3 linkages.
- They are used for intravenous infusion, as plasma volume expanders in the treatment of hypovolemic shock.
- Dextrans are also used as food additives and cryo-preservatives

B. Heteropolysaccharides

Heteropolysaccharides **(heteroglycans)** are the **polymers of nonidentical monosaccharide units**, also referred to as **glycosaminoglycans** (GAGs). Glycosaminoglycans, **originally designated as mucopolysaccharides**, are large complexes of negatively charged heteropolysaccharides associated with a small amount of protein, forming proteoglycans. These are the gel-forming components of the extracellular matrices. According to their monomeric composition, type of glycosidic linkage, and degree and location of sulfate units, GAGs are divided into several classes.

i. Hyaluronic acid: Hyaluronic acid is composed of repeating disaccharide units of **D-glucuronic acid** and **N-acetyl-D-glucosamine**.

- This polysaccharide chain is the longest of the glycosaminoglycans (GAGs).
- It is the only GAG which is non-sulfated.
- It is not covalently attached to protein and is not limited to animal tissues, but is also found in bacteria.
- It is an **important component of the connective tissue, synovial fluid and vitreous humor in the eye**.
- Viscoelastic behavior of hyaluronate solution makes it an excellent biological shock absorber and lubricant.
- Its concentration is decreased in osteoarthritis.

ii. Chondroitin sulfates: Chondroitin sulfates **contain glucuronic acid and N-acetyl-galactose with sulfate** on the hydroxyl group of either carbon-4 **(chondroitin-4-sulfate)** or carbon-6 **(chondroitin-6-sulfate)**.

- These are the major components of the cartilage, where they bind to collagen and hold fibers in a tight and strong network.
- They are also **found in the aorta, tendons and ligaments**.

iii. Dermatan sulfate: Dermatan sulfate is derived from chondroitin, by enzymatic epimerization of carbon-5 of its glucuronate residues to iduronate residues.

- Dermatan sulfate **contains L-iduronic acid** (with variable amounts of glucuronic acid) and **N-acetyl-galactosamine**.
- It is **found in skin, blood vessels, tendon and heart valves**.

iv. Heparan sulfate: Heparan sulfates consist of **glucuronic or iduronic acid and glucosamine**. Some glucosamines are acetylated and may also have N- or O-sulfate groups.

- It is a ubiquitous cell-surface component as well as an extracellular substance **present in blood vessel walls and brain**.
- Some heparan sulfates, which function directly at the cell surface, interact with a variety of proteins, including some growth factors and growth-factor receptors (such as fibroblast growth factors and their receptors).
- Formation of the ternary complexes of heparan sulfate with fibroblast growth factor and fibroblast growth-factor receptor initiate signaling processes.

v. Heparin: Heparin consists of **glucuronic or iduronic acid and glucosamine**. Most of its glucosamine units are **N-sulfated**. Sulfate is also bound to the hydroxyl group on carbon-2 of uronic acid residues and carbon-3 or carbon-6 of glucosamine residues.

- It is a highly charged polymer that is **found in the intracellular granules of the mast cells** that occur in arterial walls, especially in liver, lungs and skin.

- Heparin is widely **used clinically**, to inhibit blood clotting, e.g. in postsurgical patients.
- Suitably modified low-molecular weight heparin is used in the prophylaxis and **treatment of deep vein thrombosis**.

vi. Keratan sulfates: Keratan sulfate is the most heterogeneous group of glycosaminoglycans, as its sulfate content is variable. It also contains small amounts of fucose, mannose, N-acetylglucosamine and sialic acid. The repeating disaccharide, generally, is **N-acetylglucosamine and galactose**. Sulfate content is variable and may be present on hydroxyl group at carbon-6.

- Keratan sulfates are linked to proteins either by N-linked (keratan sulfate I) or O-linked (keratan sulfate II) oligosaccharides.
- Keratan sulfate I is **found in cornea** while keratan sulfate II occurs in **loose connective tissue proteoglycan aggregates** with chondroitin sulfate.

Some Important Questions

1. **Define carbohydrate. Giver their classification explain stereoisomerism of carbohydrates.**
2. **What are polysaccharides? Classify them.**
3. **Differentiate between starch and glycogen.**
4. **Write notes on:**
    I. Cellulose
    II. Anomerism
    III. Epimerism
    IV. Inulin
    V. Homopolysaccharides
    VI. Heteropolysaccharides

Chapter
2

Lipids

Lipid (Greek, *lipos* means fat) is a heterogeneous group of hydrophobic organic molecules found in cells.

- Lipids are **not soluble**, or are only sparingly soluble, **in water** but are soluble in organic solvents, such as acetone, ether, alcohol and chloroform.
- Due to this reason, lipids can be easily separated from other biological material after their extraction with some organic solvent.

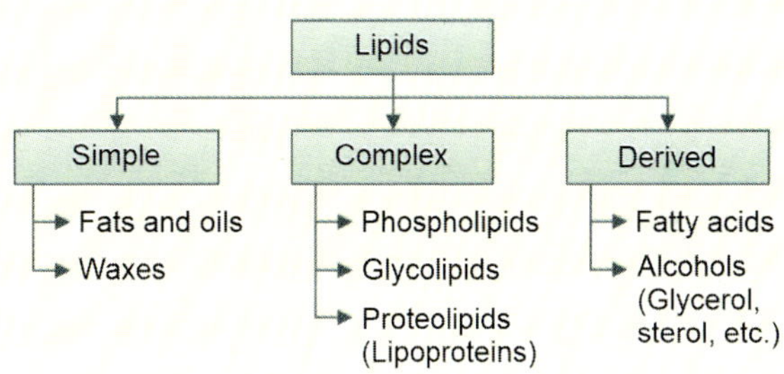

Fig. 2.1: Classification of lipids

BIOLOGICAL IMPORTANCE OF LIPIDS

- Due to their **high calorific value**, fat forms an important dietary constituent of food.
- Dietary lipids serve as a **source of fat-soluble vitamins** and **essential fatty acids**.
- Fat is the **storage form of energy** in adipose tissue.
- Fat presents in the subcutaneous tissues **acts as an insulating material**.
- Lipids, in the form of a bilayer together with proteins, form important **components of biological membranes**.
- Lipids also **act as signaling molecules**.
- Nervous system is very rich in lipids, which are essential for its proper functioning.
- Lipoproteins are the carriers of triglycerides, cholesterol and phospholipids in the body.

CLASSIFICATION OF LIPIDS

Lipids exhibit great structural variability. They constitute a category of substances that are hydrophobic in nature and are soluble in nonpolar solvents. Lipids are classified into three groups (Fig. 2.1).

1. Simple lipids

Simple lipids are the **esters of fatty acids with alcohol.** These include **neutral fats, oils and waxes**. Neutral fats and oils are the mixtures of triacylglycerols (also called triglycerides) whose fatty acids composition may vary with the source. They differ from each other in the way that fats are solid while oils are liquid at room temperature.

i. **Neutral fats** are obtained from animal sources. They have, comparatively, a greater number of saturated fatty acids and have higher melting points.

ii. **Oils** are obtained from plant seeds. They are usually rich in unsaturated fatty acids and have low melting points.

iii. **Waxes** are the esters of long chain fatty acids with high molecular weight mono-hydroxy aliphatic alcohols. They are used in the manufacturing of wax-polish.

2. Complex Lipids

In addition to fatty acids and alcohol, complex lipids **also contain an amphipathic group**. For example, lipids conjugated with phosphoric acid are called **phospholipids**, lipids conjugated with sugars are referred to as **glycolipids**, etc.

3. Derived Lipids

Derived lipids are obtained after the hydrolysis of the simple and compound lipids. They include fatty acids, glycerol, etc.

FAT AND FATTY ACIDS

Fat, mainly, comprises **triacylglycerols,** also called triglycerides or neutral lipids. These are the fatty acid tri-esters of glycerol (glycerin, a tri-hydric alcohol).

Glycerol with one molecule of fatty acid is called **monoacylglycerol**, with two molecules of fatty acids as **diacylglycerol** and with three molecules of fatty acids as **triacylglycerol** (Fig. 2.2).

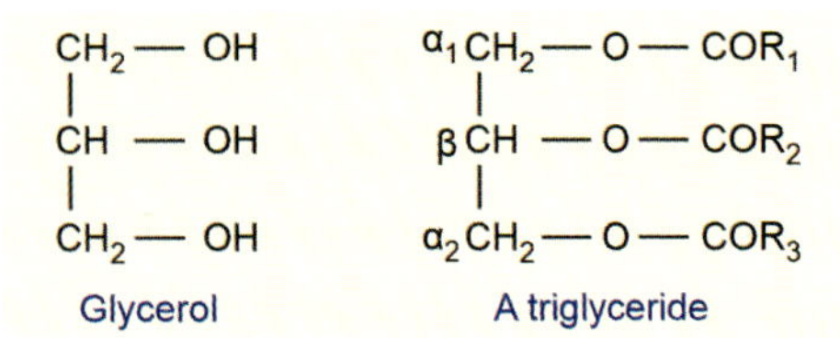

Fig. 2.2: Glycerol and a triacylglycerol

- A molecule of triacylglycerol may have **three similar or dissimilar fatty acids**, which **may be saturated and/or unsaturated**.
- All the natural fats and oils, generally, have three dissimilar fatty acids, both saturated as well as unsaturated. These are referred to as **mixed triacylglycerols**.
- **Plant oils are**, usually, **rich in unsaturated fatty acids.**
- **Triacylglycerols are transported in plasma, in chylomicrons** and very low-density lipoproteins (VLDL).
- **Nomenclature of triglycerides is done according to the presence of fatty acids** which are **attached to glycerol**, e.g. a triacylglycerol having palmitic acid at carbon-1, arachidonic acid at carbon-2 and stearic acid at carbon-3 of glycerol is called 1-palmitoyl-2-arachidonoyl-3-stearoyl-glycerol.
- Generally, **a saturated fatty acid is found at the primary alcoholic group**, i.e. at **α-position** of glycerol (position number 1 or 3) and an **unsaturated fatty acid** is found **at the β-position** (position number 2).

FATTY ACIDS

Fatty acids are the **carboxylic acids with a long hydrocarbon side chain** that may be **saturated or unsaturated** (having one or more double bonds).

- **Major source of the circulating free fatty acids is adipose tissue.**
- After **hydrolysis of the triacylglycerols** in chylomicrons and VLDL, **free fatty acids enter plasma** and serve an important source of energy for many tissues.
- Since free fatty acids have limited solubility in water, they are **transported in plasma, bound to albumin** which has specific binding sites for free fatty acids.
- Most of the naturally occurring fatty acids **have even number of carbon atoms**, since they are **synthesized from acetyl CoA,** i.e. from two carbon units.
- According to their chain length, fatty acids are **divided into three groups**, referred to as:
  - **Short chain fatty acids**, which contain **4 to 8 carbon** atoms
  - **Medium chain fatty acids**, which contain **10 to 14 carbon** atoms, and
  - **Long chain fatty acids**, which contain **16 or more carbon** atoms.
- All types of fatty acids **have different physico-chemical properties** and are metabolized in the body in different ways.
- In **plants and higher animals**, predominant fatty acids are those **containing 16 and 18 carbon atoms**, e.g. palmitic acid, oleic acid, linoleic acid, stearic acid, etc.

CLASSIFICATION OF FATTY ACIDS

Fatty acids are classified into two groups as:

- **Saturated fatty acids:** Saturated fatty acids have a **suffix '-anoic'** after the name of the hydrocarbon chain, e.g. **octadecanoic acid**, a saturated fatty acid **having 18 carbon atoms.**
  - Saturated fatty acids are highly flexible molecules and can assume a wide range of conformations because there is relatively **free rotation around the C–C bond**.
  - They are commonly **found in fats**, which are obtained **from the animal source**, such as butter.

Saturated fatty acids of common biological significance are listed in Table 2.1.

Table 2.1: Saturated fatty acids

Fatty acids	*Number of carbons*	*Formula*	*Sources*
Acetic acid	2	CH_3–COOH	Fermentation of carbohydrates
Butyric acid	4	CH_3–$(CH_2)_2$–COOH	Butter
Caproic acid	6	CH_3–$(CH_2)_4$–COOH	Butter, fat from plant sources
Caprylic acid	8	CH_3–$(CH_2)_6$–COOH	-do-
Capric acid	10	CH_3–$(CH_2)_8$–COOH	-do-
Lauric acid	12	CH_3–$(CH_2)_{10}$–COOH	Coconut oil
Myristic acid	14	CH_3–$(CH_2)_{12}$–COOH	-do-
Palmitic acid	16	CH_3–$(CH_2)_{14}$–COOH	Animal and plant fats
Stearic acid	18	CH_3–$(CH_2)_{16}$–COOH	-do-
Arachidic acid	20	CH_3–$(CH_2)_{18}$–COOH	Peanut oil

- **Unsaturated fatty acids:** Unsaturated fatty acids have a **suffix '-enoic'** after the name of the hydrocarbon chain, e.g. **octadecanoic acid**, an **unsaturated fatty acid having 18 carbon atoms** and **one double bond**. It is also called **oleic acid**.

Unsaturated fatty acids **may have one or more double bonds**.

Nomenclature of Unsaturated Fatty Acids

Widely used convention to represent an unsaturated fatty acid, is to indicate the **number of carbon atoms**, followed by the **number of double bonds with their positions** in the hydrocarbon chain. For example, **octadecanoic acid**, a fatty acid with **18 carbon atoms** and **one double bond** present **after carbon atom number 9** (i.e. between carbon atoms number 9 and 10), is represented as **18:1; 9** (Fig. 2.3).

$$\overset{18}{CH_3}-(CH_2)_7-\overset{10}{CH}=\overset{9}{CH}-(CH_2)_7-\overset{1}{COOH}$$

Fig. 2.3: Oleic acid—an unsaturated fatty acid (18:1;9)

An unsaturated fatty acid **may be identified either by the delta or the omega system of nomenclature**.

Delta System of Nomenclature

According to the delta (δ) system of nomenclature, carbon atoms in the fatty acid chain are **numbered from the carboxy-terminal end**. This carbon atom (–COOH) is labeled as carbon atom number 1. The carbon atom next to the carboxyl group, i.e. **the α-carbon atom**, is referred to as carbon atom **number 2**, and so on.

Accordingly, an unsaturated fatty acid is represented by:

- A **number showing the number of carbon atoms**, followed by the **symbol colon (:)** and **another number**, which represents the **number of double bonds**.
- This is **followed by the symbol 'Δ'** and some **other numbers as superscript**, which indicate **positions of the double bonds**.

For example, **linoleic acid**, a **fatty acid with 18 carbon** atoms and **two double bonds**, which are present **after carbon atoms number 9 and 12**, is represented as **18:2** $\Delta^{9,12}$ (Fig. 2.4).

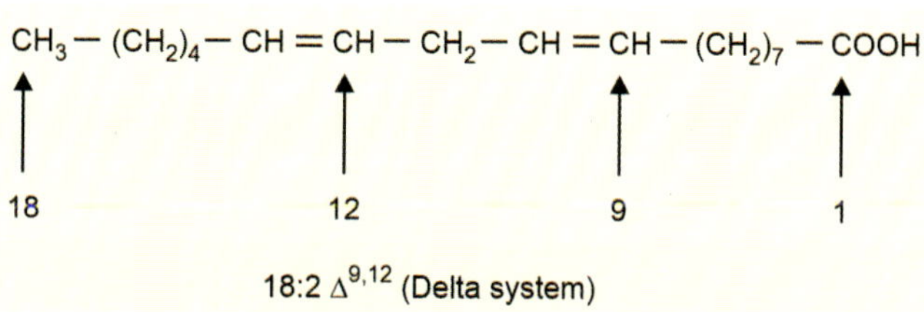

Fig. 2.4: Linoleic acid

Omega System of Nomenclature

According to the omega (ω) system of nomenclature, carbon atoms are numbered from the methyl end. This carbon is referred to as omega (ω) carbon. Accordingly, an unsaturated fatty acid is represented by the **omega symbol** (ω), **followed by a number** represents the **number of the carbon atom** immediately after which the first double bond appears from the methyl end.

For example, in **linoleic acid**, since the **first double bond from the ω-end is present after the sixth carbon atom**, it is, thus, referred to as ω-6 fatty acid (Fig. 2.5).

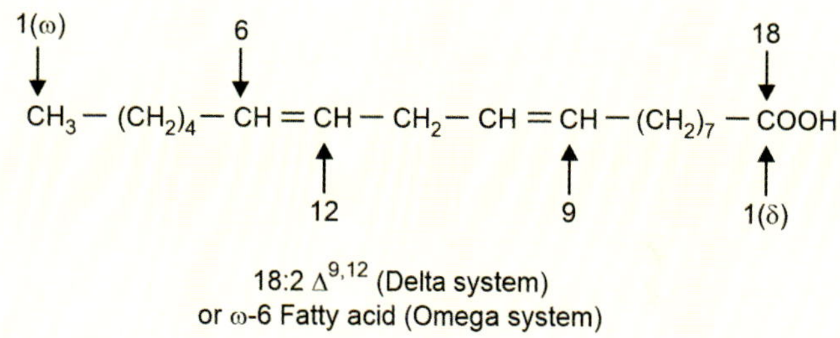

Fig. 2.5: Linoleic acid

Polyunsaturated Fatty Acids

Unsaturated fatty acids having **two or more double bonds** are referred to as polyunsaturated fatty acids **(PUFA)**. They are obtained from plant seed oils, e.g. **soybean oil, sunflower oil, groundnut oil**, etc. PUFA perform various **functions**:

- PUFA form an important **constituent of biological membranes**.
- They are essentially required for the **esterification of cholesterol**, and, thus, help in its transport and metabolism. Particularly, consumption of fat containing ω**-6 fatty acids helps in lowering plasma cholesterol level**.
- Diet rich in ω**-3 fatty acids helps in lowering plasma level of triacylglycerols**.
- **Arachidonic acid** also **acts as a precursor** of some pharmacologically important compounds, such as **prostaglandins, thromboxanes and leukotrienes**. These are referred to as **eicosanoids**.

Essential Fatty Acids

Linoleic acid and linolenic acid are referred to as essential fatty acids since they form an essential component of the diet and are necessary for growth and normal health. These are **not synthesized in our body** and serve a number of important functions, like:

i. Synthesis of prostaglandins.
ii. Serve as structural element of mitochondrial membrane.
iii. Help in the prevention of fatty liver.
iv. Play an important role in vision.

COMPOUND LIPIDS

Compound lipids mainly include a variety of phospholipids. **Phospholipids** are a **heterogeneous group of compounds**, which contain an alcohol and one or more phosphoric acid molecules.

- A phospholipid **has one or two long chain fatty acids** that are **linked to an alcohol**.
- In addition, they have a molecule of **phosphoric acid** that may be **attached to some polar group**, which may be some **nitrogenous compound or a polyhydroxy alcohol**.
- Thus, phospholipids are **amphipathic** in nature, i.e. they **have a hydrophilic head** and a long **hydrophobic tail**.

Hydrophobic and Hydrophilic Groups

Any substance that has an **affinity for water** is said to be **hydrophilic** (from the Greek *hydro* means water and philios means loving).

On the other hand, there are substances that **do not have an affinity for water**. These substances are termed **hydrophobic** (from the Greek *phobos* means fearing).

Hydrophilic and hydrophobic molecules are also known as **polar** molecules **and nonpolar molecules**, respectively.

Structure of a Phospholipid

A phospholipid, as mentioned above, has two components, i.e. a **phosphate group and a lipid**. The phosphate group is referred to as the hydrophilic head.

- Due to its negative charge, this **phosphate group is hydrophilic** (polar).
- The **phosphate** group and the **lipid are connected by a glycerol** group.
- Most phospholipids **have two lipid tails** made of hydrocarbon fatty acids which are **bound to the glycerol by an ester linkage**.
- These tails are referred to as hydrophobic tails and are nonpolar.
- The **hydrophilic domain interacts with the aqueous environment** and **comprises** an **alcohol**, a **phosphate** group **and some polar compound**, such as serine in phosphatidylserine, ethanolamine in phosphatidylethanolamine or choline in phosphtidylcholine, also called lecithin (Fig. 2.6).
- The **hydrophobic domain forms non-aqueous environment** and **contains long chain fatty acid**(s) or a fatty acid-derived long hydrocarbon chain.

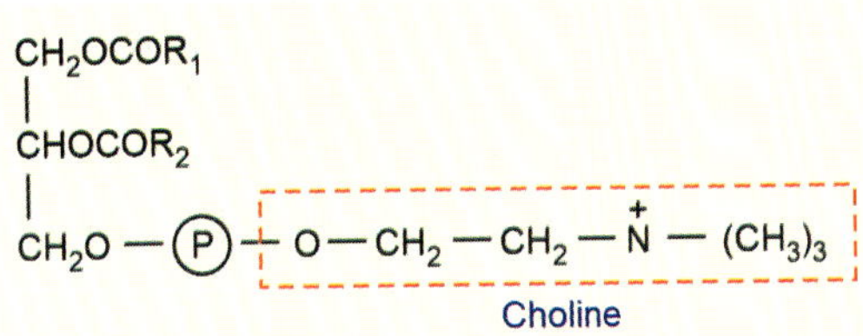

Fig. 2.6: Lecithin

Biological Importance of Phospholipids

- Phospholipids are the predominant lipids of a **cell membrane**.
- Membrane phospholipids also function as a reservoir for the **intracellular messengers**.
- They also serve as **anchors for some proteins** in cell membranes.
- Phospholipids also function as **lung surfactants**.
- They also form an **essential component of bile** and help in the regulation of serum cholesterol.
- They also have a role in **blood coagulation, lipid absorption** in intestine **and transport** of lipids from the intestine.
- They also act as a **cofactor** in the activity of the enzyme **lipases**.

Classification of Phospholipids

Phospholipids are classified into several groups (Table 2.2).

Table 2.2: Classification of phospholipids

Glycerophospholipids
• Lecithins (phosphatidylcholine)
• Cephalins (phosphatidylethanolamine and phosphatidylserine)
• Phosphatidylinositols
• Cardiolipins and plasmalogens
Sphingolipids
• Sphingomyelins
• Cerebrosides
• Gangliosides

CHOLESTERL

Cholesterol is a **derivative of** the **cyclopentano-perhydrophenanthrene ring**, also called **steroid nucleus**, which consists of four fused, nonpolar rings that are labeled as A, B, C and D.

- Cholesterol **has 27 carbon atoms** with **a hydroxyl group on carbon number 3**, a **double bond between carbon numbers 5 and 6, two methyl groups** attached to **carbon numbers 18 and 19**, and a **side chain** that is attached to **carbon number 17**.

> ***Note:*** Cholesterol, also referred to as free cholesterol, is hydrophilic in nature and thus, is not soluble in water. Due to this reason, it cannot be transported in plasma in free form.

- Due to the presence of the –OH group at carbon number 3, cholesterol reacts with a long chain fatty acid and **forms cholesterol esters**.
- Cholesterol is packaged in lipoproteins and travels in blood via emulsification.

BILE SALTS

Bile salts are **glycine and taurine conjugates of bile acids**. Bile acids contain 24 carbons with two or three hydroxyl groups and a side chain that has a carboxyl group, which is not fully ionized at physiological pH. They are **amphipathic** in nature.

- Bile acids are **synthesized in the liver**, from cholesterol. Most common bile acids that are synthesized in the liver are called **cholic acid and chenodeoxycholic acid**. These are referred to as **primary bile acids**.
- Before they leave the liver, they get **conjugated with** a molecule of either **glycine or taurine** (derived from cystine) by an amide bond, which is formed between the carboxyl group of the bile acid and the amino group of glycine/taurine.
- The conjugates of bile acids, i.e. **glycocholate and glycol-chenodeoxycholate** as well as **taurocholate and tauro-chenodeoxycholate** are referred to as bile salts.
- Bacteria in the intestine remove glycine and taurine from bile salts and regenerate bile acids.
- These bacteria also remove a hydroxyl group from primary bile acids, producing **deoxycholic acid** (from cholic acid) and lithocholic acid (from chenodeoxycholic acid), which are referred to as **secondary bile acids**.
- Because of their enhanced amphipathic nature, **bile salts are** more effective detergents than bile acids and are essential for the digestion and absorption of lipids.

MICELLE AND BIMOLECULAR LEAFLET

Micelle is a **spheroidal aggregate** where a large number of amphiphilic molecules, e.g. soaps and detergents, are **arranged** in such a way that **their hydrophilic groups** (at the globular surface) **interact with the aqueous solvent** while the **hydrophobic groups are associated at the center**, i.e. away from the solvent (Fig. 2.7).

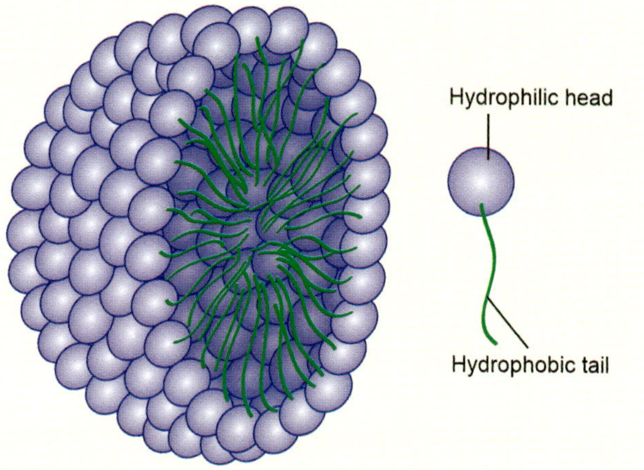

Fig. 2.7: A micelle

Micelles are formed when the cross-section of the hydrophilic head group exceeds that of the hydrophobic tails. This molecular arrangement eliminates unfavorable contact between water and hydrophobic tails of amphiphiles.

Bimolecular Leaflet

A biological membrane is made of **phospholipid bilayer** sandwiched between two layers of globular proteins. The polar **(hydrophilic) heads** of phospholipids are **oriented towards the protein layers** forming a hydrophilic zone while the nonpolar **(hydrophobic) tails** of phospholipids are oriented in between polar heads forming a hydrophobic zone.

These are extremely stable structures which are held together by noncovalent interactions of the hydrocarbon chains and ionic interactions of the charged head groups with water. Lipophilic molecules such as cholesterol intercalate between fatty acyl residues of phospholipids and have minimal contact with the aqueous phase. This type of structure is referred to as bimolecular leaflet and forms the key structure in biological membranes (Fig. 2.8).

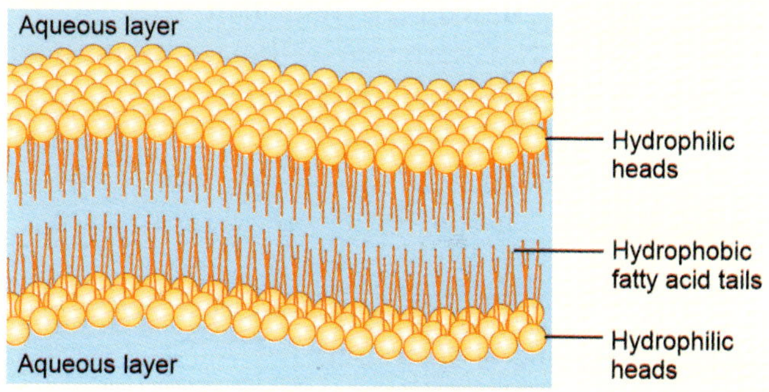

Fig. 2.8: A lipid bilayer

Some Important Questions

1. **What are lipids? Classify them. Give biological significance of lipids.**
2. **What are fatty acids? Classify them. Write biological significance of polyunsaturated fatty acids.**
3. **Describe briefly:**
   i. Classification of lipids with suitable examples
   ii. Chemistry and functions of cholesterol
4. **Write notes on:**
   i. PUFA
   ii. Triacylglycerols
   iii. Phospholipids
   iv. Bile salts
   v. Micelles
   vi. Bimolecular leaflet

Chapter 3

Proteins

Protein (Greek, *proteios* means primary) is the class of natural products, which contains nitrogen and forms an essential structural component of a cell. They are most abundant and functionally diverse molecules present in all living systems.

- All **proteins**, from whatever source it may be, **are** the **polymers of amino acids**.
- **Amino acids are the hydrolyzed products of proteins;** they are also **used in protein synthesis**.
- Though a large number of amino acids may be found in the body, only **twenty** of them are **commonly occur in all mammalian proteins**.
- Each **polypeptide has a free α-amino group on the left-hand side**, which is referred to as the **N-terminal** (amino terminal) end. A peptide also has a **free α-carboxylic group on the right-hand side**, which is referred to as the **C-terminal** (carboxyl terminal) end.
- Large polypeptides are referred to as proteins (Fig. 3.1).

$$H_2NAA_1 - AA_2 - AA_3 \text{ ---------- } AA_{n-1} - AA_nCOOH$$

N-terminal end C-terminal end

Fig. 3.1: A polypeptide

Biological Functions of Proteins

Proteins serve a variety of functions (Table 3.1):

- **Structural proteins:** Some of the proteins, e.g. **collagens** (found in bone and cartilage), **keratins** (found in hair and nail), etc. form an essential part of the particular structure within the body.
- **Enzymes:** Some of the proteins, such as **pepsin**, catalyze biological reactions and act as enzymes.
- **Hormones:** Some of the proteins act as hormones, e.g. **insulin**. They regulate metabolic processes within the cell.
- **Transporters:** Several proteins serve as a carrier for the transport of a substance within the body. For example, **hemoglobin** is important for the transport of oxygen, ceruloplasmin transports copper, etc.
- **Protein receptors:** Some of the proteins, such as **hormone receptors**, act as receptors for certain hormones and play an important role in signal transduction.
- **Storage of substances:** Some of the proteins bind to a substance for its storage in different tissues in the body, e.g. **ferritin**. Ferritin stores Fe^{3+}.
- **Antibodies:** Some proteins, such as **γ-globulin,** act as antibodies and provide immunity.

Table 3.1: Biological functions of proteins

Biological function	*Examples of proteins*
As structural proteins	Collagen, keratins, etc.
As enzymes	Pepsin, amylase, etc.
As hormones	Insulin
As transporters	Hemoglobin
As receptors	Hormone receptors
As storage molecules	Ferritin
In immune response	γ-Globulin

AMINO ACIDS

As mentioned above, amino acids are the **hydrolyzed products of proteins**. These are also **used in the synthesis of proteins**. All the naturally occurring amino acids are designated as **α-amino acids**, because:

- **Each amino acid has a carboxyl group** (–COOH) as well as a **primary amino group** ($-NH_2$), which are present on the α-carbon atom.
- Each amino acid also has **an atom or group**, which is **attached to the α-carbon atom**. It is called **R-group.**

General structure of an amino acid is shown in Fig. 3.2.

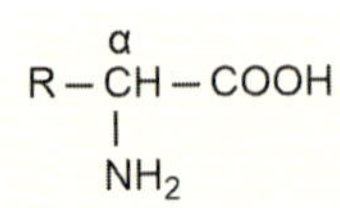

Fig. 3.2: General structure of an amino acid

Classification of Amino Acids

According to the properties of the side chain such as **charge, polarity** and **dietary requirement**, amino acids may be classified into several groups.

According to Charge

According to the net ionic charge of its acidic and basic groups, amino acids may be classified as **neutral, acidic or basic** (Table 3.2).

Table 3.2: Classification of amino acids according to charge

Amino acid	*Abbreviation**
NEUTRAL AMINO ACIDS	
Simple amino acids	
Glycine	Gly
Alanine	Ala
Branched chain amino acids	
Valine	Val
Leucine	Leu
Isoleucine	Ile
Hydroxy amino acids	
Serine	Ser
Threonine	Thr
Aromatic amino acids	
Phenylalanine	Phe
Tyrosine	Tyr
Tryptophan	Trp
Sulfur-containing amino acids	
Cysteine	Cys
Methionine	Met
ACIDIC AMINO ACIDS	
Aspartic acid	Asp
Glutamic acid	Glu
Amides of the acidic amino acids	
Asparagine	
Glutamine	Asn
	Gln
BASIC AMINO ACIDS	
Lysine	Lys
Arginine	Arg
Histidine	His

* Three letters abbreviation is widely used. This, generally, includes first three letters of an amino acid.

i. Neutral Amino Acids

These amino acids have **one amino group** ($-NH_2$) and **one carboxyl group** (–COOH). Thus, they may also be referred to as **monoamino-monocarboxylic acids.** They are neutral in reaction. These amino acids may be **aliphatic or aromatic** in nature.

Aliphatic amino acids

Aliphatic amino acids are further subdivided into various groups, as follows:

- **Simple aliphatic amino acids:** These include **glycine,** which has hydrogen (H), and **alanine,** which has a methyl group ($-CH_3$) as the R-group (Fig. 3.3).

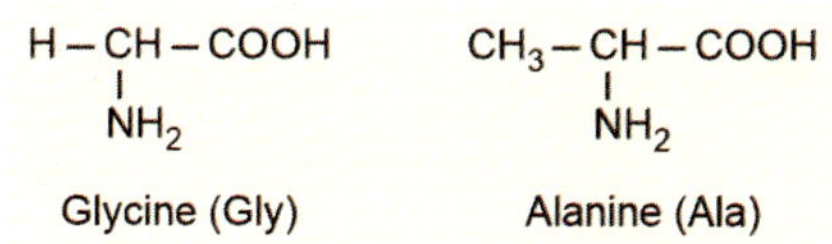

Fig. 3.3: Glycine and alanine

- **Branched chain amino acids:** These amino acids have an **aliphatic side chain, which is** not straight, but is **branched.** These include **valine, leucine** and **isoleucine** (Fig. 3.4).

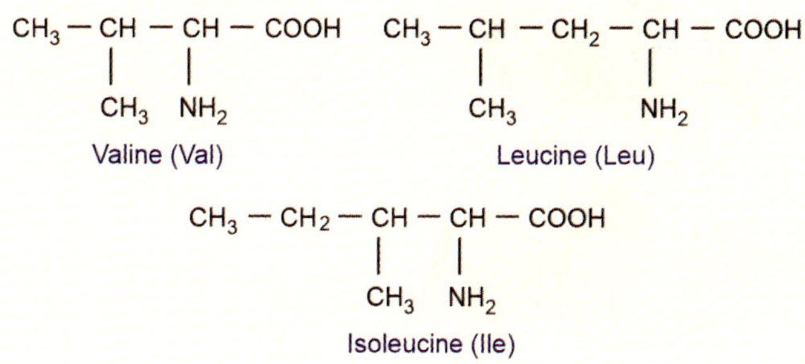

Fig. 3.4: Branched chain amino acids

- **Hydroxyl group-containing amino acids:** These amino acids have a **hydroxyl** (–OH) **group in the aliphatic side chain** (R group). These include **serine** and **threonine** (Fig. 3.5).

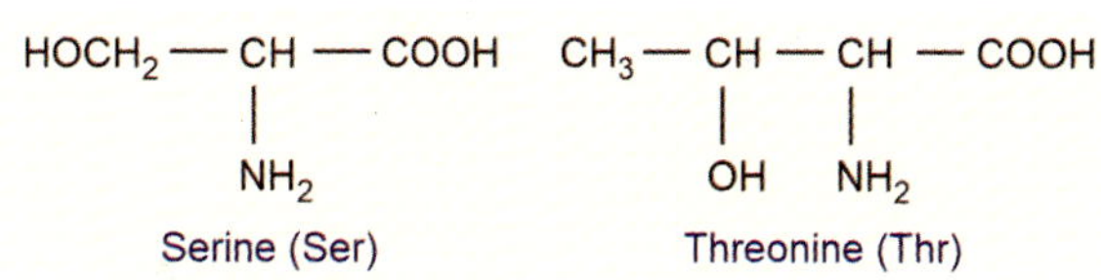

Fig. 3.5: Hydroxyl group-containing amino acids

- **Sulfur-containing amino acids:** In addition to C, H, O and N, these amino acids also **contain sulfur** (S) in their side chain (R group). These include **cysteine, cystine** and **methionine.**
  - **Cysteine** has a **thiol group** (–SH) at the terminal carbon of the R group.
  - **Two molecules of cysteine**, when present at the nearby positions within the same peptide (intra-chain) or two different peptide chains (interchain), can link with each other through their –SH groups and form another amino acid called **dicysteine,** which has a disulfide linkage (–S–S–) and is also referred to as cystine.

– **Methionine** has a **methyl group attached to sulfur** (CH_3–S–) at the terminal point in R group (Fig. 3.6).

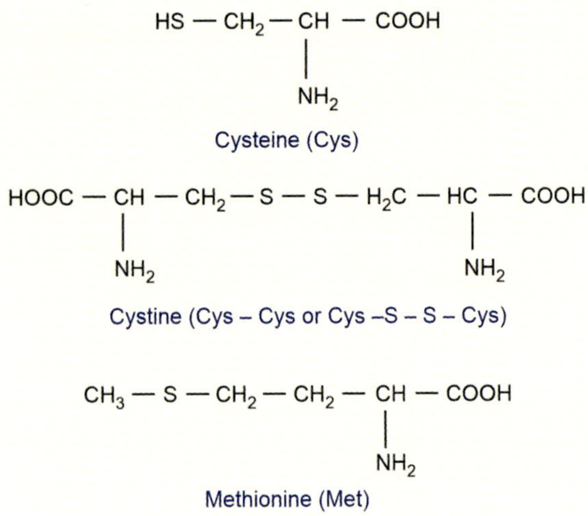

Fig. 3.6: Sulfur-containing amino acids

Aromatic amino acids

These amino acids have an aromatic ring in the side chain. Aromatic amino acids include **phenylalanine** (alanine attached to a phenyl group), **tyrosine** (4-hydroxyphenylalanine, also called p-hydroxyphenylalanine) and **tryptophan** (alanine attached to an indole ring; Fig. 3.7).

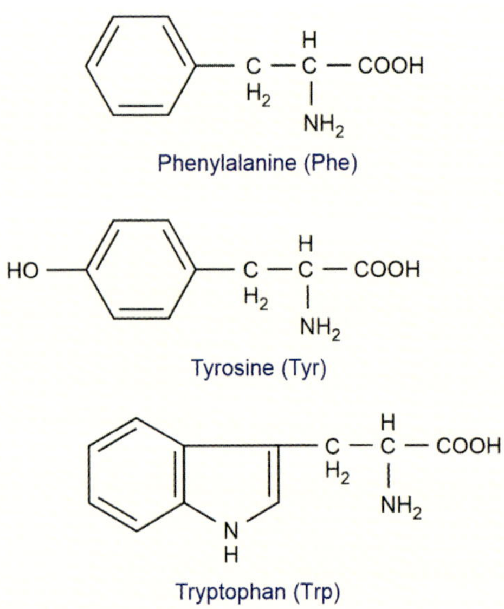

Fig. 3.7: Aromatic amino acids

ii. Acidic Amino Acids

These amino acids have one amino group but two carboxyl groups. Hence, these amino acids can also be referred to as monoamino-dicarboxylic acids. These include **aspartic acid** and **glutamic acid**.

Amides of the acidic amino acids: There are two amino acids which are actually not acidic in reaction but are the amides of the acidic amino acids. These include **asparagine** and **glutamine**. In these amino acids, an additional amino group is attached to the terminal carboxyl group of the acidic amino acid and forms an amide group (Fig. 3.8).

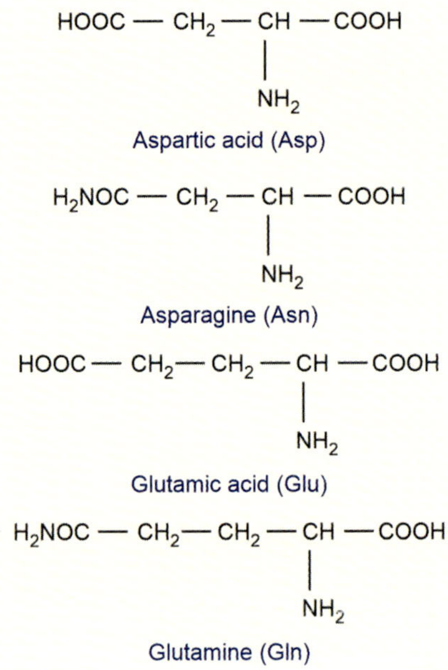

Fig. 3.8: Acidic amino acids (aspartic acid and glutamic acid) and their amides (asparagine and glutamine)

iii. Basic Amino Acids

They have one carboxyl group and either more than one amino group in the aliphatic side chain or a heterocyclic ring that is basic in reaction. These include lysine, arginine and histidine.

- **Lysine** has two –NH_2 groups. One amino group is attached to the alpha carbon atom while the other one is attached as the terminal carbon atom of the aliphatic side chain.
- **Arginine** has a guanidino group which is basic in reaction.
- **Histidine** has a heterocyclic ring, called imidazole ring, which is basic in nature (Fig. 3.9).

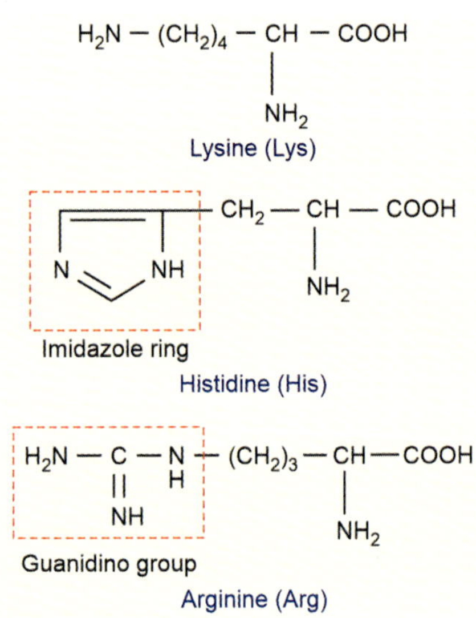

Fig. 3.9: Basic amino acids

Imino acid

In addition to the various amino acids, as discussed above, some of the proteins, such as collagen, contain an imino acid, referred to as proline (Fig. 3.10).

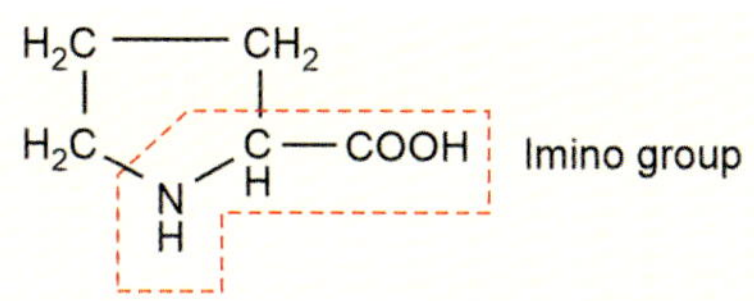

Fig. 3.10: Proline—an imino acid

- **Proline:** Proline (Pro) does not **contain** a primary α-amino group ($-NH_2$) but has a **secondary amino group** (–NH–), called imino group, which forms a part of the heterocyclic ring. Hence, proline is not actually an amino acid but is an imino acid. However, for uniformity, proline is included in the list of the α-amino acids.
- **4-Hydroxyproline:** Proline is incorporated into the peptide chain during collagen synthesis. When the immature collagen, called protocollagen, undergoes post-translational modifications, some of its proline residues get hydroxylated and converted to 4-hydroxyproline (HO-Pro), which is found in collagen. Thus, in addition to proline, 4-hydroxyproline is also found in the blood.

According to Polarity

According to polarity, amino acids are classified into different groups, as follows (Table 3.3).

Table 3.3: Classification of amino acids according to polarity

Nonpolar	*Polar*	
	Uncharged	*Charged*
• Glycine • Alanine • Valine • Leucine • Isoleucine • Methionine • Phenylalanine • Tryptophan • Proline	• Serine • Threonine • Asparagine • Glutamine • Tyrosine • Cysteine	• Lysine • Arginine • Histidine • Aspartate • Glutamate

i. Polar Amino Acids

These amino acids have a polar group in the side chain, which may be charged or uncharged.

- **Uncharged polar amino acids** have a polar side chain which does not bear any charge and is neutral in reaction. For example, –OH group-containing amino acids **serine, threonine** and **tyrosine**. Their –OH group also serves as a site for the attachment of phosphate, monosaccharide or oligosaccharide.
- **Charged polar amino acids** have a side chain which has a charge, e.g. acidic amino acids (aspartate and glutamate), their amides (**asparagine** and **glutamine**) and basic amino acids (**lysine, arginine** and **histidine**).

ii. Nonpolar Amino Acids

They have a side chain, which is nonpolar. These amino acids neither release proton nor participate in hydrogen/ionic bond formation and are referred to as nonpolar amino acids. These are **glycine, alanine, valine, leucine, isoleucine, methionine, phenylalanine, tryptophan** and **proline**.

According to Dietary Requirement

According to dietary requirement, amino acids are classified into three groups, referred to as essential, semi-essential and nonessential amino acids (Table 3.4).

Table 3.4: Classification of amino acids according to dietary requirement

Essential	*Semi-essential*	*Nonessential*
• Methionine • Threonine • Tryptophan • Valine • Isoleucine • Leucine • Phenylalanine • Lysine	• Arginine • Histidine	• Glycine • Alanine • Serine • Cysteine • Tyrosine • Aspartate • Glutamate • Asparagine • Glutamine • Proline

i. Essential Amino Acids

Out of the 20 amino acids, commonly found in proteins, eight amino acids, i.e. **methionine, threonine, tryptophan, valine, isoleucine, leucine, phenylalanine** and **lysine** can not be synthesized in human beings. These are called essential amino acids and have to be supplied in the diet.

ii. Semi-essential Amino Acids

Besides the above eight amino acids, there are two amino acids, i.e. **arginine** and **histidine**, which are not essential for normal adult human beings but become dietary essential under certain conditions when either their demand is increased (such as during growth, pregnancy or lactation) or in hypercatabolic states (like high grade fever and chronic infections). Hence, these two amino acids are referred to as semi-essential amino acids.

iii. Nonessential Amino Acids

All the remaining amino acids which can be synthesized by human beings are not dietary essential and are referred to as nonessential amino acids.

FORMATION OF PEPTIDE BONDS

Peptides are biologically occurring short chains of amino acid monomers, which are linked by peptide (amide) bonds. When two amino acids join together, they form a peptide bond (–CO–NH–). During this process, carboxyl group of one amino acid reacts with the amino group of the other amino acid. This is a condensation reaction and results in the formation of amide linkage, called peptide bond (Fig. 3.11).

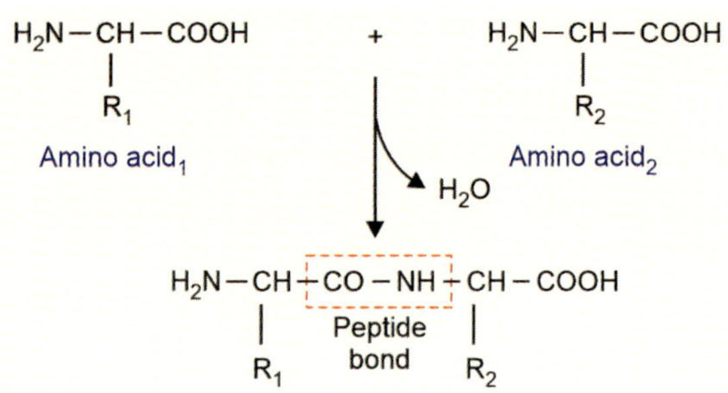

Fig. 3.11: Formation of a peptide bond

When several amino acids join to each other, it forms a polypeptide or protein. As discussed above, one end of the peptide has a free carboxyl group, which is referred to as C-terminus while the other end has a free amino group and is referred to as N-terminus (Fig. 3.1).

CLASSIFICATION OF PROTEINS

Depending upon their solubility and physical properties, proteins are classified into three groups (Table 3.5).

Table 3.5: Classification of proteins based on solubility and physical properties

Simple proteins	*Conjugated proteins*	*Derived proteins*
• Albumins • Globulins • Prolamines • Glutelins • Scleroproteins • Histones	• Nucleoproteins • Glycoproteins • Phosphoproteins • Metalloproteins • Lipoproteins	• Primary derived proteins • Secondary derived proteins

1. Simple Proteins

Based on their solubility, simple proteins are further divided into different groups, as follows:

i. **Albumins:** Albumins are soluble in water and neutral salt solutions. For example, **serum albumin, lactalbumin, egg albumin**, etc.
ii. **Globulins:** These are sparingly soluble in water, but are soluble in a neutral salt solution. Generally, globulins are found with albumins, e.g. **serum globulins, lactglobulin, egg globulin**, etc.
iii. **Prolamines:** Prolamines are insoluble in water, but are soluble in 60–80% of alcohol. For example, **gliadin** of wheat, **zein** of maize, etc.
iv. **Glutelins:** Glutelins are soluble in dilute acid or alkali, e.g. **gluten** of wheat, **oryzenin** of rice, etc.
v. **Scleroproteins:** These are highly insoluble and are **found**, mostly, **in** the supporting tissues such as **bone and cartilages**, and the protective tissues like **skin, hair, nail,** etc.
vi. **Histones:** Histones are soluble in water. They are rich in basic amino acids, e.g. **nucleohistones.**

2. Conjugated Proteins

These are the proteins, which are conjugated with some nonprotein substance called prosthetic group. These include:

i. **Nucleoproteins:** Proteins are **conjugated with nucleic acids**, e.g. histones.
ii. **Glycoproteins:** Proteins are **conjugated with carbohydrates**, e.g. **mucin**.
iii. **Phosphoproteins:** Proteins are **conjugated with phosphoric acid**, which is attached through the –OH group of serine, threonine or tyrosine, e.g. **casein** (a milk protein).
iv. **Metalloproteins:** Proteins are **associated with some metal**. They are also called metal-containing proteins. For example, **ceruloplasmin** (copper-containing protein), **hemoglobin** (iron-containing protein), etc.
V. **Lipoproteins:** Proteins **conjugated with lipids**, e.g. **chylomicrons, very low-density lipoproteins** (VLDL), etc.

3. Derived Proteins

These are the derivatives of simple proteins. They include:

i. **Primary derived proteins:** These are **obtained as a result of denaturation or coagulation** of a protein.
ii. **Secondary derived proteins:** These are **obtained as a result of the hydrolysis of proteins**, i.e. by the cleavage of the peptide bonds.

PROPERTIES OF PROTEINS

Acid–Base Properties

Amino acids may acquire either positive or negative charge, hence exhibit acid–base properties.

- At low pH, an amino acid exists in the cationic form as its amino group is protonated, i.e. in the form of $-NH_3^+$.
- As the pH rises, carboxyl group loses its proton and the amino acid is present as an ampholyte (Fig. 3.12).
- With further increase in pH, an amino group is deprotonated, thereby exhibiting the anionic form.

Isoelectric pH: Isoelectric pH, is **the pH at which a particular molecule carries no net charge**. The standard nomenclature to represent the isoelectric pH is

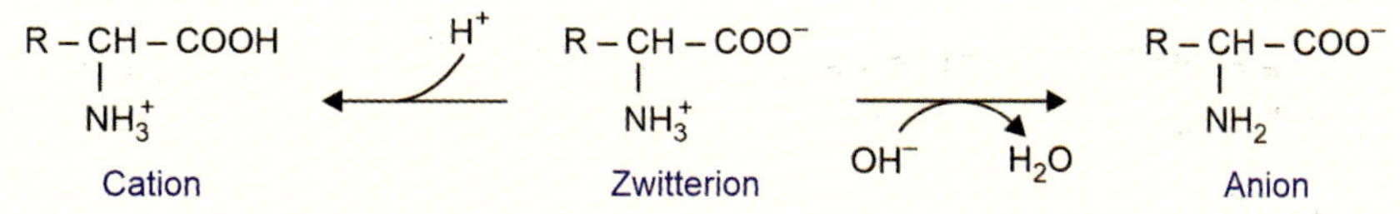

Fig. 3.12: Various ionic forms of an amino acid

isoelectric point (pI). The **pI** value can affect solubility of a molecule at a given pH.

Buffer Action

Amino acids, in an aqueous solution, contain weakly acidic α-carboxyl groups and weakly basic α-amino groups. In addition, acidic and basic amino acids also contain an ionizable group in its side chain. Hence, **amino acids also act as buffers**.

STRUCTURAL CONFORMATION OF PROTEINS

Variations in the number and the order of amino acids, i.e. the manner in which various amino acids are arranged in a polypeptide chain reflect **structure conformation of proteins**.

There are four levels of protein structure conformation, referred to as primary, secondary, tertiary and quaternary conformation of protein structure.

Primary Structure of Proteins

- Primary structure of a protein refers to the order and sequence of amino acids in a protein chain.
- Protein with a primary structure is a single polypeptide chain that has N-terminal and C-terminal ends, and various amino acids are linked together by the peptide linkages (Fig. 3.13).
- Some of the polypeptides may be synthesized as large peptides that are cleaved into two or more small peptides. These peptides may be linked together by the disulfide bonds, e.g. insulin.
- Thus, primary structure of a protein has peptide linkages and disulfide bonds. A change in the sequence or number of amino acids may cause some abnormality, which, in turn, may also affect functions and properties of the protein.

Secondary Structure of Proteins

Secondary structure of a protein refers to folding and twisting patterns of the polypeptide chain, i.e. spatial arrangement of the polypeptide. Secondary structures include **α-helix** and **β-sheet structures**.

Helix structure: As we know, helix is formed by twisting the backbone of the straight chain of a macromolecule such as protein or nucleic acids.

α-Helix

It refers to the right-handed folding of the protein chain (Fig. 3.14).

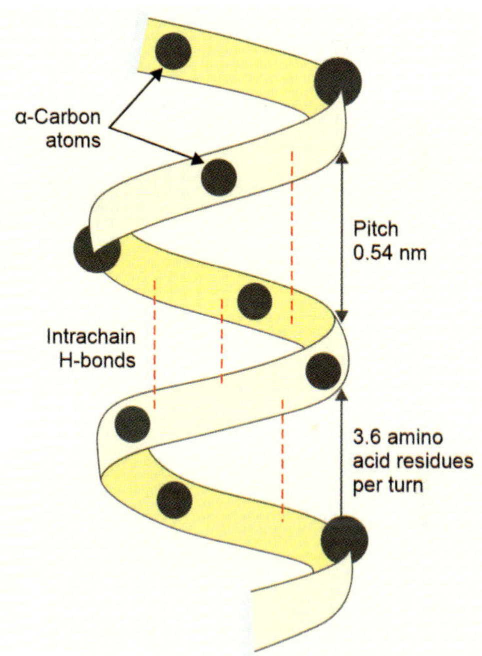

Fig. 3.14: Secondary structure of protein: α-helix (right-handed helix)

It is the most stable conformation, which is observed in a peptide chain, e.g. keratin. These have **intrachain peptide linkages**.

β-Pleated sheet structure

The second regular structural organization found in proteins is referred to as β-pleated sheet structure. It is referred to as β, since it was described after the discovery of the α-helix structure.

- β-Pleated sheet structure has **rippled or pleated edge**, therefore, this conformation is also called **pleated sheet-like structure**.

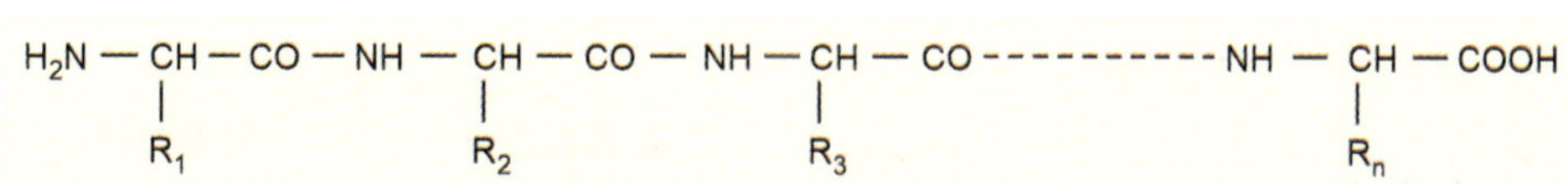

Fig. 3.13: Primary structure of a protein

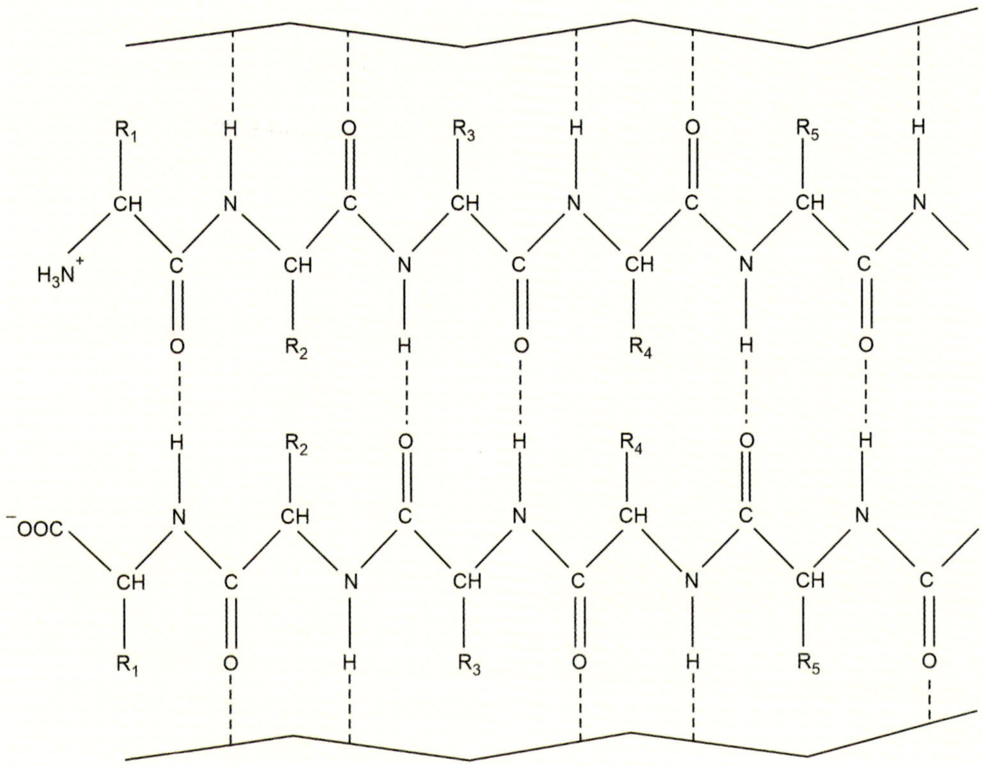

Fig. 3.15: Secondary structure of protein: β-pleated she

- β-Pleated sheet-like structure is **formed due to the stretching of the polypeptide chains**. These have **interchain peptide linkages** (Fig. 3.15).

Tertiary Structure of Proteins

Tertiary structure of a protein refers to the **intramolecular folding of the polypeptide chain**, thereby, **forming** a compact **three-dimensional structure that has a specific shape**.

- **Electrovalent linkages, hydrogen bonds, disulfide bridges, van der Waals forces and hydrophobic interactions** are responsible for the stabilization of the tertiary structure of proteins (Fig. 3.16).
- Depending upon their overall morphology, proteins having tertiary level of structures may exhibit **globular or fibrous shapes**.

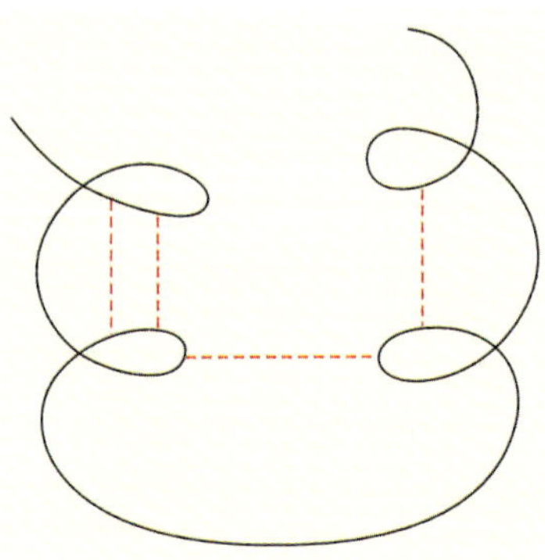

Fig. 3.16: Tertiary level of protein structure

- **Globular proteins**—globular proteins have a **spheroidal shape** with varying sizes.
  - Globular proteins are **highly soluble** in water, and weak acids and bases.
  - They **perform various functions** such as **catalysis, transport of substances, regulation of metabolic pathways and gene expression.**
  - They have several types of secondary structures and their shape is a result of the complex interaction between the secondary, tertiary and sometimes, may be, quaternary structures.
  - Most common globular proteins include **myoglobin, hemoglobin, immunoglobulins,** etc.
  - **Hemoglobin** consists of heme that is surrounded by four globular protein subunits, due to which it **has a globular structure**.
- **Fibrous proteins**—fibrous proteins exhibit special mechanical properties. They contain large amount of the regular secondary structures and have long cylindrical (rod-like) shapes.
  - They have low solubility in water.
  - Fibrous proteins have protective, connective or supportive role in the living organisms.
  - They are found as the components of skin, connective tissue, blood vessel walls, and sclera and cornea of the eye, e.g. **collagen, keratin, tropomyosin**, etc.
  - **Keratin is a fibrous protein** since it is an elongated strand-like protein, insoluble in water, and weak acids and bases.

Quaternary Structure of Proteins

Proteins having quaternary structure have several identical and/or different peptide chains. Each of its peptide chain is referred as a subunit. Several subunits are associated with a specific geometry (Fig. 3.17).

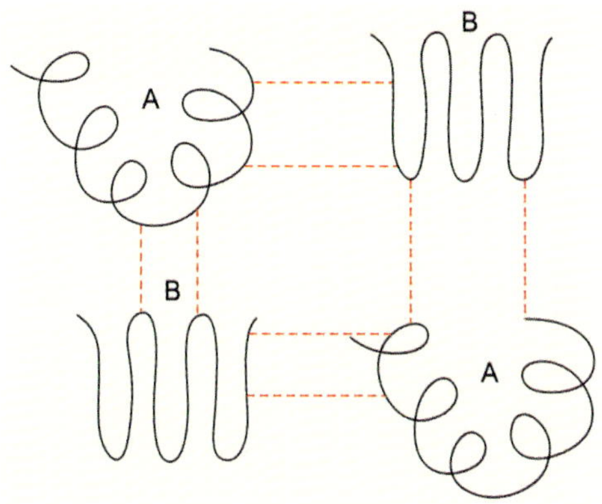

Fig. 3.17: Quaternary level of protein structure

Proteins with more than one subunit are called **oligomeric proteins,** e.g. hemoglobin.

Hemoglobin is an oligomeric protein. It has four subunits, i.e. 2α and 2β chains (α2β2). Disintegration of the monomeric subunits of the protein having quaternary structure may result in loss of its biological activity.

PROTEIN DENATURATION

Due to their organized structure, proteins are, usually, soluble in water. On heating or by the addition of a strong acid, protein loses its native structure and gets precipitated. This is referred to as denaturation.

- **Denaturation** of a protein **results in loss of its biological activity**, due to unfolding and disorganization of its secondary and tertiary structures.
- Under ideal conditions, **denaturation may be reversible**, however, most proteins, once denatured, remain permanently disordered.
- Denatured proteins are **often insoluble** and, therefore, can be removed from the solution.
- **Denaturing agents include mechanical force, detergents, strong acids or bases, heavy metals (such as lead and mercury), alkaloidal reagents and heat.**

Denaturation by heavy metals: Proteins can also be precipitated by denaturation by the addition of the salts of heavy metals such as **lead acetate, mercuric chloride, barium chloride, zinc sulfate**, etc. This is due to the adsorption of the metallic cations by the negatively charged colloidal protein particles.

Hydrochloric acid (HCl) can also hydrolyse a peptide bond but at high temperature only (more than 100°C). HCl cannot break a peptide bond at room temperature.

Denaturation by alkaloidal reagents: Proteins can be precipitated by the addition of some alkaloidal reagent, e.g. **picric acid**. Precipitation by an alkaloidal reagent is due to the formation of an insoluble salt by the anions of the reagent and the positively charged protein particles.

Denaturation by heat: Proteins can also be denatured by the heat. This process is referred to as **heat coagulation**. Coagulation is maximum at isoelectric pH (pI).

Some Important Questions

1. **What are amino acids? Classify them.**
2. **What are proteins? Classify proteins based on their solubility.**
3. **Discuss briefly:**
   i. α-Helix
   ii. β-Sheet structure
   iii. Quaternary structure of protein
   iv. Structure conformation of protein
   v. Biological functions of proteins
   vi. Aromatic amino acids
   vii. Sulfur-containing amino acids
   viii. Essential amino acids
   ix. Branched chain amino acid
   x. Basic amino acids
   xi. Classification of amino acids according to nutritional requirement
4. **Write notes on:**
   i. Zwitter ion
   ii. Fibrous proteins
   iii. Globular proteins
   iv. Protein denaturation

Chapter

4

Nucleic Acids

Nucleic acids are the **macromolecules**, which occur in cells in association **with basic proteins**, such as histones and protamines. They are **strongly acidic** in nature, and are **negatively charged** at physiological pH.

Building Units of Nucleic Acids

Repeated monomer units, called **nucleotides**, are the building blocks of nucleic acids, as amino acids to proteins or monosaccharides to polysaccharides.

A nucleotide has 3 constituents, i.e. a **nitrogenous base**, a **pentose sugar** and **phosphoric acid.**

Nitrogenous Bases

Nitrogenous bases, found in nucleotides, are the derivatives of either a purine or a pyrimidine.

- **Purines:** A purine is a nine-member ring, containing 5 carbons and 4 nitrogen atoms (Fig. 4.1).

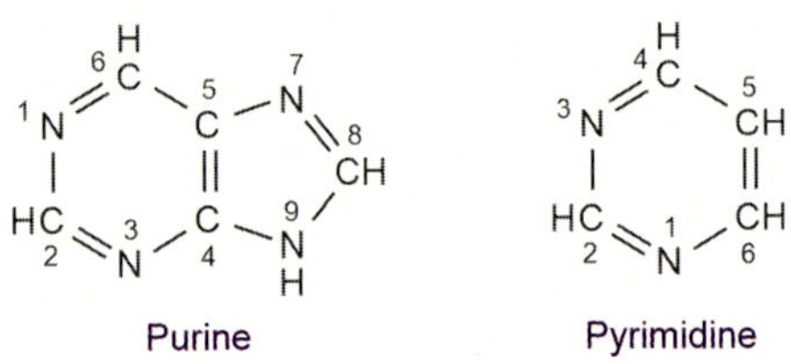

Fig. 4.1: Purine and pyrimidine rings

There are two purine bases found in nucleic acids. These are referred to as adenine (6-aminopurine) and guanine (2-amino-6-oxypurine; Fig. 4.2).

- **Pyrimidines:** A pyrimidine is a six-member ring, having 4 carbons and 2 nitrogen atoms.

Pyrimidine bases found in nucleic acids include **cytosine** (2-oxy-4-aminopyrimidine), **uracil** (2,4-dioxypyrimidine) and **thymine** (2,4-dioxy-5-methylpyrimidine, also referred as 5-methyluracil.

Out of the three pyrimidines, only two are found in a nucleic acid. Usually, cytosine and uracil are found in RNA, while cytosine and thymine are found in DNA.

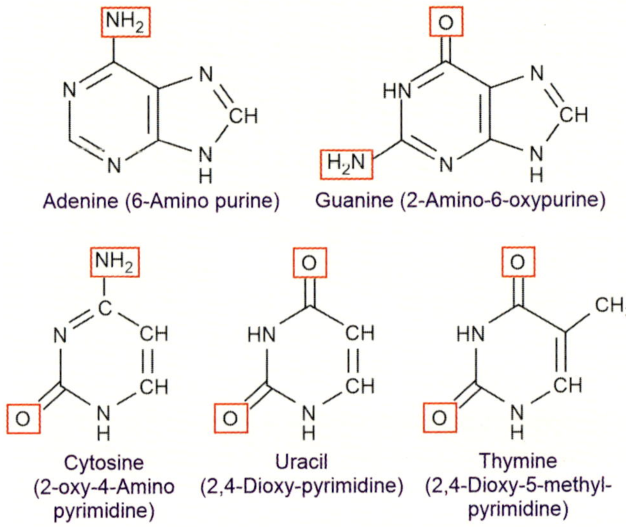

Fig. 4.2: Purine and pyrimidine bases found in nucleic acids

Pentose Sugars

Presence of the pentose sugar defines type of the nucleic acid.

There are two classes of nucleic acids, called deoxyribonucleic acid (DNA) and ribonucleic acid (RNA). As the name suggests, deoxyribonucleic acid contains deoxyribose, whereas ribonucleic acid contains ribose.

- **Ribose:** Ribose has three –OH groups, one each at carbon atoms 1, 2 and 3 of the pentose sugar.
- **Deoxyribose:** Deoxyribose does not contain oxygen at the second carbon, and, thus, it has only two –OH groups (one each at carbon numbers 1 and 3). Deoxyribose thus, is also called 2-deoxyribose (Fig. 4.3).

Molecule of the pentose sugar is linked to the nitrogenous base on one side through carbon number one (C-1) and to phosphoric acid on the other side, through carbon number five (C-5) in a nucleotide.

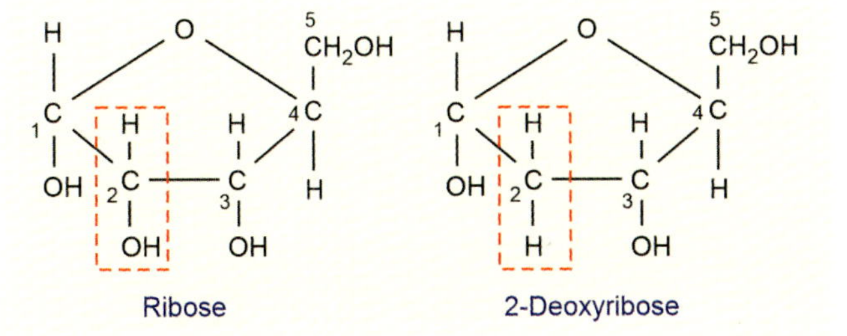

Fig. 4.3: Ribose and deoxyribose

NUCLEOSIDES

A nucleoside has two components and consists of a **nitrogenous base** and a **pentose sugar**.

- The molecule of sugar (ribose or deoxyribose) is linked to the nitrogenous base with the N-glycosidic linkage.
- To differentiate the carbon of the sugar from the carbon of the nitrogenous base, position of the carbon of the sugar molecule is shown with a prime sign ('), such as C-1', C-5', etc. On the other hand, carbons and nitrogen of the nitrogenous bases are written without the prime sign, as N-1, C-2, etc.
- In a nucleoside, generally, carbon at the first position of the sugar, i.e. C-1', is linked to N-1 of the pyrimidine or N-9 of the purine, as shown below:

Base-N (1/9) - C-1′-Sugar

According to the presence of the pentose sugar, nucleosides are classified as ribonucleosides and deoxyribonucleosides.

- **Ribonucleosides:** Nucleosides containing ribose are called ribonucleosides. The ribonucleosides of adenine guanine, cytosine and uracil are designated as **adenosine, guanosine, cytidine** and **uridine**, respectively (Fig. 4.4).

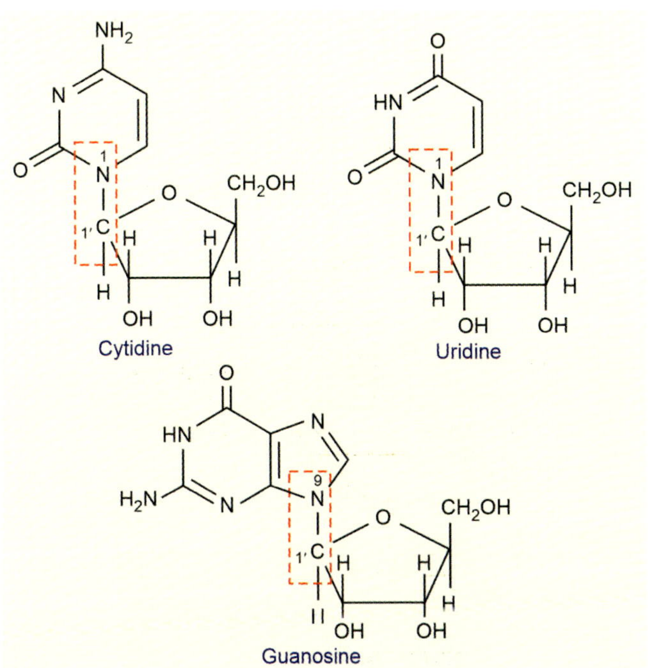

Fig. 4.4: Ribonucleosides

- **Deoxyribonucleosides:** Nucleosides containing deoxyribose are designated as deoxyribonucleosides. These are written with a prefix deoxy- (or d-). Thus, **deoxyadenosine, deoxyguanosine, deoxycytidine** and **deoxythymidine** are the nucleosides containing deoxyribose with adenine, guanine, cytosine and thymine, respectively. Since thymine is usually found in DNA only and is, generally, linked to deoxyribose, deoxythymidine can simply be referred to as **thymidine** (Fig. 4.5).

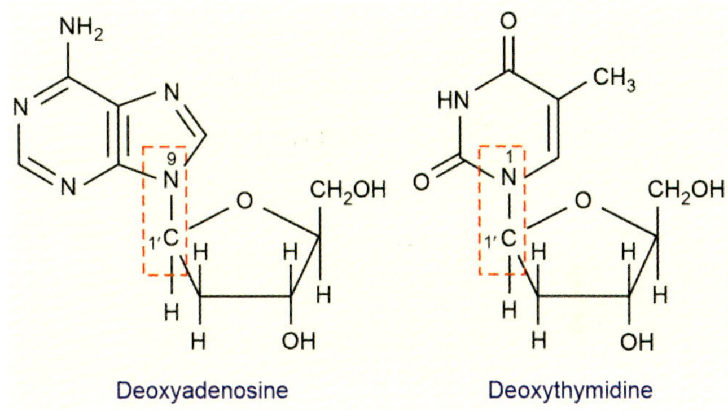

Fig. 4.5: Deoxyribonucleosides

NUCLEOTIDES

In addition to base and sugar (nucleoside), a nucleotide also has a molecule of phosphoric acid. The sugar molecule (ribose or deoxyribose) is, generally, linked to the nitrogenous base on one side and to phosphoric acid on the other side, e.g. C-1' of a sugar is linked to the nitrogenous base through N-1 of a pyrimidine or N-9 of a purine. Though any hydroxy group (–OH) of a sugar may be esterified with phosphoric acid, generally, C-5′of a sugar is linked to phosphoric acid (also referred to as phosphate), as shown below:

Base-N (1/9) - C-1′-Sugar-C-5′-P

According to the presence of the type of sugar, nucleotides are classified as ribonucleotides and deoxyribonucleotides.

- **Ribonucleotides:** Nucleotides of the ribose are called ribonucleotides. Four ribonucleotides are generally obtained on hydrolysis of RNA. These are designated as **adenosine monophosphate** or **adenylate (AMP), guanylate (GMP), cytidylate (CMP)** and **uridylate (UMP).** Some of these are shown in Fig. 4.6).
- **Deoxyribonucleotides:** Deoxyribonucleotides are obtained on the hydrolysis of DNA and are designated as **dAMP, dGMP, dCMP** and **dTMP** (Fig. 4.7).

Various nitrogenous bases, nucleosides and nucleotides, which are commonly obtained on the hydrolysis of nucleic acids, are given in Table 4.1.

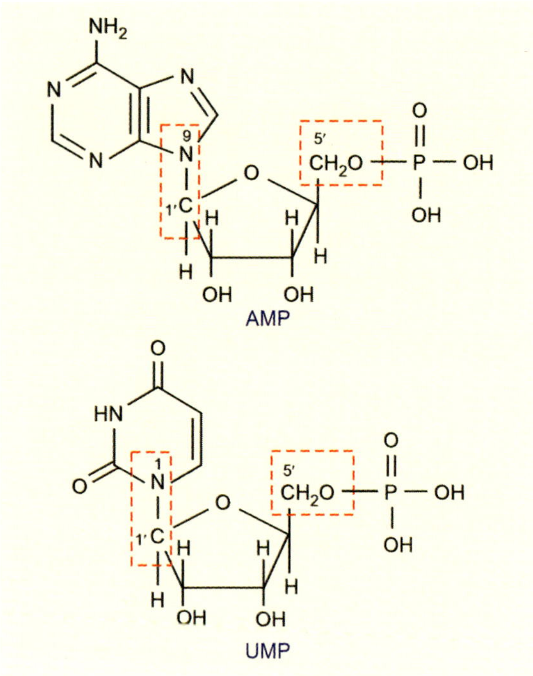

Fig. 4.6: Ribonucleotides

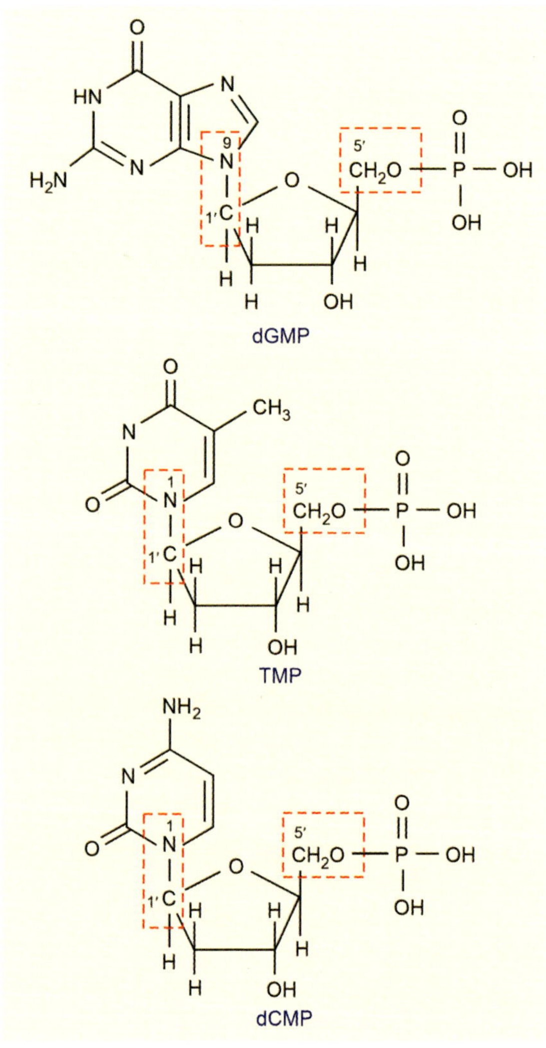

Fig. 4.7: Deoxyribonucleotides

Table 4.1: Various nitrogenous bases, and the corresponding nucleosides and nucleotides found in RNA and DNA

Nitrogenous bases	*Nucleosides (Base + Sugar)*	*Nucleotides (Base + Sugar + P)*
RNA		
Adenine	Adenosine	AMP
Guanine	Guanosine	GMP
Cytosine	Cytidine	CMP
Uracil	Uridine	UMP
DNA		
Adenine	Deoxyadenosine	dAMP
Guanine	Deoxyguanosine	dGMP
Cytosine	Deoxycytidine	dCMP
Thymine	Thymidine	dTMP

NUCLEIC ACIDS

Two types of nucleic acids are found in nature, these are called deoxyribonucleic acid **(DNA)** and ribonucleic acid **(RNA)**.

DEOXYRIBONUCLEIC ACID

Deoxyribonucleic acid **(DNA)** stores genetic information in the cell and is called the chemical basis of heredity. DNA is a large molecule, which occurs in various sizes, with few hundred to several million nucleotides. It is a double-stranded polymer of deoxyribonucleotides, which are linked together by phosphodiester bonds.

Structure of DNA

Watson and Crick described various features of the DNA molecule, hence, the most commonly referred structure of DNA is called **Watson-Crick model of DNA** (Fig. 4.8).

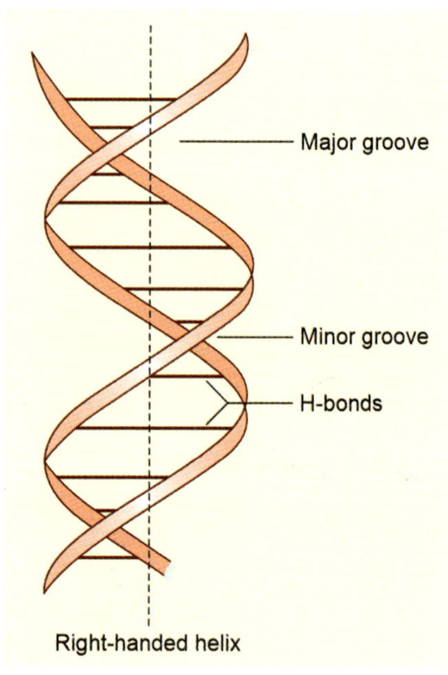

Fig. 4.8: Watson-Crick model of DNA

- DNA is a polynucleotide of deoxyadenylate **(dAMP)**, deoxyguanylate **(dGMP)**, deoxycytidylate **(dCMP)** and thymidylate **(TMP)**.
- **Information** content of DNA **resides in the sequence**, in which various deoxyribonucleotides are arranged.
- The polymer **possesses a polarity**. Its **left-hand terminal** has a **free hydroxyl group or phosphate** and is called **5′-terminus**. On the other hand, the **right-handed terminal** is referred to as **3′-terminus**.
- DNA is a **double-stranded molecule**, i.e. it has two strands (polynucleotide sequences or chains), which run **antiparallel to each other**. Whereas, its one strand runs in the 5′→3′ direction while the other one runs in the opposite direction, i.e. in 3′→5′ direction.
- Both the polynucleotide chains are wound around a common axis, forming **right-handed helix**, which is nearly 20Å in diameter.
- This helix has a **pitch of 34 Å** with 10 base-pairs (bp) per turn.
- The **two strands** of the helix are **held together by hydrogen bonds**, which are formed between a purine and a pyrimidine. This base pairing is very specific, as A is always linked to T with two hydrogen bonds while G is linked to C with three hydrogen bonds.
- Thus, a DNA molecule has **equal number of adenine and thymine** residues as well as **guanine and cytosine** residues. This relationship is known as **Chargaff's rule**.
- Bases occupy core of the helix while sugar-phosphate chain runs along the periphery. This, in turn, forms two grooves of unequal width. They are called the **major groove** and the **minor groove**.

RIBONUCLEIC ACIDS

Three main classes of **RNA** are known to occur in cells. They are known as messenger RNA, ribosomal RNA and transfer RNA. Though all the three types of RNA are involved in protein biosynthesis, they differ from each other with respect to their size, composition, location within the cell and functions.

Types of RNAs

Messenger RNA

Messenger RNA (mRNA) is a **group of RNAs**, which is most **heterogeneous**. They are highly elongated but **short-lived** molecules, which are **synthesized within the nucleus**, as a result of **transcription**.

- The mRNA transcript has 5′→3′ polarity, which is **complementary to the coding strand of gene** (DNA molecule) with the only difference that mRNA contains uracil in place of thymine, which is found in DNA (Fig. 4.9).
- The molecule of mRNA **conveys message** (information) **from gene to the protein-synthesizing machinery**.

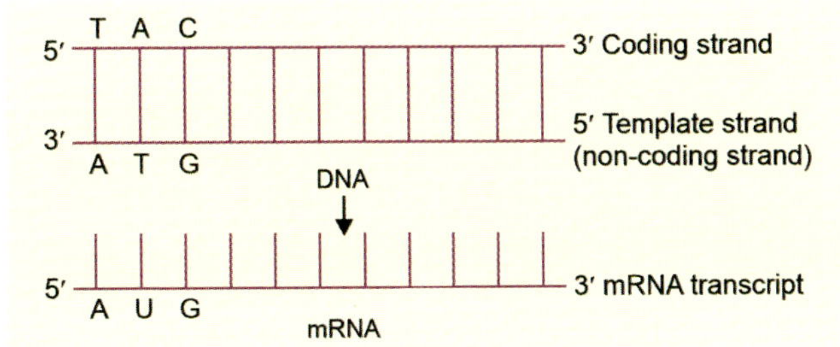

Fig. 4.9: Representation of DNA and the corresponding mRNA

This information is present in mRNA in the form of sequences of nucleotides, as **triplets**, called **codons**.

- Each mRNA molecule serves as a template on which a specific sequence of amino acids is polymerized to form a specific protein, the ultimate product of gene.
- The mRNAs are, generally, stable in eukaryotes but quite unstable in prokaryotes.
- **In mammalian cells**, the transcription product of DNA is a large molecule called **heterogeneous nuclear RNA** (hnRNA) that **undergoes post-transcriptional changes** and gets **converted to mRNA**, which is released into cytosol and is **used for protein biosynthesis**.

Transfer RNAs

Transfer RNA (tRNA) molecules are much smaller in size and consist of **75 to 90 ribonucleotides** only. Total tRNA comprises about 15 per cent of the cellular RNA. The tRNA is **also known as soluble RNA (sRNA)** because it is **found in the soluble fraction of the cell**.

- There are about **50 different types of tRNAs**, each one of which fulfils its role as an adapter molecule and has a sequence of three nucleotides, called **anticodon**.
- Each tRNA **binds an amino acid** and **locates itself at the correct codon**, for the translation of information. This information is present in the sequence of nucleotides on mRNA and is **translated into the sequence of amino acids**, thereby, **forming a peptide chain**.
- **Various tRNAs**, though differ from each other with respect to their nucleotide sequences, as a class **have many common features**:
  - The nucleotide sequence (primary structure) allows extensive **folding and intramolecular base-pairing** to form a secondary structure, which gives it a **cloverleaf-like structure**.
  - All tRNA molecules, in addition to the four bases, i.e. A, G, C and U, also **contain several unusual (modified) bases**, e.g. 7-methylguanine, thymine, dihydrouracil, pseudouracil, hypoxanthine, etc.
  - All tRNA molecules **have different** intramolecular foldings, called arms:
    - ❑ **Amino acid acceptor arm:** It has **7 base-paired stem** that has **CCA sequence in the 5′→3′** direction at the terminal. Its **adenosyl moiety** (A) **accepts the particular amino acid.** In this process, the carboxyl group of amino acid forms

an ester linkage with the 3′-hydroxyl group of the adenosyl moiety.

- **Anticodon arm: It has 5 base-pairs and a loop.** Its loop **has a triplet**, i.e. a sequence of three nucleotides called **anticodon**. Hence, this arm is called anticodon arm. The anticodon has a sequence which is **complementary to the sequence of three nucleotides of the codon.** It is **responsible for the specificity of the tRNA molecule.**
- **DHU-arm:** It **has an unusual base** called dihydrouracil (**DHU** or UH2), in its loop. Hence, it is called DHU arm. Besides DHU, it has 3 to 4 base pairs.
- **TψC-arm:** It **has a sequence of thymine** (T), **pseudouracil** (ψ) and cytosine (C) in its loop. Hence, it is called TψC arm. Besides, it also has 5 base pairs.
- **Extra arm:** In addition to the above, each tRNA also has one small arm, called **extra arm**, which has a **small loop of 3–5 base pairs** (Fig. 4.10).

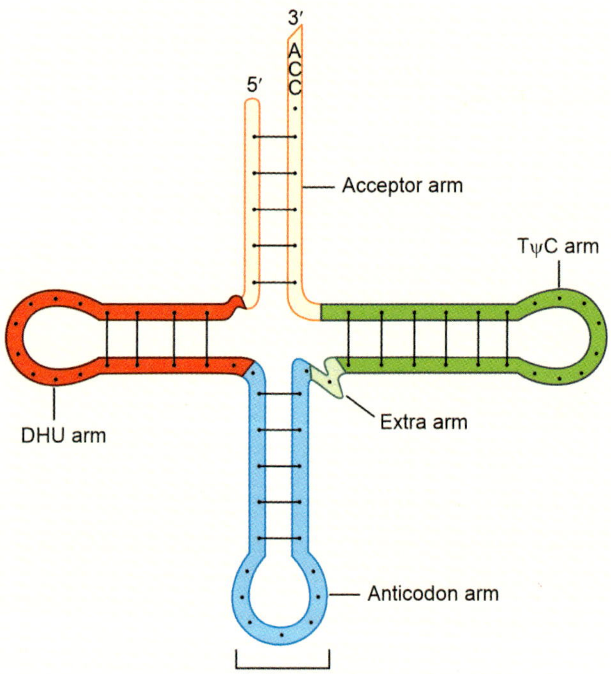

Fig. 4.10: tRNA

Ribosomal RNA

Ribosomal RNA (rRNA) molecules are **present in ribosomes, in association with several polypeptides.**

- Ribosomes are **found in cytosol** of the cell and contain nearly 80% of the total RNA, found in the cell.
- Both, **mRNA and tRNA interact on ribosomes**, to translate the information, which is transcribed from gene, into a specific protein.
- **Mammalian ribosomes** are very complex in nature with a sedimentation velocity of **80S**. Each of the ribosome **has** 2 subunits, which are referred to as **large subunit (60S)** and **small subunit (40S).**
- The large subunit contains 3 different types of rRNA, which are designated as **5S, 5.8S and 28S rRNA.** It also has more than 50 polypeptides. The **small subunit has 18S rRNA** and nearly 30 polypeptides (Fig. 4.11).

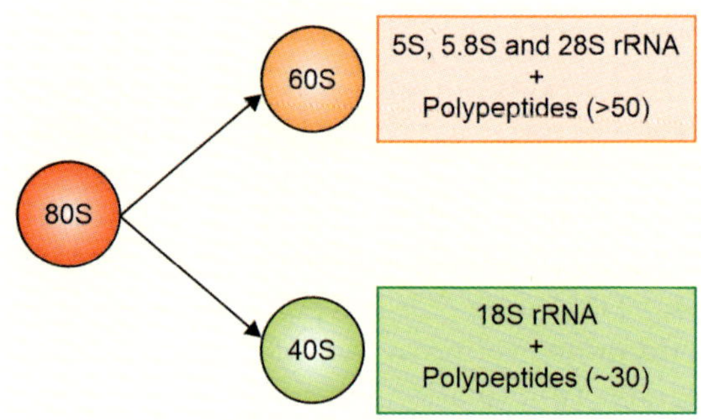

Fig. 4.11: Mammalian ribosome particles and their contents

DIFFERENCES BETWEEN DNA AND RNA

As shown in Table 4.2, DNA differs from RNA in several aspects.

Table 4.2: Differences between DNA and RNA

	DNA	*RNA*
Sugars	Deoxyribose	Ribose
Bases	A, G, C and T	A, G, C and U
Strands	Double-stranded	Usually single-stranded
Purine/pyrimidine ratio	A = T and G = C Also, A + G = C + T	No ratio

Some Important Questions

1. **Describe various features of the Watson-Crick Model of DNA.**
2. **Describe various types of RNAs with their functions.**
3. **What is a nucleotide? Name different nucleotides found in DNA.**
4. **Write notes on:**
   - i. Structure and functions of tRNA
   - ii. Differences between DNA and RNA
   - iii. Various nitrogenous bases found in nucleic acids
   - iv. Nucleosides
   - v. Nucleotides
   - vi. hnRNA
   - vii. Structural features of tRNA
   - viii. Messenger RNA

Chapter

5

High-energy Compounds

High-energy compounds include **compounds** such as phosphate esters and mixed anhydrides, **which have a high-energy bond** whose **hydrolysis yields** large amount of **energy**.

Most of the high-energy compounds have high-energy phosphate bonds (called **high-energy phosphate compounds**) while others may be the **thioesters**.

HIGH-ENERGY PHOSPHATE COMPOUNDS

High-energy phosphate compounds include active phosphate carriers such as various **nucleoside triphosphates (ATP, GTP, CTP, UTP,** etc.); **phosphorylamidines,** e.g. creatine phosphate; and **enolphosphates,** like 1, 3-bisphosphoglycerate, phosphoenolpyruvate, etc.

Adenosine Triphosphate

Adenosine triphosphate **(ATP)** is an organic compound, a **ribonucleotide, comprising of adenine, ribose** and 3 phosphate molecules. The last two of the phosphate groups are joined as **high energy phosphate bonds,** referred to as β **and** γ **bonds.**

When the γ-bond of ATP is hydrolyzed, it provides nearly 7.3 kcal of the useable energy in metabolism (Fig. 5.1).

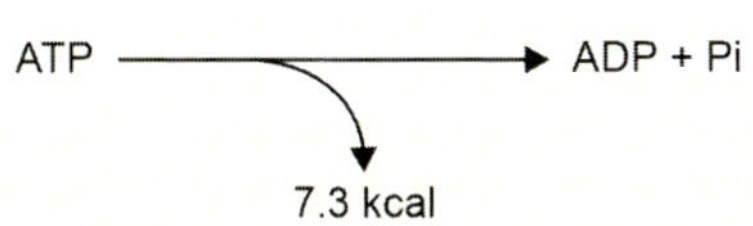

Fig. 5.1: Hydrolysis of ATP with release of energy

ATP Requiring Metabolic Processes

All the cellular and metabolic processes require ATP to meet their energy requirements. As mentioned above, during these cellular processes ATP transfers its energy (high energy phosphate) to phosphorylate other compounds.

In the cell, ATP is used in various processes such as DNA replication, active transport of substances, muscle contraction and various synthetic processes:

- **Growth and repair:** Increase of cell size and replacement of the damaged tissue requires ATP.
- **Movement:** The contraction of muscle fibers, in order to generate movement in organisms, also requires ATP.
- **Nerve transmission:** The generation and transmission of a nerve impulse (action potential) too needs ATP.
- **Active transport:** Moving molecules against their concentration gradient, or by cytosis, also require ATP.
- **Biosynthesis of macromolecules:** Building complex organic molecules from the simpler subunits (anabolism) also require ATP.
- **Emission of light:** Some of the cells may be capable of luminescence, and this process also requires ATP.

Molecular Unit of Currency

Energy, in living cells, is stored and released in the chemical form of ATP (adenosine triphosphate). **ATP** provides energy to derive and support various metabolic processes in the body. Thus, it is also referred to as **molecular unit of currency** for the intracellular transfer of energy from one molecule to another.

ATP serves as the molecular unit of energy currency in the cell. After the hydrolysis of the phospho-anhydride bond, ATP can be regenerated by coupling its formation to a more exergonic metabolic process, such as by the direct transfer of a phosphoryl group from another high-energy compound, like phosphoenolpyruvate.

Thus, **ATP is an energy carrier** and not a store of energy. There is a continuous flow of energy from high energy phosphate compounds (such as 1,3-bisphosphoglycerate) to form ATP, and from ATP to low energy phosphate compounds (such as glucose-6-phosphate and glycerol-3-phosphate) whose free energy of hydrolysis is much below than the preceding high energy compound. Since, it is continually hydrolyzed as well as regenerated, ATP occupies a middle rank with respect to the standard free energy of phosphate hydrolysis of various high energy and low energy phosphorylated compounds (Table 5.1).

Table 5.1: Phosphorylated compounds of biological significance

Phosphorylated compound	*Free energy of hydrolysis ($\Delta G^{o\prime}$; kcal/mol)*
Phosphoenolpyruvate	14.8
1,3-Bisphosphoglycerate	11.8
Creatine phosphate	10.5
ATP	**7.3***
Glucose-1-phosphate	5.0
Glucose-6-phosphate	3.3
AMP	2.2

*ATP occupies a central position, hence it is also called universal cellular energy currency.

ATP Generation

ATP cannot be synthesized as it is only a carrier of the high-energy phosphate bond, but is regenerated by the transmembrane enzyme ATP synthase, via cell respiration.

Our body recycles ATP, nearly, equivalent to our body weight, daily. Since it is a continuous process, nearly 10 g of ATP is needed in the body at any given time to meets all the energy needs.

The complex organic food macromolecules, i.e. carbohydrates, lipids and proteins, are the rich sources of energy for cells, because much of the energy used to form these molecules is, literally, stored within the chemical bonds that hold them together. Cells release this energy (stored in the food molecules) through a series of metabolic processes.

Biochemical processes involved in the generation of ATP—eukaryotic cells use three major processes to transform the energy held in the chemical bonds of food molecules into more readily usable forms, often energy-rich carrier molecules.

1. **The first process** in the eukaryotic energy pathway **is glycolysis,** which, literally, means sugar splitting. It is a series of ten chemical reactions that requires the input of two ATP molecules. This input is used to generate four new ATP molecules, which means that glycolysis results in a net generation (gain) **of two ATP**.
   - During glycolysis, a molecule of **glucose is split** and, ultimately, converted **into two molecules of pyruvate, which enters the second process of energy generation, called citric acid cycle** (tricarboxylic acid cycle or **TCA**).
   - **Besides** two ATP, **two molecules of NADH are also generated** in glycolysis, which serve as electron carriers **to enter the third process of energy generation** called **electron transport chain (ETC)** and are also used for other biochemical reactions in the cell.
2. **The second process is called TCA cycle.** It is an **aerobic process.**

   In this process, **pyruvate** produced as above, **enters mitochondria** and **is converted to acetyl CoA** (two-carbon energy carrier compound). This in turn also **generates NADH.**

   Thereafter, **acetyl CoA enters TCA** cycle where it is oxidized to CO_2 and water, and **generates three NADH, one $FADH_2$** and **one GTP** (*see* Chapter 12).
3. **The third major energy generation process** in the eukaryotic energy pathway involves an **electron transport chain** which is catalyzed by several protein complexes located in the mitochondrional inner membrane. This process called **oxidative phosphorylation** transfers electrons from NADH and $FADH_2$ through the membrane protein complexes to oxygen and form water. As electrons travel through the protein complexes in the chain, a gradient of hydrogen ions, or protons, is formed across the mitochondrial membrane. Cells harness the energy of this proton gradient to create three additional ATP molecules for every electron that travels along the chain (*see* Chapter 11).

   Together these processes that occur inside the mitochondria, i.e. the TCA cycle and oxidative phosphorylation, **are referred to as respiration.**

Nucleoside Triphosphates other than ATP

Besides ATP, **other nucleoside triphosphates** such as CTP, GTP, UTP or the deoxy-nucleoside triphosphates (dATP, dGTP, dCTP and TTP) are also referred to as high-energy phosphate compounds. These can be synthesized from the corresponding nucleoside diphosphates and ATP.

PHOSPHORYLAMIDINES

Phosphorylamidines, phosphoguanidines or phosphogens include high energy compounds such as phosphocreatine and phosphoarginine which have phosphoryl group transfer potentials. For example, phosphocreatine acts as ATP reservoir in cells, such as muscle and nerve cells, which contain creatine phosphokinase and have high ATP turnover.

Intracellular concentration of the reactants and the products, however, operate close to equilibrium ($\Delta G = 0$). Accordingly, when the cell is in a resting state and that ATP concentration is relatively high, reaction proceeds towards the synthesis of phosphocreatine. On the other hand, at the time of high metabolic activity, when ATP concentration is low, the equilibrium shifts so as to yield ATP from phosphocreatine and ADP.

THIOESTERS

Thioesters include high energy compounds such as acetyl CoA and succinyl CoA.

Coenzyme A

Coenzyme A (HSCoA or CoA) functions as a carrier of the acetyl and other acyl groups.

In acetyl CoA, acetyl group is linked by the thioester linkage to the sulfhydral-portion of the β-mercapto-ethylamine. Acetyl CoA is also a high-energy compound.

The ΔG^{o}/for the hydrolysis of its thioester bond is 7.8 kcal/mol, which makes this reaction slightly more exergonic than the hydrolysis of ATP.

Succinyl CoA

Cleavage of the succinyl CoA also releases sufficient free energy to synthesize GTP from GDP and Pi.

ENOL PHOSPHATES

There are several compounds called enol-phosphates such as 1,3-bisphospho-glycerate, which have phosphoryl group transfer potentials. They can directly transfer their phosphoryl-group to ADP and generate ATP. Such compounds rank above ATP and are called **high-energy phosphate donors**.

On the other hand, there are some other compounds, such as glucose-6-phosphate and glycerol-3-phosphate whose free energy of hydrolysis is lower than ATP. These are formed by the transfer of a phosphoryl-group from ATP. Such compounds rank below ATP and are referred to as **low energy phosphate acceptors**.

Some Important Questions

1. Discuss various high-energy compounds.

2. Write notes on:

i. ATP
ii. Phosphocreatine
iii. Thioesters
iv. Enol phosphates
v. ATP as cellular currency of energy

Chapter
6

Enzymes

Enzymes are **organic molecules,** which are produced in living organisms and **increase rate of a biochemical reaction** without being utilized in the overall process. These are **nondialyzable colloidal particles,** which are **thermolabile proteins** with highly specific catalytic activity.

CLASSIFICATION OF ENZYMES

Enzymes are, usually, **named by the suffix "-ase"** with the name of the substrate, or the catalytic action of the enzyme, e.g. lipase (which catalyses hydrolysis of lipids), fatty acid synthase (which catalyses synthesis of fatty acids), etc. These names are called trivial names. However, while assigning a trivial name to an enzyme, no systematic rules were followed.

International Union of Biochemistry and Molecular Biology (IUBMB) adopted a scheme for rational system of naming each enzyme and suggested their functional classification.

- **According to IUBMB,** each enzyme is assigned **four-digit systematic code,** commonly known as **Enzyme Commission number** (EC number).
- **First digit** of the code denotes **main class of the enzyme,** which is assigned according to type of the chemical reaction it catalyzes.
- **Second digit** of the EC number characterizes **sub-class,** which is based on the nature of the chemical group removed or transferred, or any bond splitted or formed.
- Its **third digit** indicates **sub-sub-class** and describes detailed subdivision of the sub-class.
- **Last digit** of the EC number indicates **serial number of the enzyme** in the sub-sub-class.

For example, **1.1.1.1** denotes the enzyme **alcohol dehydrogenase,** which belongs to **class 1,** i.e. oxidoreductases. Sub-class 1 of the class 1 (oxidoreductases) includes enzymes, called **dehydrogenases. Sub-sub-class** 1, of the class 1 (oxidoreductases), of the sub-class 1 (dehydrogenases) includes those **dehydrogenases which require NAD^+ as a coenzyme.** Accordingly, **alcohol dehydrogenase** is the **first enzyme,** which is a **NAD^+ requiring dehydrogenase** that belongs to the class **oxidoreductases.**

According to the enzyme commission enzymes are classified into six classes (Table 6.1).

Table 6.1: Classification of enzymes with examples

Class of enzyme	*Examples*
Oxidoreductases	Alcohol dehydrogenase, xanthine oxidase, catalase
Transferases	Glutamate pyruvate transaminase, serine hydroxymethyl transferase, hexokinase
Hydrolases	Glucose-6-phosphatase, carboxypeptidase, pepsin
Lyases	Pyruvate decarboxylase, aldolase, histidase
Isomerases	Phosphotriose isomerase, phosphoglucomutase, alanine racemase
Ligases	Glutamine synthetase, acetyl-CoA carboxylase, glutathione synthetase

1. Oxidoreductases

Oxidoreductases are involved in the oxidation and/or reduction of a substrate, i.e. they catalyze addition of oxygen, removal of hydrogen or removal of electrons. Their sub-classes include dehydrogenases, oxidases, oxygenases, etc. Examples of the class oxidoreductases include alcohol dehydrogenase, xanthine oxidase, glutathione reductase, etc.

2. Transferases

Transferases catalyze transfer of a particular group from one substrate to another. On the basis of the group being transferred, they are sub-classified as aminotransferases, phosphotransferases, etc. Glutamate oxaloacetate transaminase, hexokinase, glucose-1-phosphate uridyl-transferase are some of the examples of transferases.

3. Hydrolases

Hydrolases catalyzes the hydrolysis of a substrate with a molecule of water. According to nature of the group or bond hydrolyzed, hydrolases are sub-classified as peptidases, glycosidases, etc. Examples of the class hydrolases include glucose-6-phosphatase, amylase, pepsin, etc.

4. Lyases

Lyases catalyze splitting of a substrate into two products without water. They are sub-classified on the basis of the linkage removed, e.g. breakdown of the C– C, C–N or C–S bond, etc. Examples of the class lyases include fumarase, pyruvate decarboxylase, histidase, etc.

5. Isomerases

Isomerases convert one isomeric form of a substrate to other, i.e. they catalyze isomerization of the substrate. Racemases, epimerases and mutases, etc. are the sub-classes of isomerases. Examples of the class isomerases include phosphohexose isomerase, phosphoglucomutase, alanine racemase, etc.

6. Ligases

Ligases catalyze synthesis of a product from two different substrates. This requires energy, which is coupled to the hydrolysis of a high-energy bond. Its various sub-classes include ligases, which form C–C, C–N or C–S bonds. Examples of the class ligases include glutamine synthetase, acetyl-CoA carboxylase, glutathione synthetase, etc.

ENZYME SPECIFICITY

Enzymes are highly specific in nature, i.e. they interact with only one or a few substrates and catalyze a specific type of reaction only. The extent of substrate specificity varies from enzyme to enzyme, as given in the following example.

Absolute Specificity

An enzyme has absolute specificity for its substrate and will not act upon any other substrate, e.g. urease is specific for urea only.

Relative Specificity

An enzyme may be specific either to a particular group or type of bond, e.g. protease (hydrolyzes peptide bond of protein), glycosidase (hydrolyzes glycosidic bond of polysaccharide), esterase (hydrolyzes ester bond of triacylglycerols), etc.

ACTIVE SITE OF ENZYME

The specificity of an enzyme is located in a particular region called active site or active center (Fig. 6.1).

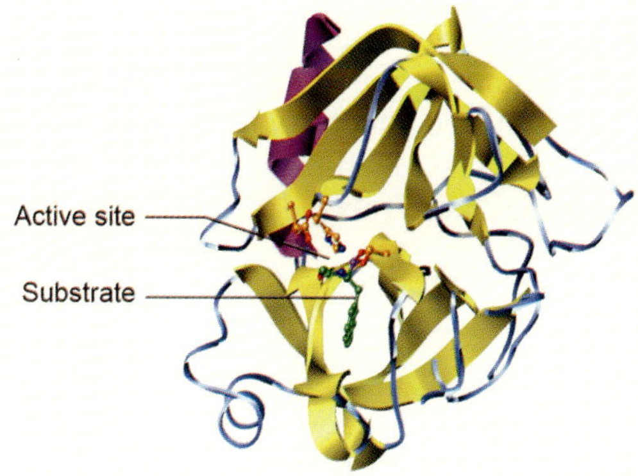

Fig. 6.1: Active site/center of an enzyme is a small cleft in the tertiary structure

Salient features of the active site

- Active site of an enzyme has a small cleft in the tertiary structure of the enzyme molecule, which is made up of:
  - **Substrate binding site:** This is the site where a substrate binds to the enzyme through various noncovalent forces such as van der Waals forces, electrostatic forces, hydrogen bonds and hydrophobic interactions.
  - **Catalytic site:** It is lined by specific amino acids, called catalytic residues, most commonly serine (others include cysteine, aspartate, histidine, tyrosine, arginine, lysine, etc.).
    - Catalytic residues are spatially close but actually distant from each other in the primary structure.
    - Cofactors are a part of the catalytic site.
    - Specific nucleotides are present in ribozymes.
- Binding of the substrate with the active site is explained by the lock-and-key model (assumes a rigid character of active site) or induced-fit model (assumes a flexible character of active site).
- It may be inactivated by alterations in temperature and pH.
- It may be blocked by various compounds resembling the substrate (reversible competitive enzyme inhibition) or by unrelated substances (irreversible enzyme poisoning).

COFACTORS AND COENZYMES

Some of the enzymes require the presence of certain small nonprotein factors, such as an organic molecule (coenzyme) or a metal ion (cofactor) for their activity.

Cofactors

The **inorganic ions**, such as Mg^{2+}, Zn^{2+} or Cl^-, etc. required for the catalytic activity of an enzyme, are called cofactors. Depending upon the attachment of the metal ion with the enzyme, such enzymes may be divided into two groups:

- **Metal-activated enzymes:** When the cofactor (metal ion) is **loosely associated** with the enzyme, it forms a **metal-enzyme complex.** For example, Cl^- (chloride ions) are required for the activation of the enzyme salivary amylase. Such enzymes are called metal-activated enzymes (Table 6.2).

Table 6.2: Metal-activated enzymes

Enzymes	*Ion required for activity*
Lipase, ATPase, succinate dehydrogenase	Ca^{2+}
Phosphorylase, enolase, DNA polymerase	Mg^{2+}
Arginase, phosphoglucomutase, choline esterase	Mn^{2+}
Salivary amylase	Cl^-
Pyruvate kinase	K^+

- **Metalloenzymes:** When the metal ion **forms an integral part** of the enzyme, such enzymes are called **metalloenzymes.** For example, Zn^{2+} (zinc) forms an integral part of several enzymes such as carbonic anhydrase, LDH, etc. (Table 6.3).

Coenzymes

These are the **organic low molecular weight substances,** which are dialyzable and thermostable. These are instead called coenzymes. The coenzyme may also act as a **co-substrate.**

Table 6.3: Metalloenzymes

Enzymes	*Integrated metal*
Cytochromes, peroxidases, catalase	Fe
Ascorbic acid oxidase, cytochrome oxidase, tyrosinase	Cu
Aldehyde oxidase, xanthine oxidase, nitrate reductase	Mo
Carbonic anhydrase, lactate dehydrogenase, carboxypeptidase	Zn
Glutathione peroxidase	Se

The coenzyme may also form a **prosthetic group** of the enzyme proteins. In such cases, the enzyme (protein) is referred to as **apoenzyme.** Such an enzyme, however, is not active. It becomes catalytically active only after the enzyme t binds to the coenzyme. This **apoenzyme–coenzyme complex** is called **holoenzyme.**

Holoenzyme = Apoenzyme + Coenzyme
(active) (inactive) (inactive)

Coenzymes are the derivatives of the B complex group of vitamins. These are chemically changed by the enzymatic reaction in which they participate. For example, NAD^+ (the coenzyme form of the vitamin niacin) is reduced to NADH in a dehydrogenase reaction (Table 6.4).

Table 6.4: Coenzymes, their precursor vitamins along with the type of reaction in which the coenzyme participates

Vitamin	*Coenzyme form(s)*	*Reactions catalyzed*
Thiamin	TPP	Pyruvate → Acetyl-CoA α-Ketoglutarate → Succinyl-CoA
Riboflavin	FMN FAD	L-Amino acids → α-Keto acids Succinate → Fumarate
Niacin	NAD^+ $NADP^+$	Lactate → Pyruvate Glucose-6-P → 6-P-Gluconolactone
Pyridoxine	Pyridoxal-5-P	Alanine + α-Ketoglutarate → Pyruvate + Glutamate Tyrosine → Tyramine
Pantothenic acid	CoA	Pyruvate → Acetyl-CoA Fatty acid → Fatty acyl-CoA
Biotin	Carboxybiotin	Acetyl CoA → Malonyl-CoA Pyruvate → Oxaloacetate
Folate	Tetrahydrofolate	Glycine → Serine Homocysteine → Methionine
B_{12}	Deoxyadenosylcobalamin Methylcobalamin	Methylmalonyl-CoA → Succinyl-CoA Homocysteine → Methionine
Lipoic acid	Lipoic acid	Pyruvate → Acetyl-CoA α-Ketoglutarate → Succinyl-CoA

FACTORS AFFECTING ENZYME ACTIVITY

An enzyme exhibits maximum activity only under optimal conditions. Enzyme activity is markedly affected, *in vitro*, by several factors such as pH, temperature, pH, enzyme concentration, concentration of the substrate or the presence of the inhibitor.

pH

The pH of the reaction medium also affects reaction velocity. The **pH at which enzyme activity is maximum** is defined as its **optimum pH.** Relationship of enzyme activity to pH is represented by a bell-shaped curve, which has its peak at optimum pH of the enzyme (Fig. 6.2).

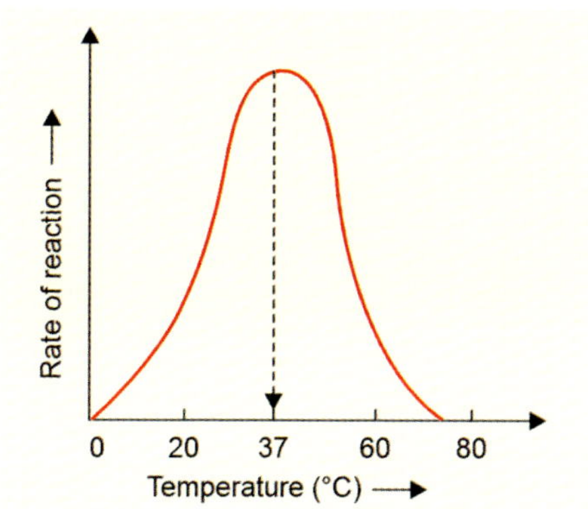

Fig. 6.2: Effect of temperature on enzyme activity

Optimum pH of an enzyme depends upon ionization state of the enzyme as well as its substrate. Change in pH affects ionization state of the enzyme, thereby decreasing the number of active sites. Hence, at extremely low or high pH, enzyme gets denatured. **Optimum pH for most of the enzymes** is in the neutral range, i.e. around **7.0.** However, optimum pH for pepsin is about 2.0 while for the enzymes of the pancreatic juice optimum pH is near 8.0.

Temperature

Rate of an enzyme catalyzed reaction increases with increase in temperature of the reaction mixture. It is, however, possible up to certain temperature only, which is called **optimum temperature**.

Optimum temperature of an enzyme is defined as the **temperature at which its activity is maximum.** For **most of the enzymes,** optimum temperature is near body temperature, i.e. **37°C.** With rise in temperature of the reaction mixture beyond optimum temperature of the enzyme, being protein, enzyme gets denatured and loses its biological activity.

Relationship of enzyme activity to a change in temperature is represented by a bell-shaped curve, peak of which represents an optimum temperature of the enzyme (Fig. 6.3).

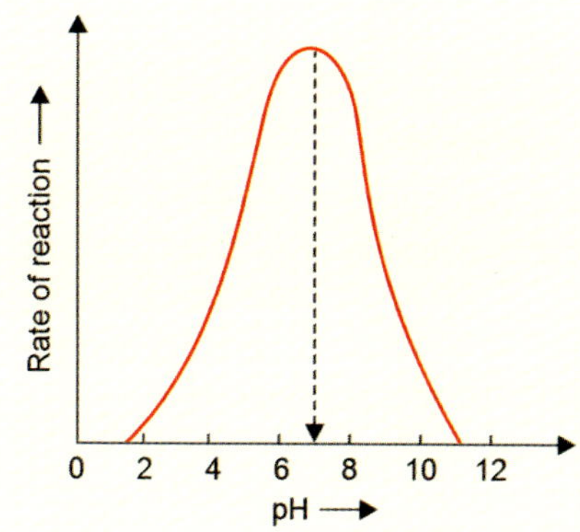

Fig. 6.3: Effect of pH on enzyme activity

Substrate Concentration

With a fixed quantity of enzyme, reaction rate is proportional to concentration of the substrate. This is, however, true only up to a certain point, i.e. the point at which its velocity is maximum (V_{max}). Further increase in substrate concentration, beyond this point, will not increase rate of the reaction (Fig. 6.4).

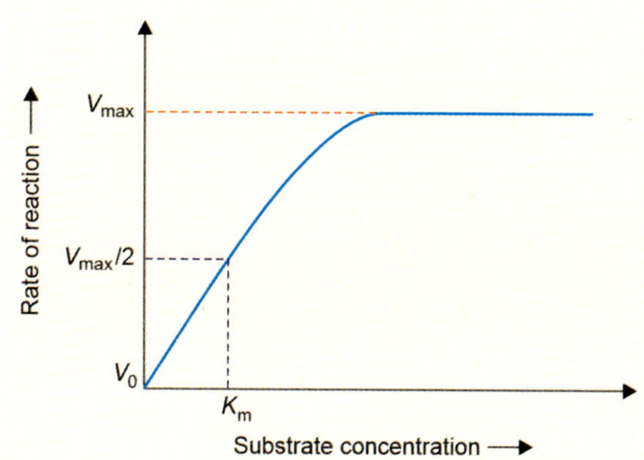

Fig. 6.4: Effect of substrate concentration on enzyme activity

To confirm it, Michaelis and Menten derived a **relationship between substrate concentration and reaction velocity** by an equation, called **Michaelis-Menten equation,** which is as follows:

$$V_0 = V_{max} [S]/K_m + [S]$$

where, V_0 is initial reaction velocity, V_{max} is maximum velocity of the reaction, $[S]$ is concentration of the substrate and K_m is a constant, referred to as **Michaelis constant.**

K_m is defined as the **substrate concentration at which reaction velocity is half of the maximum velocity,** i.e.

$$K_m = V_{max}/2$$

Enzyme Inhibition

Phenomenon of **decrease in rate of an enzymatic reaction** brought about **by the addition** of a substance other than the substrate **(inhibitor)** is called enzyme inhibition. An inhibitor may affect enzyme activity either competitively or noncompetitively.

Competitive Inhibitors

A competitive inhibitor **competes with the substrate**, for **binding at the active site** of the enzyme. **Chemical structure** of a competitive inhibitor, closely, **resembles the substrate**. For example, malonate (which inhibits the action of succinate dehydrogenase) has structure closely similar to the substrate, i.e. succinate.

A competitive inhibitor forms complex with the **enzyme, called enzyme-inhibitor (EI) complex**, and **inhibits action of the enzyme**. Binding of the enzyme with the competitive inhibitor, and the substrate, depends upon relative concentrations of the two. It is, usually, a reversible process. By increasing concentration of the substrate, degree of inhibition is reduced.

Presence of a **competitive inhibitor increases K_m without any change in V_{max}** of the enzymatic reaction (Fig. 6.5).

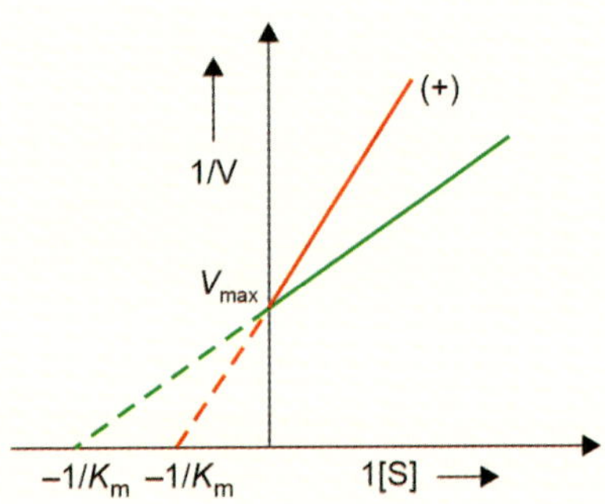

Fig. 6.5: Effect of a competitive inhibitor (+) on enzyme activity

Some of the enzymes, their substrates and competitive inhibitors are given in Table 6.5.

Table 6.5: Some enzymes, their substrates and competitive inhibitors

Enzyme	*Substrate*	*Competitive inhibitor*
Succinate dehydrogenase	Succinate	Malonate
Carbonic anhydrase	Carbonate	Acetazolamide
Dihydrofolate reductase	Dihydrofolate	Amethopterin (methotrexate)
Histidase	L-Histidine	D-Histidine
Xanthine oxidase	Hypoxanthine	Allopurinol
HMG-CoA reductase	HMG-CoA	HMG

Drugs Act as Competitive Inhibitors

Several drugs are known to be used as competitive inhibitors. Due to their structural similarity with the substrates, several drugs act as inhibitors of some of the specific enzymes. For example, **sulfanilamide** (a sulfa drug) is an antibacterial agent and **resembles p-aminobenzoic acid**, structurally. It is used as a **competitive inhibitor of** the enzyme **dihydropteroic acid synthase**, in bacteria. Similarly, **methotrexate**, a **structural analogue of folate**, competitively **inhibits dihydrofolate reductase**. It is used in the treatment of childhood leukemia (Fig. 6.6).

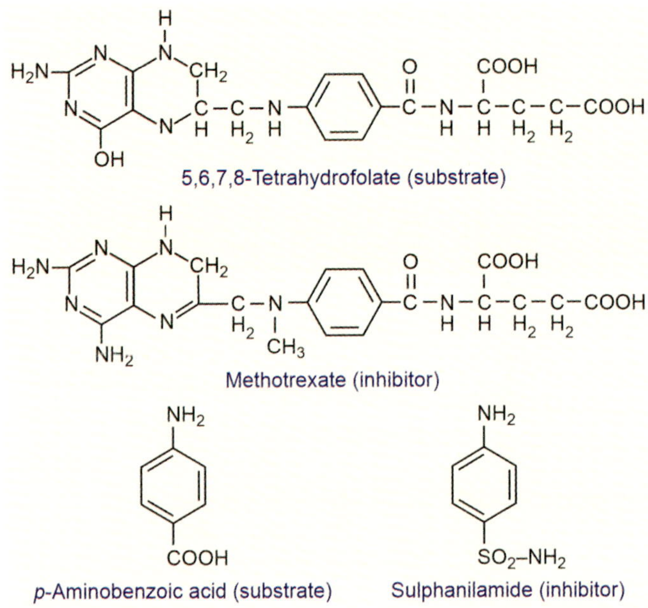

Fig. 6.6: Some drugs (structural analogs) as competitive inhibitors

Noncompetitive Inhibitors

Several substances react covalently with the functional groups on the active site of the enzyme. This, in turn, inactivates the enzyme, noncompetitively. For example, enzymes which have free SH-groups in their molecules are inhibited by substances like iodoacetate or p-chloromercurobenzoate, which binds SH-groups, oxidizes cysteine molecules and inactivates the enzyme. **Heavy metals** like Hg^{2+} or Ag^{+} denature protein and **inactivate enzymes**.

This type of inhibition is, usually, irreversible and makes active sites of the enzyme ineffective. A noncompetitive inhibitor may even bind at a site other than the substrate-binding site. In such cases, either the enzyme or the enzyme-substrate complex binds with the inhibitor. As a result of it, both, binary (EI) as well as ternary (ESI) complexes may be formed. Under these conditions, ESI is converted to product but at a slower rate.

A reversible noncompetitive inhibitor **decreases V_{max} but not K_m** (Fig. 6.7).

Drugs as Noncompetitive Inhibitors

Several drugs are known to be used as noncompetitive inhibitors. These compounds are, generally referred to as **antimetabolites**.

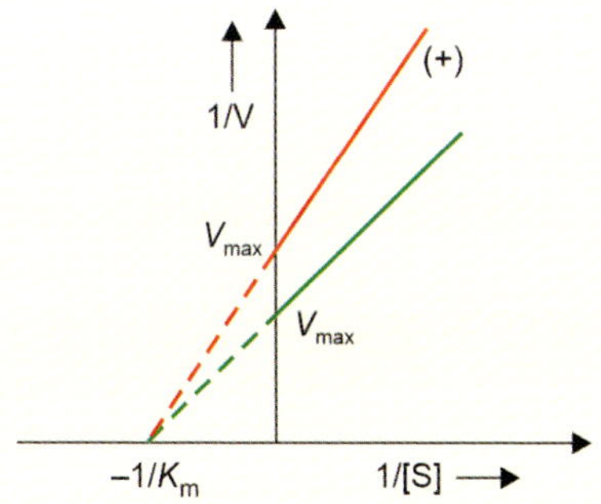

Fig. 6.7: Effect of a noncompetitive inhibitor (+) on enzyme activity

Antimetabolites include certain derivatives of the purines and pyrimidines and act as noncompetitive inhibitors. These are also **used as chemotherapeutic agents**, e.g. **5-fluorouracil**, an **analogue of thymine, inhibits thymidylate synthetase**, noncompetitively (Fig. 6.8).

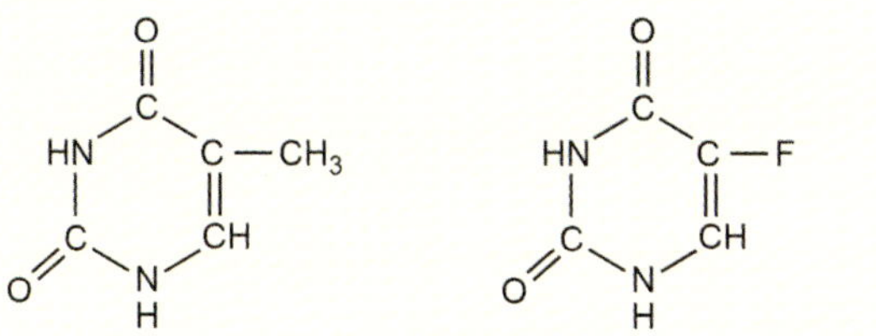

Fig. 6.8: Thymine and its structural analog 5-fluorouracil

PROENZYMES

Several enzymes are secreted in the inactive form, called **zymogen** or proenzyme (**precursor of the enzyme**).

Zymogen is **converted to its active enzyme (zymase) by** some **activating agent, such as H^+** (HCl), other enzyme or the active form of the zymogen. For example, gastric juice secretes **pepsinogen** (a zymogen), which is **converted to pepsin by HCl** of the gastric juice. Once pepsin is formed, it acts on pepsinogen and catalyzes its conversion to pepsin.

Hydrochloric acid (HCl), however, in the stomach cannot break peptide bonds, but can hydrolyse peptide bonds at high temperature only (more than 100°C).

Some of the proenzymes, their activators and active enzymes are given in Table 6.6.

Table 6.6: Some of the proenzymes, their activators and active enzymes

Proenzyme	*Activator*	*Active enzyme*
Pepsinogen	H^+, pepsin	Pepsin
Trypsinogen	Trypsin, enterokinase	Trypsin
Chymotrypsinogen	Trypsin	Chymotrypsin
Procarboxypeptidase	Trypsin	Carboxypeptidase
Proelastase	Trypsin	Elastase

ISOENZYMES

Enzymes which **occur in** a number of **different forms**, and differ from each other with respect to their **chemical, immunological** and **electrophoretic** properties are called isoenzymes or **isozymes** (or more generally as **multiple forms of an enzyme**).

Isozymes are present in the serum and tissues of mammals, amphibians, birds, insects, plants and unicellular organisms.

Properties of Isoenzymes

- Isoenzymes are **multiple forms of an enzyme** that **have different amino acid sequences** and, therefore, different **shapes, sizes** and **electrical charges,** but **perform the same function**, i.e. they **catalyze the same reaction** but can be **distinguished by physical methods**, such as **electrophoresis**, or **immunological methods**.
- They display **different kinetic parameters** as well as **regulatory properties**. For example, isozymes have **different K_m** and V_{max} values, and can be **distinguished** from one another **by biochemical properties** such as electrophoretic mobility.
- The difference between some isozymes is due to differences in the quaternary structure of the enzymes, e.g. lactate dehydrogenase **(LDH)**. It exists in **five isozymic forms**. The isozymic forms of LDH are **tetramers**; each is made up from two types of units H and M. Only the tetrameric molecule possesses catalytic activity.
- Isozymes are encoded by different genes and expressed in a distinct organelle, or at a distinct stage of development. Different isozymes appear in specific regions of the body; differing in specifics organelles or tissues.
- Isozymes, in general, can be used to meet metabolic needs of different tissues and developmental stages, e.g. LDH. The H isozyme is expressed more in the heart, whereas the M isozyme is expressed more frequently in the skeletal muscle.
- Isozymes may also be **utilized to diagnose tissue damage** such as damaged heart muscle cells during a **heart attack** or **myocardial infarction**. When heart muscle cells are damaged, they release cellular material such as the H isozyme. When taking blood samples, if the H isozymes appear in increased levels, then there is a possibility that the heart cells are damaged.

Isoenzymes of Clinical Significance

Lactate Dehydrogenase

Lactate dehydrogenase is a **tetramer**, i.e. it **has four polypeptide subunits**. Its each subunit may be one of the two types, known as the **H** (heart) type and the **M** (muscle) type. LDH, thus, exists in serum in five distinct forms (isoenzymes) with different proportions of the H and the M subunits.

LDH_1 has four polypeptide chains of the H type **(H_4)** while **LDH_5** has four subunits of the M type **(M_4)**. Other forms include HHHM **(H_3M)**, HHMM **(H_2M_2)** and HMMM **(HM_3)**.

LDH_1 and LDH_2 are predominant in the myocardium and erythrocytes while LDH_4 and LDH_5 are predominant in the liver and skeletal muscle. LDH_1 increases between 12 to 24 hours following myocardial infarction. LDH_5 is diagnostic of secondary congestive liver involvement.

Creatine Phosphokinase

Creatine phosphokinase **(CPK)**, also referred to as creatine kinase **(CK)** has three isoenzymes. Each of its isoenzyme is a **dimer**, i.e. **composed of two** subunits which may either be of **M** (muscle) type or **B** (brain) type.

CPK has **three isoenzymes**, which are called CPK_1 (CK_1 or CK-BB) that is mainly **found in the brain; CPK_2 (CK-MB)** found **in the myocardium**; and CPK_3 (CK-MM) found **in skeletal muscle**.

Normally, **CK-MB** is present in very small amount in serum. Its **level rises within 4 hours, reaching a maximum value within 24 hours of myocardial infarction.**

Alkaline Phosphatase

Alkaline phosphatase **exists in three forms**. Different tissues contain a distinct form of the enzyme.

- Major portion of the enzyme in serum is from liver whose level rises in post-hepatic jaundice.
- In growing children, the serum enzyme is mainly from bone and is related to increased osteoblastic activity.
- During the last trimester of pregnancy, there is an increase in serum alkaline phosphatase, which is primarily of the placental origin. This form of the enzyme is heat-stable; hence, placental enzyme is also called heat-stable alkaline phosphatase.

REGULATION OF ENZYME ACTIVITY

Regulation of enzyme activity is essential for the coordination of the numerous metabolic processes. Besides changes in the substrate concentration, enzyme activity is also regulated by modifying the activity of the existing enzyme molecules by a number of processes which include allosteric regulation, covalent modifications and induction/repression.

Allosteric Regulation

Oligomeric enzymes, having two or more subunits, have two different sites, which are called the **catalytic site** or regulatory site (also known as the allosteric site) and the **substrate-binding site** (active site). These two sites are located apart from each other on two different subunits of the oligomeric enzymes. Such enzymes are called **allosteric enzymes** or **regulatory enzymes**.

Allosteric enzymes frequently catalyze committed step that is generally present in the beginning of the pathway, e.g. HMG CoA reductase (a regulatory enzyme of cholesterol biosynthesis), aspartate transcarbamoylase (of pyrimidine synthesis), etc.

Certain substances, called **allosteric modulators** or **effectors, bind reversibly to** such an enzyme at the **allosteric site** and regulate its activity. An interaction with the effector molecule brings about conformational changes at the catalytic site of the enzyme. An effector molecule may either activate an enzymatic reaction (called positive effector or allosteric activator), or inhibit it (called allosteric inhibitor), and is referred to as allosteric regulator.

Due to interaction between the substrate and the activator/inhibitor, a characteristic sigmoid curve (S-shaped curve) is obtained. Presence of an allosteric activator (+) shifts the curve to the right whereas an allosteric inhibitor (–) shifts the curve to the left (Fig. 6.9).

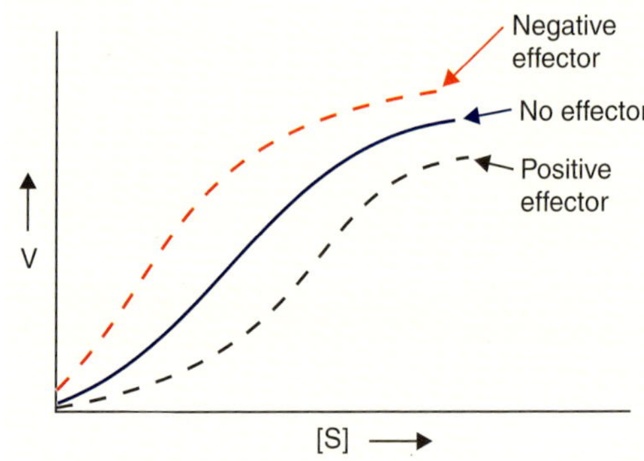

Fig. 6.9: Allosteric regulation

Table 6.7 lists some of the enzymes that are allosterically regulated along with their allosteric activators/inhibitors.

Table 6.7: Some allosteric modulators

Enzyme	*Allosteric activator*	*Allosteric inhibitor*
Hexokinase	ADP	Glucose-6-P, ATP
Isocitrate dehydrogenase	ADP	Glucose-6-P, ATP
Glutamate dehydrogenase	ADP	ATP, NADH
Pyruvate carboxylase	Acetyl CoA	ADP

Regulation by Covalent Modification

Several enzymes are regulated by covalent modification, most frequently by the addition or removal of a phosphate group from serine, threonine or tyrosine residues of the enzyme. Protein kinases catalyze

Unit I: Chemistry of Bio-organic Molecules 6

phosphorylation of enzymes while phosphoprotein phosphatases remove phosphate groups from the phosphorylated enzymes. Depending upon the specific enzyme, either the phosphorylated (such as for glycogen phosphorylase) or the dephosphorylated (e.g. glycogen synthase) enzyme is active.

Regulation by Induction/Repression

Cells can also regulate the amount of an enzyme, usually by altering its rate of synthesis. Increased (induction) or decreased (repression) synthesis of the enzyme in turn regulates its activity. Enzymes that are required only at one stage of development or under selected physiological conditions are regulated in this way. For example, elevated levels of insulin, as a result of high blood glucose level, cause increased synthesis of the key enzymes that are involved in glucose utilization.

SERUM ENZYMES IN DIAGNOSIS

Several enzymes are extensively used as markers of various pathological conditions, e.g. creatine kinase (CK or CPK), alanine transaminase (ALT or GPT), aspartate transaminase (AST or GOT), acid phosphatase (ACP), alkaline phosphatase (ALP), etc. They are used as markers in conditions such as myocardial infarction, jaundice, pancreatitis, cancer as well as in neurodegenerative disorders and provide insight into the disease process in diagnosis, prognosis and assessment of response to therapy (Table 6.8).

Table 6.8: Diagnostic significance of enzymes

Enzyme	*Principle source*	*Clinical situation in which altered*
Acid phosphatase	Prostate, RBC	Increases in carcinoma of prostate
Alkaline phosphatase	Liver, bone, placenta, kidney	Increases in obstructive jaundice, rickets, Paget's disease, hyperparathyroidism
Aldolase	Skeletal muscle, heart	Increases in muscular dystrophies, acute liver disease
Amylase	Salivary glands, pancreas, ovaries	Increases in acute pancreatitis, intestinal obstruction, acute parotitis Decreases in acute liver diseases
Ceruloplasmin	Liver	Increases in cirrhosis Decreases in Wilson's disease
Choline esterase	Liver	Increases in nephrotic syndrome, organophosphorus poisoning Decreases in acute liver diseases
Creatine phosphokinase	Skeletal muscle, brain, heart	Increases in myocardial infarction, muscular dystrophies
Glutamate oxaloacetate transaminase (GPT)	Liver, skeletal muscle, heart, kidney, RBCs	Increases in myocardial infarction, toxic liver cell necrosis, acute liver disease, muscle disease
γ-Glutamyltransferase	Liver, kidney	Increases in alcoholism, hepatobiliary disease
Lactate dehydrogenase	Heart, liver, skeletal muscle, RBCs, platelets	Increases in acute myocardial infarction, acute hepatitis, muscle disorders
Lipase	Pancreas	Increases in acute pancreatitis, pancreatic carcinoma Decreases in liver disease, diabetes mellitus
5′-Nucleotidase	Hepatobiliary tract	Increases in liver disease, obstructive jaundice, hepatic carcinoma
Trypsin	Pancreas	Increases in acute pancreatic disease

Some Important Questions

1. **What are enzymes? Classify them. Discuss factors affecting enzyme activity.**
2. **Define enzyme, cofactor and coenzyme. Discuss role of B vitamins as coenzymes.**
3. **Define enzyme. What are isoenzymes? Discuss importance of isoenzymes in clinical diagnosis.**
4. **Give brief account of factors affecting enzyme activity.**

5. Discuss briefly:

i. Various types of enzyme inhibition, giving examples.
ii. Apoenzyme, holoenzyme and coenzyme, with examples.
iii. Classification of enzymes with examples.

6. Write notes on:

i. Noncompetitive inhibition of enzyme activity
ii. Isoenzymes and their importance
iii. Proenzymes
iv. Competitive inhibitors
v. Specificity of enzyme action
vi. Coenzymes
vii. Classification of enzymes
viii. Allosteric regulation
ix. Covalent modification
x. Induction and repression of enzyme activity
xi. Serum enzymes in diagnosis

Unit II

Macronutrients Digestion and Absorption

Chapter

7

Energy Requirements

Energy is a prime requisite for body functions and growth. Energy is also required for doing physical work. Body gets energy from the combustion of carbohydrates, fat and proteins. Energy, present in these macronutrients is locked in chemical bonds, and is released when food is metabolized. Thus, body converts chemical energy present in food to mechanical, electrical or heat energy.

Energy requirements (needs) of an individual is defined as the **level of energy intake in relation to energy expenditure** (output). Energy intake and energy output of normal healthy individuals are finely balanced.

UNIT OF ENERGY

The unit of energy is **calorie**. A calorie is defined as the **quantity of heat, required to raise the temperature of 1 g of water** by 1°C, more specifically from **14.5°C to 15.5°C**. Its large unit is **kilocalorie**, which is equal to one-thousand g calories (based on one kg of water).

In the context of **nutrition**, the large unit, i.e. kilocalorie **(kcal)**, is used. The calorie value, we see on a food package is, actually, in kcal or 1000 calories.

The **SI unit of energy is joule** (J). One calorie is approximately 4.2J.

COMPONENTS OF ENERGY REQUIREMENT

Total energy requirement, for different categories of people, is made up of three components, which include:

1. Basal Requirement

Basal requirement depends upon **basal energy expenditure**. It is the total **amount of energy used, over** the period of **24 hours**, in the state of **complete physical and mental rest**, at comfortable environment (temperature and humidity), is referred to as **energy requirement during resting condition**. It is also referred as **basal energy expenditure**.

It is the **amount of energy spent by the body for** performing various activities, which are necessary to sustain normal body functions and homeostasis, such as **respiration, blood circulation, synthesis of several substances for use in the body, pumping of ions across the membranes as well as maintenance of body temperature**.

It is expressed in terms of basal metabolic rate **(BMR)**.

BASAL METABOLIC RATE

Basal metabolic rate (BMR) is the **amount of energy expenditure at rest**, in a neutrally temperate environment, in the post-absorptive state, by indirect calorimetry in the laboratory setting. The amount of energy at complete physical and mental rest meets the requirement for the functioning of vital organs, i.e. the heart, lungs, kidneys, nervous system, intestine, liver, sex organs, muscles and skin, etc.

Determination of BMR

BMR is measured, when a person is lying **at complete rest but awaken**, from a normal overnight sleep, **10 to 12 hours after the last meal**, and **performing no physical activity**. BMR remains constant throughout the day under normal conditions and constitutes about 50–75% of the total energy expenditure by an individual. It is **expressed in terms of kcal/hr**.

Factors Affecting BMR

Several factors affect BMR (Table 7.1).

Table 7.1: Factors affecting BMR

Factors that increase BMR	*Factors that decrease BMR*
Total body weight	Growing age
Increased lean body mass	Female gender
Large body surface area	Starvation
Rapid growth	Hot temperature
Cold temperature	Sleep
Stress	Hypothyroidism
Hyperthyroidism	
Caffeine	
Pregnancy and lactation	
Smoking	
Fever	

- **Body mass:** Lean body mass refers to the portion of the body, exclusive of the stored fat, i.e. the fat-free mass (metabolically active tissue). Muscles, various other organs, bones and body fluids, make up most of the lean body mass. An individual, with a **large lean body mass** has **higher resting energy expenditure** than the one with same weight but having higher proportion of body fat.
- **Age:** BMR is highest during the period of rapid growth, mainly **within first two years of life**. It is **reduced thereafter, but again reaches a peak during puberty and adolescence**. BMR is further **reduced**, by about 2 to 3% per decade, **in adults**. This is due to the reason that whereas lean body mass tends to decrease, fat content increases with age.
- **Sex:** Metabolic rate is **higher in men** (by about 50 kcal per day) **than women**. This is due to the reason that women have less active muscle mass, for each kg of body weight. Women generally have less lean body mass. Resting metabolic rate also varies during menstrual cycle. It fluctuates from the low point from about one week before ovulation to the high point, just before the onset of menstruation.
- Other factors: These factors, however, may be less consistent of shorter duration and limited to individual situations:
  - BMR **falls** by about 10% **during sleep**.
  - It **rises during the period of rapid growth**, such as in infancy and adolescence.
  - Hormones, especially, **thyroxin and norepinephrine**, regulate **BMR. Hypothyroidism slows BMR**, while hyperthyroidism increases BMR.
  - **Excitement and stress**, which cause release of epinephrine, increase cellular activity and, thus, **BMR**.
  - BMR is decreased in early stages of pregnancy, whereas **later in pregnancy BMR is increased** because of uterine, placental and fetal growth.
  - **Fever increases BMR** by about 7%, for each degree increase in body temperature above 37°C.
  - Environment temperature also affects BMR. During **exposure to cold, BMR increases**. People living in tropical climate, usually, have higher BMR than those living in the temperate areas.
  - **During starvation BMR declines**, as body slows basic functions to conserve energy.
  - Some unknown **genetic factors** have also been attributed to the variations in BMR.

2. Requirements for Physical Activities

It is the most variable component of energy expenditure. Energy expenditure for physical activities varies from 30 to 100% of the basal requirement. It depends upon the duration, type and intensity of physical activity, including the energy expenditure for occupational work. According to the type of occupational work, various individuals are classified into 3 categories as:

- **Light workers** (such as those doing office work)
- **Moderate workers** (like a student)
- **Heavy workers** (such as those performing manual physical labor, rickshaw pullers, etc.).

Amounts of energy expenditure for different types of physical activities, as per National Institute of Nutrition, Indian Council of Medical Research (NIN–ICMR, 2011) are shown in Table 7.2.

3. Requirement on Account of Specific Dynamic Action

Specific dynamic action **(SDA)** is also referred as **diet-induced thermogenesis** or **thermogenic effect of food**. It is the amount of energy expenditure associated with the consumption of food. Our body spends some energy to digest, absorb and metabolize dietary nutrients which depends upon the type and amount of various nutrients consumed.

Table 7.2: Energy expenditure for different types of physical activities

Activity zones	*Type of activities*	*Energy expenditure* (kcal/min)*
1	Sleeping, resting or relaxing	1.0
2	Sitting, sitting (light activities); eating, reading, writing, listening or talking	1.5
3	Standing, standing (light activity); washing face, shaving, combing, or watering plants	2.3
4	Walking (slow), driving, dusting, bathing. dressing, marketing or childcare	2.8
5	Light manual work, sweeping, cleaning utensils, washing clothes or other house chores	3.3
6	Warm-up and recreational activities, walking up/down stairs, cycling or fetching water	4.8
7	Manual work (moderate pace), loading/unloading, walking with load, harvesting, carpentry or plumbing	5.6
8	Practice of non-competitive sport/games, cycling (15 kmph), gymnastics, swimming or digging	6.0
9	High intense manual work and sports activities—tournaments, wood cutting, carrying heavy loads, running or jogging	7.8

*NIN-ICMR (2011)

SDA value is more after the consumption of carbohydrates and proteins than fat. This is due to the reason that fat is metabolized more efficiently compared to proteins. On an average, for a mixed diet, SDA value constitutes about 10% of total energy expenditure.

DAILY ENERGY INTAKE

As discussed above, several factors determine energy intake (requirement) such as basal metabolic rate, level and duration of physical activity, age and physiological state (pregnancy and lactation), and SDA (processes involved in the extraction of energy from food). Besides, daily energy intake also varies and depends upon the source of energy.

Main sources of energy in our diets are carbohydrates including dietary fiber, fat and proteins which provide different levels of energy.

Average metabolizable energy available from different dietray components is shown in Table 7.3.

Table 7.3: Average metabolizable energy available from different components

Dietary component	*Available energy (kcal/g)**
Carbohydrates	4
Fat	9
Protein	4
Fiber	2

*ICMR-NIN 2020

According to ICMR-NIN (2020), average daily energy requirement for different age groups and type of work performed by an adult is shown in Table 7.4.

It is suggested that on an average, a moderate male worker (e.g. a student) requires 2710 kcal/day while a female performing the same type of work needs 2130 kcal/day.

It is suggested that 55–60% of dietary energy should be derived from carbohydrates, 20–30% from fats and 10–15% from proteins.

DIETARY SOURCES OF ENERGY

CARBOHYDRATES

Carbohydrates are the **cheapest source of energy** and are easily available dietary sources. They are the main sources of energy for the body. Carbohydrates, in addition to the supply of energy also serve as the components of cell membrane and receptors. Carbohydrates are synthesized in our body from non-carbohydrate sources.

Carbohydrates are classified according to their number of sugar units as monosaccharides (such as glucose and fructose), disaccharides (such as sucrose and lactose) and polysaccharides (such as starch, glycogen and cellulose).

- **Monosaccharides**, i.e. glucose and fructose (found in fruits, vegetables and honey), and **disaccharides**, i.e. sucrose (found in sugar, also called table sugar)

Table 7.4: Energy requirement (kcal/d)*

Population/group	*Category of worker/age*	*Body weight (kg)*	*Energy requirement (kcal)*
Adult men	Sedentary worker Moderate worker Heavy worker	65	2110 2710 3470
Adult women	Sedentary worker Moderate worker Heavy worker	55	1660 2130 2720
Pregnant women			(+) 350
Lactating women (during 0–6 months of lactation)			(+) 600
Lactating women (during 7–12 months of lactation)			(+) 520
Infants	0–6 Months 7–12 Months	5.8 8.5	530 660
Children	1–3 Years 4–6 Years 7–9 Years	12.9 18.3 25.3	1110 1360 1700
Adolescents	Boys 10–12 Years Boys 13–15 Years Boys 16–18 Years Girls 10–12 Years Girls 13–15 Years Girls 16–18 Years	36.4 50.5 61.4 34.9 49.6 55.7	2220 2860 3320 2060 2400 2500

* (ICMR-NIN, 2020)

and lactose (found in milk) are referred to as **simple carbohydrates**.

- **Polysaccharides**, such as **starch** (found in cereals, millets, pulses and root vegetables) and **glycogen** (found in animal foods) are referred to as **complex polysaccharides** (*see* Chapter 1).

Recommended Dietary Allowance (RDA)

As mentioned above, ICMR-NIN (2020) recommended that **55–60% of the dietary energy intake** should be derived from carbohydrates.

The **minimum requirement** for carbohydrate has been recommended to be **100 g/day**. Minimum requirement **during pregnancy** has been recommended as **135 g/day** while **during lactation** it is **155 g/day**.

Dietary free sugar should be restricted to 5–7% of energy intake.

DIETARY FIBER

Dietary fiber comprises:

- **Insoluble fiber**, also called **crude fiber** or **roughage**), include **cellulose** and hemicellulose. Their functions include:
  - **Retention of water** during intestinal transit thereby preventing constipation.
  - **Binding various dietary toxins**, thereby reducing the incidence of colon cancer.
  - **Imparting a sense of early satiety** (fullness of stomach) thereby helping to reduce calorie intake and, thus, to control obesity and diabetes mellitus.

Insoluble fibers are abundant in vegetable grains. It is worth mentioning that insoluble fibers also include some nonpolysaccharides, e.g. lignins (carrots, strawberry seeds), cutins and tannins.

- **Soluble fiber**, e.g. **gums and pectins** found in legumes, fruits and oats. Their functions include:
  - **Binding cholesterol** and bile salts, thereby reducing their enterohepatic circulation and enhancing the conversion of cholesterol into bile salts, lowering plasma cholesterol levels.
  - **Reducing gastric emptying**, thereby delaying the postprandial rise in blood glucose of diabetic patients.

Recommended Dietary Allowance (RDA)

ICMR-NIN (2020) Expert Group has suggested an **adequate intake of 15 g of dietary fiber per 1000 kcal per day**.

DIETARY LIPIDS

Lipids or fat include a group of substances which are poorly soluble, or nearly insoluble, in water but are soluble in organic solvents. Over 90% of the dietary fat includes **triacylglycerols (triglycerides)**, which consist of a molecule of glycerol (glycerin) with three fatty acids attached to it.

Fatty acid molecules contain a –COOH group attached to unbranched hydrocarbon chains connected by single bonds alone (saturated fatty acids) or by both double and single bonds (unsaturated fatty acids). Other types of dietary lipids include cholesterol, phospholipids, sterols and carotenoids).

Essential Fatty Acids

Essential fatty acids are those which cannot be synthesized in our body; hence, they should be supplied through the diet. They are **linoleic acid** and **linolenic acid** (*see* Chapter 2).

Recommended Dietary Allowance (RDA)

ICMR-NIN (2020) Expert Group has recommended that dietary fat **should contribute for 20–30% of the energy requirements**.

It is suggested that nearly **10% of energy** should be available **from visible fat**. On an average **an adult moderate worker female** should consume **25 g of visible fat per day** while a **moderate worker male** can consume **30 g of visible fat per day**. The **diet of the pregnant and lactating women should contain at least 30 g of visible fat.**

Minimum intake level for essential fatty acids to prevent deficiency symptoms should be **2.5% energy intake of linoleic acid plus 0.5% α-linolenic acid**.

DIETARY PROTEINS

Proteins are organic compounds that **consist of amino acids**, which are joined by peptide bonds. Proteins are needed for their content of certain amino acids that are essential to human body for the biosynthesis of proteins, body repair in adult, and for body building and body repair in children.

Proteins are in a constant state of flux in the body, with **continuously being synthesized and degraded**.

Nitrogen Balance

Nitrogen balance is a comparison between intake of nitrogen as protein and its excretion through various routes, chiefly, as undigested protein in feces, and urea and ammonia in urine (Fig. 7.1).

Protein status of the body can be assessed by calculating the nitrogen balance of an individual.

- A subject is said to be in **nitrogen equilibrium**, i.e. **zero nitrogen balance**, when **daily nitrogen intake equals excretion**, i.e. the output through the urine, feces and skin.
- A growing child should be in a **positive nitrogen balance**. Other conditions like pregnancy, lactation and convalescence (recovery from metabolic stress or acute illness) should also be associated with positive nitrogen balance.
- On the other hand, injury, chronic diseases (such as tuberculosis, rheumatoid arthritis, cancer), increased

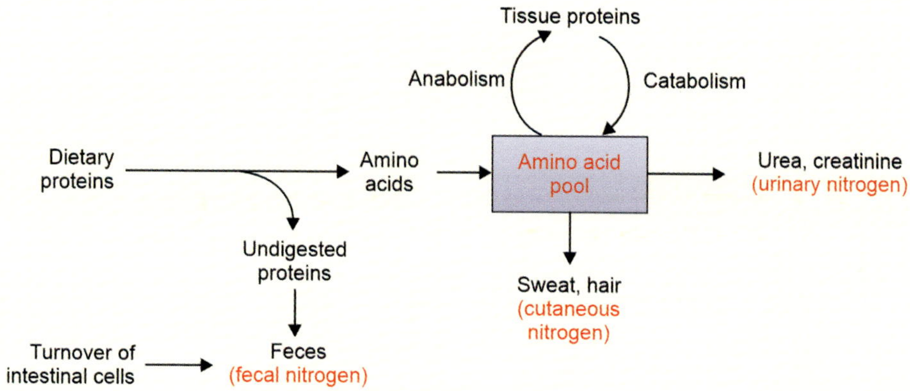

Fig. 7.1: Nitrogen balance

muscular activity, inadequate protein intake, lack of essential amino acids and increased metabolic stress leads to a negative nitrogen balance (Table 7.5).

Table 7.5: Type of nitrogen balance and examples of the prevailing conditions

Nitrogen balance	*Protein intake (I)/output (O)*	*Condition*
Equilibrium	I = O	Normal/healthy individuals
Positive	I > O	Growth, pregnancy, convalescence
Negative	I < O	↓ Protein intake, trauma, chronic illness (e.g. tuberculosis)

Foods rich in protein include meat, poultry, fishes, nuts, eggs, milk and milk products.

Essential Amino Acids

As discussed in Chapter 3, all the proteins are **made up** of only **20 amino acids**, out of which, nearly, **10 amino acids can be synthesized** in the body but the remaining once **cannot be synthesized**, hence, must be supplied in the diet. Therefore, these are known as **essential amino acids**.

An adult human body can maintain its nitrogen equilibrium on a mixture of 8 amino acids as the sole source of nitrogen, which are called essential amino acids. These include **isoleucine, leucine, lysine, methionine, phenylalanine, threonine, tryptophan and valine**. Besides, **histidine and arginine** are also needed in extra amounts by infants during growth and by females during pregnancy and lactation.

Protein Quality

Different foods contain different amounts and combinations of amino acids (building blocks of proteins). Accordingly, proteins are said to be the:

1. **High quality proteins** are, mainly, obtained from animals (e.g. meat, fish, eggs and dairy products). They contain full range of essential amino acids, needed by the body. These are also referred to as the proteins of high biological value.
2. **Low quality proteins** are obtained from plant sources. They have low biological value, since an individual protein may lack one or the other essential amino acid. Vegans and vegetarians cannot get all the amino acids they need, from a single source. However, combining the plant foods from different sources provide them good quality protein, e.g. pulses and cereals.

Quality of the dietary protein can be assessed by several criteria, such as biological value, digestibility, net-protein utilization, amino acid score or chemical score. These can be assessed by knowing the amount of protein nitrogen that is ingested, absorbed and retained by the body:

- **Biological value** (BV) **of a protein** refers to the proportion of the absorbed protein nitrogen retained by the body.
- **Amino acid score** refers to the total amino acid content in the protein relative to that present in the same quantity of a reference protein, expressed as percentage.
- **Chemical score** refers to the content of each essential amino acid in the protein relative to that present in the same quantity of a reference protein, expressed as percentage.

Recommended Dietary Allowance (RDA)

ICMR-NIN (2020) Expert Group has recommended that dietary proteins **should contribute for 10–15% of the energy requirements**.

Recommended daily allowances (RDA) of proteins vary with age, physiological status and stress, and the source of protein in diet.

Daily protein requirement for adults has been suggested to be **54 g/day for men** and **46 g/day for women**. This pre-supposes the use of first-class protein (high in essential amino acids) with adequate energy supply.

In disease conditions: In some diseases, protein intake must be controlled, e.g. **acute liver failure**, when the intake has to be restricted, in order to avoid hepatic coma, and in uremia, in which the capacity to excrete nitrogenous end products is limited.

PROTEIN ENERGY MALNUTRITION

Protein energy malnutrition **(PEM)**, also called **protein calorie malnutrition (PCM)**, refers to the form of malnutrition due to **inadequate intake of calories and/or protein**. PEM, though, can occur at any stage of life, it is most **common during childhood**, when extra protein is needed for rapid growth. PEM occurs in all parts of the world, but is most common in Southeast Asia, Africa, South and Central America, and Middle East countries. It is seen, most often, in population living in poverty, elderly people and hospitalized patients having some associated condition, such as anorexia nervosa, AIDS, cancer or malabsorption syndrome.

Two common forms of PEM include kwashiorkor and marasmus. This classification of PEM is based on deficit in body weight for age and presence or absence of edema (Fig. 7.2).

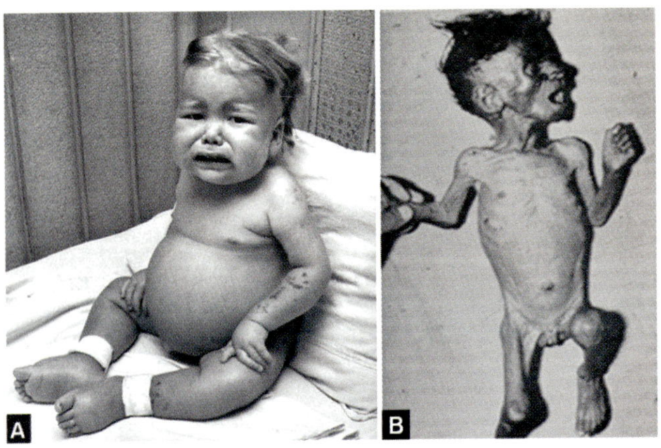

Fig. 7.2: The two extremes of the spectrum of protein energy malnutrition. (A) Kwashiorkor; (B) Marasmus

KWASHIORKOR

The term kwashiorkor comes from a word used in Ghana, which means a disease of a baby deposed from the breast when the next one is born. It is said that kwashiorkor, usually, **develops when a baby is weaned from the protein-rich breast milk and switched to a protein-poor food**. Today, it is the most serious and prevalent form of malnutrition in the world, especially, in industrially underdeveloped countries.

Kwashiorkor, typically, occurs **at about 1 year of age**, after infants are weaned from breast milk to a **protein-deficient diet**, but can develop at any time during the formative years.

Signs and symptoms of kwashiorkor include:

- Edema with swollen legs
- Pot belly (enlarged liver)
- Mild-to-moderate growth retardation
- Some weight loss and low subcutaneous fat
- Muscle atrophy
- Round face (moon face)
- Dry, flaky peeling skin
- Thin, dry and easily plucked hair

MARASMUS

Marasmus occurs due to the **deficient intake of both protein and calories**, i.e. total food, generally, **due to early weaning**.

Marasmus differs from kwashiorkor with respect to the subcutaneous fat, which disappears in marasmus but not in kwashiorkor. An infant with marasmus, thus, generally, has a **thin, wasted appearance** and is **small for age**. Marasmus occurs most often in infants and children **between 6 and 18 months of age**, particularly, in those who are given diluted milk.

Signs and Symptoms of marasmus include:

- Severe weight loss
- No edema
- Severe growth failure
- Severe loss of subcutaneous fat
- Weight loss up to 40%
- Severe muscle atrophy
- Wrinkled face (old man's face)
- Rare skin changes
- Common hair changes

BALANCED DIET

A balanced diet is defined as the **diet that contains all the food constituents in proper proportion, to meet energy and nutritional requirements of an individual**. A balanced diet is good for our physical and mental health.

Components of a balanced diet vary depending upon age, sex, physiological needs such as pregnancy and lactation, and nature of physical activity. While designing the quality and quantity of a balanced diet, total calories must be distributed among three classes of foodstuffs, in the following proportion:

- **Carbohydrates** (the energy yielding substances): **55–60%**
- **Fat** (to yield energy and act as insulating materials): **20–30%**
- **Proteins** (to act as building materials, and bear the wear and tear of the body): **10–15%.**

In addition, a balanced diet should also provide other non-nutrients, such as **dietary fiber, antioxidants** and **phytochemicals**, which have positive health benefits.

- **Dietary fiber**, includes **complex carbohydrates**, such as those obtained from whole grains, fruits, vegetables, beans and legumes. They are low or moderate in calories, and are devoid of refined grains and sugar. Dietary fiber promotes healthy bowel movement and decreases the risk of chronic diseases, such as coronary heart disease and diabetes.
- **Antioxidants** such as vitamins C, vitamin E, beta-carotene, riboflavin and selenium, protect our body from the damage caused by free radicals. Besides, spices like turmeric, ginger, garlic, cumin and cloves, etc., are also rich in antioxidants.
- **Phytochemicals** such as polyphenols, flavones, etc. also give protection against oxidative damage.

PLANNING OF A BALANCED DIET

Balanced diet may be planned according to the kind of food produced in the region, economic capacity, religion, customs, taste and habit of the people.

- **According to the kind of the food produced:** The diet must contain various groups of foodstuffs such as energy yielding foods, body building foods and protective foods, in correct proportions.
  - **Energy yielding foods**—energy yielding foods should include:
    - **Cereals, roots and tubers**—cereals provide proteins, certain minerals and vitamins in addition to energy in the diets of the low-income groups, whereas roots and tubers provide some amounts of proteins, minerals and vitamins.
    - **Pure carbohydrates and fats**—pure carbohydrates and fats provide only energy.
  - **Body building foods:** These contain high protein and are divided into two groups:
    - Milk, egg, meat and fish
    - Pulses, oilseeds and nuts
  - **Protective foods:** These are rich in proteins, vitamins and minerals. These are classified into two groups:
    - Foods rich in vitamins, minerals and proteins of high biologic value, e.g. milk, egg, fish and liver.
    - Foods rich in certain vitamins and minerals only, e.g. green-leafy vegetables and some fruits.
- **According to economic capacity:** According to economic capacity, balanced diet may be planned for high cost, moderate cost or low cost, as follows:
  - **Balanced diets at high cost:** Balanced diets at high cost may include large amounts of costly foods such as milk, eggs, meat, fish and fruits, and moderate quantities of cereals, pulses, nuts and fats.
  - **Balanced diets at moderate cost:** Balanced diets at moderate cost may include moderate amounts of milk, egg, meat, fish, fruits, fat, and large amounts of cereals, pulses, nuts and green-leafy vegetables.
  - **Balanced diets at low cost:** Balanced diets at low cost may include small amounts of milk, egg, meat, fish, fat, and large amounts of cereals, pulses, nuts and green-leafy vegetables.

Some Important Questions

1. **Define basal metabolic rate. Discuss factors affecting BMR.**
2. **What is a balanced diet?**
3. **Write notes on:**
   i. SDA
   ii. Dietary sources of carbohydrates.
   iii. Dietary fiber
   iv. Essential fatty acids
   v. Significance of dietary lipids
   vi. Nitrogen balance
   vii. Essential amino acids
   viii. Protein calorie malnutrition
   ix. Significance of dietary fiber

Chapter

8

Digestion and Absorption of Dietary Macronutrients

Digestion (enzymatic hydrolysis) of dietary carbohydrates begin in the mouth, where salivary amylase hydrolyses starch to smaller polysaccharides and maltose.

- **Chewing stimulates production of saliva and mixes salivary amylase with the food.** Only about 5% of the starch in food is broken down by the time the food is swallowed. When carbohydrate enters the stomach, acidity of the stomach stops the action of salivary amylase by denaturing the enzyme. Amylase will not hydrolyze cellulose, because cellulose has α-1→4 glycosidic linkages.
- As stomach contents enter **small intestine**, the pancreas secretes **pancreatic amylase** through the pancreatic duct into the small intestine. Pancreatic amylase **continues the digestion of starch, breaking it to maltose**.
- Meanwhile, brush border **disaccharidases** hydrolyze various disaccharides into monosaccharides (Table 8.1).

Table 8.1: Effect of various enzymes on dietary carbohydrates

Enzyme	*Site of action*	*Catalytic action*
Salivary amylase	Mouth	Starch/glycogen → partially hydrolyzed dextrins, oligosaccharides, isomaltose and maltose
Pancreatic amylase	Small intestine	Partially hydrolyzed dextrins/oligosaccharides → dextrins, maltose, isomaltose and maltotriose
α-Dextrinase	Small intestine	α-Limit dextrins → maltotriose and glucose
Disaccharidases	Small intestine	
Sucrase		Sucrose → glucose and fructose
Lactase		Lactose → glucose and galactose
Maltase		Maltose/maltotriose → glucose
Isomaltase		Isomaltose → glucose

- **Dietary fiber moves to the large intestine**, where bacteria, partially ferment these undigested carbohydrates and produce gas, and a few short-chain fatty acids.
- **Soluble fiber softens the stool** and makes it easier to pass.
- Insoluble fiber resists bacterial activity and passes unchanged to add bulk to stool.

> ***Note:*** Cellulose cannot be digested by human beings because we lack cellulase, i.e. the enzyme which is required to hydrolyze β-1→ 4 glycosidic linkages.

As amylase hydrolyses α-1 → 4 glycosidic bonds only, so, amylase cannot hydrolyse cellulose which has β-1 → 4 linkages.

Absorption of Monosaccharides

- After the enzymatic hydrolysis of dietary carbohydrates (polysaccharides and disaccharides) to monosaccharides, different monosaccharides are absorbed into the mucosal cells lining the small intestine, by two mechanisms:
  - **Fructose** is absorbed **by facilitated diffusion**
  - **Glucose and galactose** are absorbed **by** the process of **active transport**, with the help of **sodium-linked glucose transporter** 1 (SLGT1).
- In the villi, absorbed monosaccharides pass through the intestinal mucosal cells and enter liver, via portal vein.
- In the liver, galactose and fructose are also converted to glucose.

LIPIDS

Digestion of Dietary Lipids

- Dietary lipids mainly include triacylglycerols. Digestion of triglycerides is **initiated in the mouth** with the of food **chewing**, and by the action of the **lingual lipase**.

- Thereafter, with the action of **gastric lipase**, and **churning and contraction by the stomach**, nearly 30% of the dietary triglycerides get degraded to diglycerides and free fatty acids, with in 2 to 3 hours.
- Contents from the stomach **pass into the small intestine**. Presence of fat in the small intestine, **stimulates the release of** two hormones, i.e. **cholecystokinin** (CCK) **and secretin**, from the duodenal cells.
- **CCK signals** the **gallbladder** to contract and **release bile**, down the bile duct and **into the duodenum**. Bile contains large quantity of bile salts and lecithin.
- **Secretin signals the pancreas** to **release pancreatic juice**, which is rich in pancreatic lipase.
- **Bile emulsifies fat** and **breaks fat globules** (clumps of triglycerides) into small pieces and **keep them suspended in solution**. This, in turn, increases total surface area for the action of **pancreatic lipase**.
- **Pancreatic lipase hydrolyses** all the accessible **triglycerides**, within minutes, **into monoglycerides** and **free fatty acids**.
- **Bile salts** surround the hydrolysed products of fat digestion and **form water-soluble globules** with a fatty core called **micelles**.
- **Micelles transport monoglycerides and free fatty acids** through the watery intestinal environment **to the brush border of the intestinal mucosal cells** for absorption.
- Similarly, **phospholipases hydrolyse phospholipids** and release monoglycerides, free fatty acids, phosphate, and a nitrogenous substance (Table 8.2).

Absorption of the Hydrolyzed Products of Lipids

Most of the triacylglycerols are absorbed **in the duodenum or jejunum of the small intestine**.

- **Micelles** carry monoglycerides and long chain fatty acids to the surface of the microvilli in the brush border and **diffuse into the intestinal cells**.
- The **unabsorbed bile salts return** to the interior of the small intestine for the transport of more monoglycerides and fatty acids.
- **Bile salts are absorbed in the ileum and return**, via the portal vein, **to the liver**, where they are **again secreted into the bile**. This recycling pathway for bile, i.e. from the liver to the intestine and from the intestine to the liver is called **enterohepatic circulation**.
- As **monoglycerides and fatty acids** pass into the intestinal cells, they **reform triglycerides**.
- Most of the **triglycerides** as well as **cholesterol and phospholipids combine with apoproteins** and **form chylomicrons**.
- Chylomicrons make their way **to the central lacteal of the villi** where they **enter the lymph system** to be propelled through the thoracic duct and **emptied into vein in the neck** (Fig. 8.1).
- **Glycerol and medium and short chain fatty acids are absorbed directly into the blood stream.**

Absorption of fat is drastically reduced in the absence of bile salts. As a result of it, bulk of the unabsorbed fat is excreted in the stool. The production of stool with an abnormally high amount of fat is referred to as **steatorrhea**. Steatorrhea may follow diseases of malabsorption, such as **cystic fibrosis**, radiation therapy, or digestive tract surgery. In such conditions triglycerides with medium chain fatty acids are often given in the diet. This is due to the reason that medium chain fatty acids are comparatively more water-soluble than long-chain fatty acids and thus can be emulsified more readily. Breast milk is a rich source of medium and short chain fatty acids.

PROTEINS

Digestion of Dietary Proteins

Digestion (enzymatic hydrolysis) of proteins **begins in the gastrointestinal tract** and is carried out by **proteases secreted by the stomach, the pancreas and the small intestine:**

- Digestion of proteins starts **in the stomach** by the action of proteolytic enzyme **pepsin**, at pH of the gastric juice. Pepsin is secreted by the cells of the gastric mucosa in the form of a zymogen (proenzyme) called **pepsinogen** which is activated by hydrogen ions of the gastric juice (HCl) and later autocatalytically by pepsin itself.

Table 8.2: Digestion of dietary lipids

Enzyme	*Site of action*	*Action of the enzyme*
Lingual lipase (important in neonates)	Mouth	Triglycerides → Fatty acids, monoglycerides, glycerol
Lipase/colipase	Pancreas	Triglycerides → Fatty acids, monoglycerides, glycerol
Phospholipase A/B	Pancreas	Lecithin → Fatty acid, lysolecithin
Cholesterol esterase	Pancreas	Cholesterol ester → Cholesterol, fatty acid
Retinyl ester hydrolase	Pancreas	Retinyl ester → Retinol, fatty acid
Monoglyceride lipase	Small intestine	Monoglyceride → Glycerol, fatty acid
Lecithinase	Small intestine	Lecithin → Fatty acids, glycerol, phosphoric acid, choline

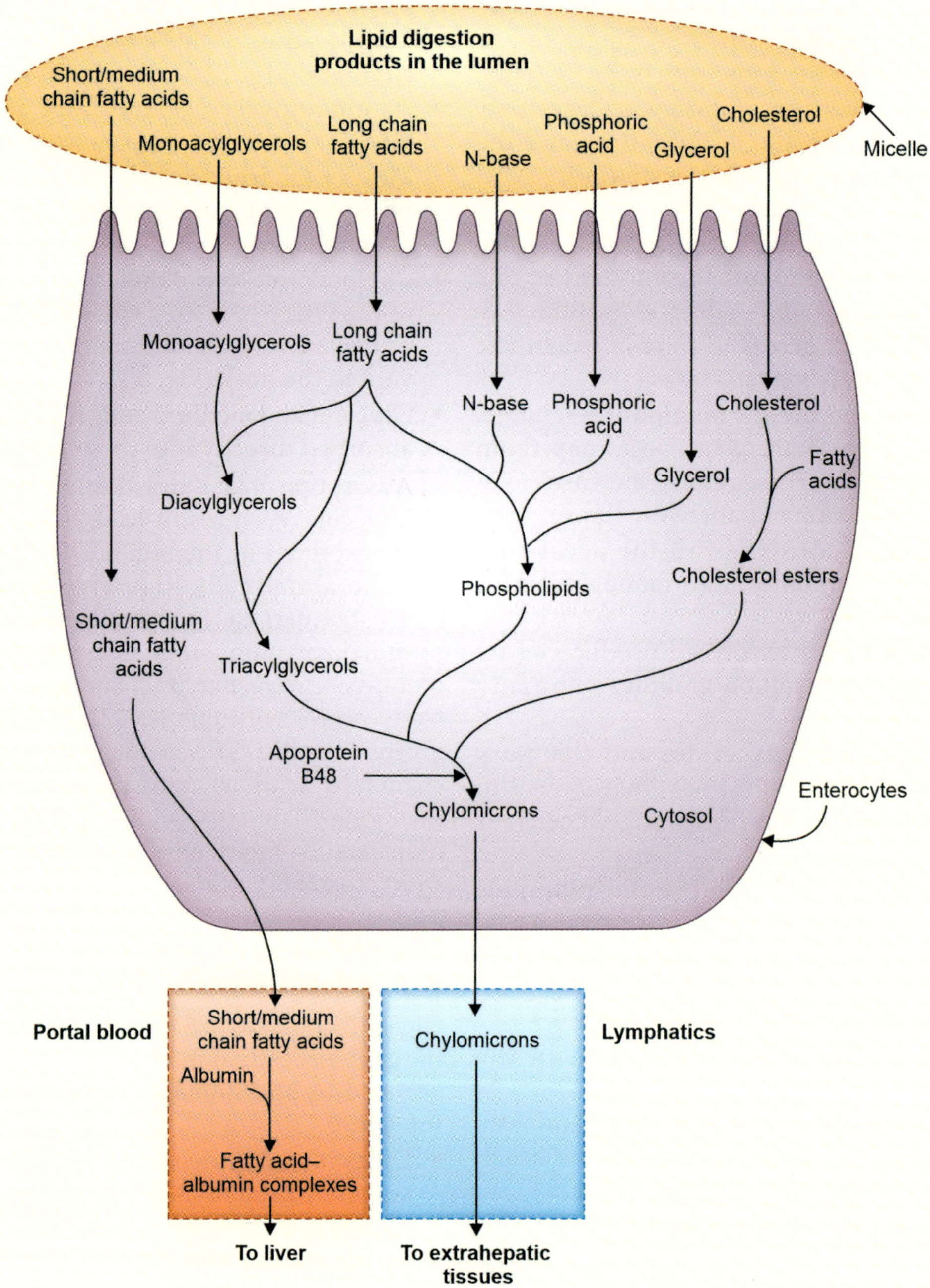

Fig. 8.1: Absorption of the hydrolyzed products of lipids

- **Proteolytic products of pepsin** pass on to the **small intestine**, where they **are attacked by** proteases that are secreted by the pancreas, i.e. **trypsin, chymotrypsin and carboxypeptidases.**
- **Trypsin** is secreted in the zymogen form as **trypsinogen** which is converted to trypsin by another enzyme called enterokinase (enteropeptidase). Once trypsin is formed, it acts on trypsinogen and converts it to trypsin, autocatalytically.
- **Chymotrypsin** is also synthesized and secreted as a zymogen designated as **chymotrypsinogen**. It is activated by trypsin.
- Pancreatic juice also contains **collagenase** and **elastase**, which specifically act on collagen and elastin, respectively.
- In addition, **procarboxypeptidase A** and **procarboxypeptidase B** (also activated by trypsin) attack peptide linkages, specifically those having a free carboxyl group.
- **Carboxypeptidase A hydrolyzes the C-terminal** amino acid in peptides, particularly, of those where the terminal amino acid is an **aromatic or aliphatic amino acid**.

- **Carboxypeptidase B hydrolyzes the terminal** peptide bond of the **basic amino acid** (arginine or lysine).
- The digestion of proteins, thereafter, is completed by the action of **aminopeptidases** and **dipeptidases** which are secreted by mucosa of the small intestine.
- Any part of the protein that is not hydrolyzed in the small intestine enters the large intestine and excreted in the feces.

Absorption of Amino Acids

Amino acids are **absorbed from the small intestine** into the portal blood. Absorption of L-amino acids is a **Na^+-dependent active transport** and **requires ATP and specific transport proteins. Pyridoxal phosphate (vitamin B_6) is also required** for the absorption of amino acids.

There are several **transport systems for the uptake of different amino acids**. These include:

- A transport system for neutral amino acids with short or polar side **chains** such as Ala, Ser and Thr;
- For **neutral amino acids with an aromatic or hydrophobic side chain** such as Phe, Tyr, Met, Val, Leu, Ile;
- For **imino acids**, i.e. Pro and hydroxyproline (HO-Pro);
- For **Lys, Arg and Cystine** (Cys-Cys);
- For **acidic amino acids**, i.e. Asp and Glu;
- For **β-amino acids**, e.g. β-Ala and taurine; and
- For **dipeptides**, e.g. peptide-1 (pep-1), glycyl-sarcosine, etc. These dipeptides are absorbed through the intestinal cells where they are hydrolysed by dipeptidases to the constituent amino acids.
- Besides, the small intestine of the foetus and the neonate can absorb intact proteins by endocytosis (pinocytosis).

Absorption of amino acids may be affected in specific transport disorders or other diseases involving the small intestine or the immune system such as Hartnup's disease and cystinuria.

AMINO ACID TRANSPORT DISORDERS

Hartnup's disease: It is a genetic lesion in epithelial amino acid transport named after the family in which the disease was first recognized. **Transport and absorption of neutral amino acids including that of tryptophan is decreased in** the epithelial cells of the **small intestine and** proximal tubules of the **kidney**. The intestinal defect results in malabsorption of free amino acids from the diet. The inability to reabsorb amino acids by the kidney manifests in the excretion of neutral amino acids including tryptophan and other indole derivatives in the urine, resulting in **neutral amino aciduria.** Symptoms of the disease are mainly those due to tryptophan amino acid and nicotinamide deficiencies. Due to tryptophan deficiency, there are **pellagra-like features** such as dermatitis, diarrhoea and dementia. Women are more susceptible to pellagra since kynurenine hydroxylase (an enzyme of the tryptophan-niacin pathway) is inhibited by oestrogen.

Cystinuria: It involves the **defect in the carrier for** sulphur-containing amino acid **cystine** and the basic amino acids, i.e. **lysine and arginine**.

Some Important Questions

1. **Discuss the process of digestion and absorption of dietary carbohydrates.**
2. **How are triacylglycerols digested? Explain the process of the absorption of the hydrolyzed products of lipids.**
3. **Write notes on:**
   i. Enzymatic hydrolysis of dietary carbohydrates
   ii. Enzymatic hydrolysis of dietary proteins
   iii. Absorption of amino acids
   iv. Hartnup's disease

Unit III

Micronutrients

Chapter 9

Vitamins

Vitamins are the organic constituents of food, called **protective accessory food factors**. These are the **micronutrients**, which are essential for life and well-being. Vitamins, in general, cannot be synthesized by the body and have to be supplied in the diet.

Antivitamins

Substances which counteract (inhibit) the action of vitamins are referred to as antivitamins, also referred to as **vitamin antagonists**. They cause symptoms resembling vitamin deficiency. For example, phytic acid, avidin, cortisone and birth control pills, etc.

Hypervitaminosis

Abnormally high storage levels of vitamins, which can lead to toxicity, is referred to as hypervitaminosis. Hypervitaminosis is mainly caused by fat soluble vitamins (vitamin A and vitamin D), since these are stored in the body for longer durations.

CLASSIFICATION OF VITAMINS

Based on their solubility, vitamins are grouped into two categories, as **fat-soluble** vitamins and **water-soluble** vitamins.

WATER SOLUBLE VITAMINS

Water soluble vitamins include **B vitamins** (vitamin B complex) and **vitamin C**. As these are soluble in water, they are rapidly absorbed from the gastrointestinal lumen.

- Water soluble vitamins are **used as coenzymes** in various metabolic reactions.
- Due to their water solubility, most of the water-soluble vitamins are **not stored in the body**. Since, they cannot be stored, a dietary deficiency quickly becomes manifest.
- Typical deficiency symptoms, for most of the water-soluble vitamins, particularly, those of vitamin B complex, include **dermatitis, glossitis, cheilosis and diarrhea,** besides some of the neurological symptoms, such as peripheral neuropathy and malaise.
- They are susceptible to destruction by heat and alkalinity. Some cooking practices also destroy water-soluble vitamins.

B-VITAMINS

The B-vitamins or **vitamin B complex** consists of various vitamins, which are generally referred by their names. These include:

- Thiamine (vitamin B_1)
- Riboflavin (vitamin B_2)
- Nicotinic acid (vitamin B_3)
- Pantothenic acid (vitamin B_5)
- Pyridoxine (vitamin B_6)
- Biotin (vitamin B_7)
- Folate (vitamin B_9)
- Vitamin B_{12}

Most of the B-vitamins are synthesized in the GIT by the intestinal flora. As mentioned above, they, primarily, act as coenzymes, and help in catalyzing various metabolic reactions, particularly, energy producing reactions.

THIAMINE (VITAMIN B_1)

Thiamine is also referred as **vitamin B_1** as it was the first water-soluble vitamin occurs in three forms, which are referred to as thiamine, thiamin monophosphate (TMP) and thiamine pyrophosphate (TPP).

Biochemical Functions

- The **coenzyme form** of thiamine is referred to as **TPP** (thiamin pyrophosphate).
- As a component of TPP, thiamine is **used** as a coenzyme **in** several **energy yielding metabolic pathways**.
- Accordingly, thiamine **requirement is related to the amount of energy consumed**.

- Thiamine is **also involved in** the normal functioning of the **nervous system** and other excitable tissues such as **skeletal muscle** and the **heart**.

Daily Requirement

As mentioned above, its requirement depends upon carbohydrate intake and has been defined as **0.5 mg/ 1000 kcal**.

RDA for thiamine for adults has been suggested between **1.4–2.3 mg/day**.

Thiamine requirement is increased during fever, hyperthyroidism, and in alcoholics and pregnant women.

Sources

Rich sources of thiamine include **whole grain cereals, oilseeds, nuts, legumes, green-leafy vegetables, organ meats, liver, eggs and milk and milk products.**

Deficiency Symptoms

Thiamine deficiency occurs with the consumption of raw fish, which contains thiaminase that destroys thiamine.

Thiamin deficiency manifest as ***beriberi,*** *which may be:*

- **Wet beriberi:** It **affects cardiovascular system** and results in edema, and dilated heart.
- **Dry beriberi:** It, normally, **affects central nervous system** and causes peripheral neuropathy with myelin degeneration, leading to foot-drop and paralysis.

Alcoholism, particularly, in those consuming poor quality of diet with low thiamine content may lead to a condition referred to as **Wernicke- Korsakoff syndrome (Wernicke's encephalopathy)**.

Common deficiency symptoms include neuropathies and numbness, **nausea, vomiting, weakness and tenderness of the calf muscles**.

RIBOFLAVIN (VITAMIN B_2)

Riboflavin is also referred to as **vitamin B_2**. It is also called **lactoflavin**, due to its presence in milk. It is needed for the normal structure and function of mucous membranes and skin.

Biochemical Functions

- Riboflavin is a component of the **coenzymes FMN** (flavin mononucleotide) and FAD (flavin adenine dinucleotide).
- As a component of FMN and FAD, riboflavin **acts as electron and hydrogen acceptor**, and **participates in** several **oxidation-reduction reactions** in the citric acid cycle, β-oxidation of fatty acids, and oxidative deamination.
- Thus, vitamin B_2 is required to release energy from proteins, carbohydrates and fat.

Daily Requirement

RDA for riboflavin for adults has been suggested between **1.9–3.2 mg/day**.

Sources

Milk, liver, kidney, egg-white, green-leafy vegetables, mushrooms and almonds are rich sources of riboflavin.

Deficiency Symptoms

Riboflavin deficiency may be observed with malabsorption, prolonged fever, hyperthyroidism and pregnancy. Deficiency symptoms include **chelosis** (lesions at angles of the mouth), **glossitis**, and **angular stomatitis**. There may be reduced iron absorption and diminished visual activity.

NIACIN (VITAMIN B_3)

Niacin is also referred to as vitamin B_3. **Nicotinic acid** and **nicotinamide** (or **niacinamide**) refer to two similarly functioning compounds which **have niacin activity.** It is also known as **pellagra-preventive factor**, due to its role in the prevention of pellagra.

Biochemical Functions

- Niacin is a component of the **coenzymes NAD** (nicotinamide adenine dinucleotide) and **NADP** (nicotinamide adenine dinucleotide phosphate).
- Both, NAD and NADP **participate in oxidation reduction reactions**.
- **NAD** accepts electrons and hydrogen, and **is reduced to NADH**, that **carries electrons to the electron transport chain**.
- **NADP is reduced to NADPH**, which is **used in the synthesis of fatty acids, cholesterol and steroid hormones**.
- Both, NAD and NADP are catabolized to yield nicotinamide, which can be deaminated into nicotinic acid or methylated to yield 1-methyl-nicotinamide.

Daily Requirement

RDA for niacin for adults has been suggested between **11–23 mg/day**.

Sources

Nuts and oilseeds are good sources of nicotinic acid whereas nicotinamide is absorbed in the liver from animal foods.

Milk and milk products, though are not an important source of niacin, but have **high tryptophan** content and, thus, play an important role in the prevention of pellagra. This is due to the reason that **niacin can be synthesized in the liver from tryptophan**.

Sixty milligrams of tryptophan gives one mg equivalent of niacin. This is called tryptophan–niacin conversion ratio and is 60:1.

Deficiency Symptoms

Deficiency of niacin can lead to a disease called **pellagra.**

Pellagra is characterized by **3Ds**, i.e. **d**ermatitis, **d**iarrhea and **d**ementia.

- **Dermatitis** results in pain, particularly, in those parts of the body which are exposed to sunlight such as face, neck, hands and feet. These parts become bronze, resembling sunburn, and get thickened.
- **Diarrhea** is accompanied with anorexia, abdominal discomforts and other symptoms of gastrointestinal tract.
- **Dementia** is due to impaired ability of the brain to utilize carbohydrates. Symptoms like depression, confusion and psychosis are commonly observed.
- Prolonged deficiency of niacin may result in 4th D, i.e. **death**.

Niacin deficiency is **common in persons whose staple food is maize and jowar** (called millets). Such individuals develop pellagra-like symptoms, since maize and jowar are **deficient in tryptophan**. On the other hand, these millets are rich in isoleucine. Low tryptophan and high isoleucine results in amino acid imbalance, which reduces biosynthesis of niacin in the body.

PANTOTHENIC ACID (VITAMIN B_5)

Pantothenic acid is also referred to as vitamin B_5. It, **structurally**, is a combination of **pantoic acid** and β-alanine.

Biochemical Functions

- Pantothenic acid forms an **integral part of coenzyme A** (CoA) as well as **acyl carrier protein** (ACP).
- **CoA is** essentially **required in fatty acid metabolism.**
- CoA is also required in the **metabolism of proteins, carbohydrates and fats**.
- **ACP is used in fatty acid synthesis.**

Daily Requirement

RDA for pantothenic acid for normal adults has been suggested as **5 mg per day**.

Sources

Rich sources of pantothenic acid are **yeast, liver, egg, potato, whole cereals and legumes.**

Deficiency Symptoms

- Pantothenic acid deficiency, in human beings, **affects nervous and digestive systems.**
- Its deficiency has also been shown to result in **adrenal insufficiency.**
- Deficiency symptoms include **headache, fatigue, impaired motor activity, muscle cramps and gastrointestinal disturbances**.
- Pantothenic acid is also **used in burning-feet syndrome** as well as **healing of ulcers and bedsores.**

PYRIDOXINE (VITAMIN B_6)

Pyridoxine, also called vitamin B_6, refers to **three different** compounds **(vitamers)**, which include:

- Pyridoxine,
- Pyridoxal, and
- Pyridoxamine.

Biochemical Functions

- The **coenzyme form** of vitamin B_6 is called pyridoxal-5-phosphate **(PLP).**
- **PLP is used as a coenzyme** with different enzymes which are involved in the **transfer of amino group** (NH_2), **carboxyl group** (–COOH) or water from one compound to another.
- PLP also plays a role in the **synthesis of non-essential amino acids**.
- PLP also **promotes gluconeogenesis** and facilities glycogenolysis.
- **Vitamin B_6** also **helps in the production of several neurotransmitters**, such as serotonin, γ-aminobutyric acid, dopamine and norepinephrine.
- It also helps in the **conversion of tryptophan to niacin.**
- Vitamin B_6 is also important in the **synthesis of hemoglobin** and also in the **binding of oxygen to hemoglobin.**
- Dietary vitamin B_6, along **with folate and vitamin B_{12}, lowers blood homocysteine levels**, which, in turn, is associated with the risk of cardiovascular disease.

Daily Requirement

RDA for vitamin B_6 for normal adults has been suggested between **1.9–3.1 mg per day**.

Sources

Rich sources of vitamin B_6 include **nuts and seeds, poultry, chicken and liver.**

Deficiency Symptoms

Deficiency symptoms include **cheilosis, glossitis and peripheral neuritis.**

- **In infants,** deficiency of B_6 affects central nervous system and results in **convulsions, demyelination** of the peripheral nerves and **degeneration of axons.** Its deficiency also associated with hypochromic microcytic anemia.
- Pyridoxine has also been shown to be **helpful in the treatment of nausea and vomiting during pregnancy,** radiation therapy and muscular dystrophy.

Vitamin B_6 Antagonist

Deficiency of vitamin B_6 has been shown to **occur in patients** with tuberculosis, who are **taking antitubercular**

drug INH (isonicotin-hydrazide), since **INH acts as an antagonist to vitamin B_6** (Fig. 9.1).

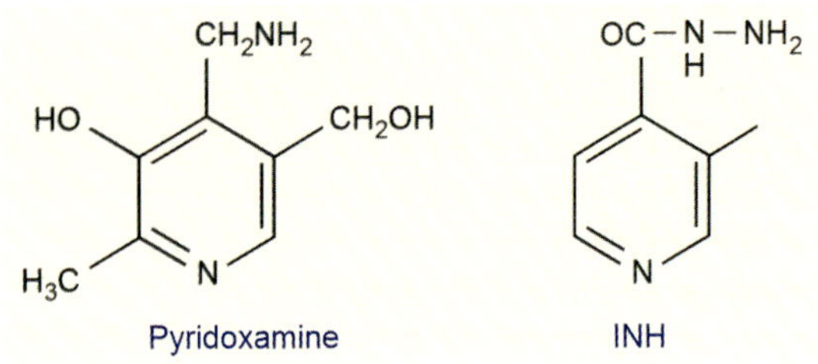

Fig. 9.1: Pyridoxamine and INH

BIOTIN (VITAMIN B_7)

Biotin is also referred to as vitamin B_7. It is involved in a wide range of metabolic processes, primarily, related to the utilization of fats, carbohydrates and amino acids.

Biochemical Functions

- Biotin forms **prosthetic group of the biotin-containing enzymes**.
- It is important **in carboxylation reactions,** where **carbon dioxide is added to the substrate,** e.g. in the conversion of pyruvate to oxaloacetate, propionyl CoA to succinyl CoA and acetyl CoA to malonyl CoA.

Daily Requirement

RDA for biotin for normal adults has been suggested as **25 μg/day**.

Sources

Rice polish, whole cereals, milk, yeast and organ meat such as liver and kidney are good sources of biotin.

Deficiency Symptoms

Deficiency of biotin may cause **mild dermatitis, nausea and loss of appetite, muscular pain and anemia.**

Avidin and Biotin

Raw egg-white contains a heat labile **biotin-binding protein** called **avidin** which binds to biotin and **inhibits its absorption**. If raw egg-white is taken in large amounts, avidin acts as **antivitamin** for biotin and causes biotin deficiency.

Heating raw egg white denatures avidin and prevents its effect.

FOLIC ACID (VITAMIN B_9)

Folic acid is also referred to as folate or vitamin B_9. It refers to a **group of derivatives of pteroylglutamic acid**. The synthetic form of folate, available commercially, is used as supplement in food fortification.

Biochemical Functions

- The **coenzyme form** of folic acid is referred to as tetrahydro-folic acid **(FH_4)**.
- Tetrahydro-folic acid is **important in one-carbon metabolism.**
- It also plays an important role in **amino acid metabolism,** particularly, in the metabolism of serine and methionine, and in **purine synthesis**.
- With vitamin B_{12}, folic acid also helps in the **formation of red blood cells.**
- It is also required for normal **cell division,** structure of the nervous system, specifically, in the **development of the neural tube**, which develops into the spinal cord and skull, in the embryo.
- With vitamin B_6 and vitamin B_{12}, folic acid is also required for the **maintenance of blood homocysteine** level.

Daily Requirement

RDA for folate for normal adults has been suggested as **220–300 μg/day**.

Sources

Green leafy vegetables such as spinach and cabbage, yeast, liver and kidney are good sources of folic acid.

Deficiency Symptoms

- Folic acid **deficiency may be seen in stressful conditions,** during pregnancy, intestinal malabsorption such as steatorrhea, and during antibiotic therapy.
- Folic acid deficiency may result in macrocytic **(megaloblastic) anemia**.
- Combined deficiency of folic acid and vitamin B_{12} may result in **psychosis and mental retardation.**
- Folic acid deficiency in early pregnancy, has also been implicated in **neural tube defects.**

Folic Acid Antagonists

Several compounds **interfere with the metabolic functions of folic acid**. These are referred to as folic acid antagonists. Most potent of these include **aminopterin and amethopterin**.

- **Amethopterin** (N10-methylfolic acid or **methotrexate**) **inhibits folic acid reductase**, thus, affects the conversion of folic acid to FH_4.
- **Aminopterin** (4-aminofolic acid) inhibits the conversion of folic acid to folinic acid and, thus, **inhibits biosynthesis of nucleic acids**.
- They act as competitive inhibitors of dihydrofolate reductase, and, thus, are **used as anticancer agents,** particularly, in the treatment of childhood leukemias.

CYANOCOBALAMIN (VITAMIN B_{12})

Vitamin B_{12}, also called **cyanocobalamin**, refers to a family of cobalamin-containing compounds, which include **cyanocobalamin** and **hydroxy-cobalamin**.

Biochemical Functions

- **Coenzyme forms** of vitamin B_{12} include **deoxyadenosyl-cobalamin** and **methyl-cobalamin**.
- Vitamin B_{12} is also important for the **metabolism of folic acid**.
- With folic acid, **deoxyadenosyl-cobalamin** plays a key **role in one-carbon metabolism.**
- **Methyl-cobalamin** is **essential in amino acid metabolism, DNA synthesis and cell multiplication.**
- It is also **required in propionate metabolism** (in the conversion of methyl-malonyl CoA to succinyl CoA).
- Vitamin B_{12} also helps to maintain myelin sheath.
- It is also important for the nervous system and formation of red blood cells.

Daily Requirement

RDA for vitamin B_{12} for normal adults has been suggested as **2.2 µg/day**.

Sources

Liver, kidney, egg, fish and milk are the good sources of vitamin B_{12}.

Deficiency Symptoms

- Vitamin B_{12} deficiency **can be seen in geriatric persons,** particularly, in those who are **strict vegetarians**.
- Its deficiency may also occur on **prolonged reduced intake, intestinal malabsorption,** atrophy of the gastric mucosa, or due to deficiency of the intrinsic factor such as in **pernicious anemia**.
- Vitamin B_{12} deficiency can result in **methylmalonic aciduria.**
- Measurement of the **urinary excretion of methylmalonic acid** is used to **confirm deficiency of this vitamin**.

VITAMIN C

Vitamin C is also called **ascorbic acid**. Due to its role in the prevention of scurvy, vitamin C is also called **anti-scurvy factor**.

- Majority of the animals can synthesize vitamin C from glucuronate, but **men**, primates, and guinea pigs **cannot synthesize it**.
- Vitamin C is **destroyed by heat**.

Biochemical Functions

Ascorbic acid performs several functions in the body. These include:

- **Collagen synthesis:** Ascorbic acid plays an important role in hydroxylation reactions. **Hydroxylation of proline** by the enzyme prolyl-hydroxylase converts it to hydroxyproline which is an important constituent of collagen.
- **Antioxidant activity:** Ascorbic acid acts as an antioxidant and **prevents damage caused by free radicals.** This, in turn, reduces the risk of certain chronic diseases such as heart disease, cancers and cataract.
- Ascorbic acid also helps in **recycling of** the oxidized form of **vitamin E** for its reuse within the cells.
- Vitamin C also **stabilizes** the reduced form of **folic acid.**
- **Absorption of iron:** As a reducing agent, vitamin C also enhances the absorption of non-heme iron from plant foods.
- **Synthesis of vital compounds:** Ascorbic acid also helps in the synthesis of various vital compounds such as **carnitine, norepinephrine, epinephrine, serotonin, thyroxin, bile acids, steroid hormones and purines.**
- **Immune functions:** Vitamin C also enables lymphocytes and other cells of the immune system to function properly. Accordingly, high doses of vitamin C may reduce severity and duration of cold-related symptoms.

Daily Requirement

RDA for vitamin C for normal adults has been suggested as **65–80 mg/day**.

Sources

Amla is the richest source of vitamin C. **Citrus fruits, green chilies, guava and tomatoes** are also good sources of vitamin C.

Deficiency Symptoms

Prolonged deficiency of vitamin C causes **scurvy**.

- Early symptoms of the disease include **swollen, spongy and bleeding gums; loosening of teeth; and pain in joints**. In severe cases there may be **multiple hemorrhages** including bleeding from nose, gastrointestinal tract and genitourinary tract.

> ***Note:*** Prolong deficiency of vitamin C inhibits prolylhydroxylase, as a result of which hydroxyproline cannot be synthesized thereby resulting in defective collagen synthesis and bleeding of gums. Thus, **low levels of vitamin C in blood increases the risk of gum bleeding** (one of the symptoms of scurvy), which can be resolved by increased intake of vitamin C.

- **Infants may lose appetite and body weight** with **painful tenderness of the extremities, bleeding from gums and mucous membrane**, and **cessation of osteogenesis of long bones**.
- Because of its role in the absorption, transport and storage of iron, vitamin C deficiency may also cause **anemia**.

Vitamin C is not normally toxic but large doses may result in **abdominal pain, diarrhea, and nausea.** More than 3 g/day may lead to **urolithiasis** (formation of oxalate stones).

Water-soluble vitamins, their coenzyme forms, major **biochemical functions, principal deficiency diseases and daily requirements** are shown in Table 9.1.

Table 9.1: Water soluble vitamins, their coenzyme forms, biochemical role, deficiency diseases and recommended daily allowances for adults

Vitamin	*Coenzyme form*	*Biochemical functions*	*Deficiency symptoms/ disorders*	*Recommended daily allowances**
Vitamin B complex				
Thiamin (B_1)	TPP	Oxidative decarboxylation	Beriberi	1.4–2.3 mg
Riboflavin (B_2)	FMN, FAD	Oxidation-reduction with flavo-proteins	Lesions on lips, cheilosis	1.9–3.2 mg
Niacin	NAD^+, $NADP^+$	Hydrogen acceptor for dehydro-genases	Pellagra	11–23 mg
Pyridoxine (B_6)	Pyridoxal-5-phosphate	Transamination, decarboxylation	Peripheral neuritis	1.9–3.1 mg
Pantothenic acid	Coenzyme A	Formation of CoA, component of the acyl carrier protein	Muscle cramps, burning feet	5 mg
Biotin	Carboxybiocytin	Cocarboxylase	Anemia, dermatitis	25 µg
Folate	Tetrahydrofolate (FH_4)	Carrier of one-C moiety	Megaloblastic macrocytic anemia	220–300 µg
Cyanocobalamin (B_{12})	Deoxyadenosyl cobalamin and methylcobalamin	Transmethylation with FH_4	Pernicious anemia	2.2 µg
Vitamin C (Ascorbic acid)	L-Ascorbate	Hydroxylation	Scurvy	65–80 mg

* ICMR-NIN (2020)

FAT SOLUBLE VITAMINS

Fat soluble vitamins include vitamin A, vitamin D, vitamin E and vitamin K. These are absorbed from the gastrointestinal lumen, in the presence of dietary fat (triacylglycerols) and bile salts.

Provitamins: Precursors of vitamin A and vitamin D are called provitamins, which are found, mostly, in plant sources.

VITAMIN A

Vitamin A refers to a group of compounds, collectively, called retinoids. These includes **retinol** (vitamin A alcohol), **retinal** (vitamin A aldehyde or retinaldehyde) and **retinoic acid** (vitamin A acid).

Provitamin A

Plants contain a group of compounds called **carotenoids.** Carotenoids are referred to as **provitamin A** (precursors of vitamin A), because they are converted to retinoids (vitamin A), when metabolized in the body.

Physiological Functions

Vitamin A is essential to the normal structure and functions of the skin and mucous membranes such as eyes, lungs and digestive system. It is, therefore, vital for vision, embryonic development, growth and cellular differentiation, and immune system. Besides:

- **Retinal** is essential for **night and color vision.**
- **Retinol** is required in **reproduction and bone health.**
- **Retinoic acid** is important for **cell growth and differentiation.**
- **Provitamin A** (carotenoids) functions as a potent **antioxidant** and **prevents damaging effects of free radicals.** Thus, carotenoids help to prevent damage from chemical carcinogens and lower the risk of certain types of cancer.

Role of Vitamin A in Visual Process

Retinal (vitamin A aldehyde), as mentioned above, is essential for vision, both in rods as well as cones:

- **In rods: Rod cells contain** a conjugated transmembrane protein called **rhodopsin**, which consists of an apoprotein **opsin** and a nonprotein prosthetic group called **11-*cis*-retinal** (11-cisretinene).

  Rhodopsin is essential for vision in dim light.
  - **When light falls on retina, rhodopsin** is bleached and **generates all-*trans*-retinal**, which cannot form a complex with opsin.
  - All-*trans*-retinal is **reduced to all-trans-retinol by** the enzyme **all-*trans*-retinol dehydrogenase** (retinene reductase).
  - It is then **transported to the liver and stored** there.
  - In the liver, it is **isomerized to 11-*cis*-retinol by** an **isomerase.**
  - After its delivery to the retina, 11-*cis*-retinol is **changed to 11-*cis*-retinal**, which again **conjugates with opsin** and **reforms rhodopsin, in dark (Fig. 9.2).**
  - This is called **vision cycle.**

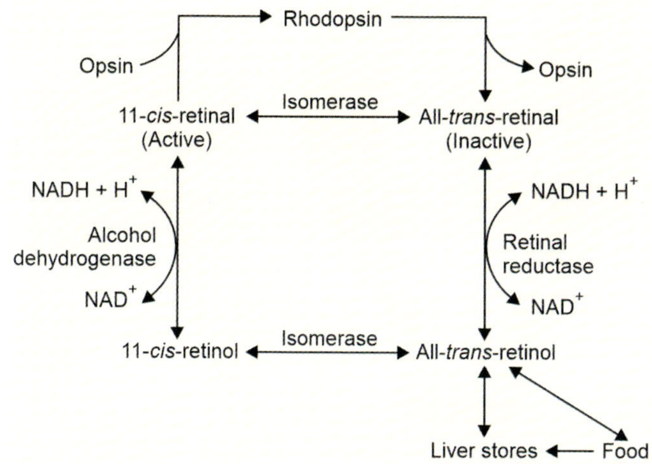

Fig. 9.2: Role of vitamin A (retinal) in the synthesis of rhodopsin

- **In cones:** Similar to rhodopsin, which is present in rods for the black and white vision, **cones contain** 3 different pigments that are sensitive to three primary colors, i.e. **porphyropsin (for red), iodopsin (for green)** and **cyanopsin (for blue)**. Prosthetic group in these pigments is the same, i.e. **11-cis-retinal**.

Daily Requirement

- RDA for **vitamin A** for normal adults has been suggested as **840–1000 µg/day**.
- Daily requirement of **β-carotene** is about **2000 µg/day**.

Sources

Liver oil, fish-liver oil, egg, milk and milk products are the good sources of **vitamin A**.

On the other hand, **papaya, carrots, sweet potato, and green leafy vegetables** are the good sources of **β-carotene**.

Deficiency Symptoms

Vitamin A deficiency is observed, primarily, due to its low intake. Its deficiency is aggravated by infections, which reduces its absorption and utilization. Vitamin A deficiency affects many tissues:

- It is most detrimental for eyes. Deficiency of the vitamin may result in **xerophthalmia**, which is characterized by **drying of conjunctiva and cornea, followed by destruction of cornea, leading to blindness**. Manifestations of xerophthalmia are shown in Fig. 9.3.
- Vitamin A deficiency also affects osteoblastic activity and results in **defective resorption of bone**, affecting growth.
- Deficiency of vitamin A also results in xerosis and keratinization of the mucous membrane, resulting in **dry and rough skin**. Keratinization of the mucous membrane increases its susceptibility to infections.
- Keratinization of the urinary tract may lead to **urolithiasis**.

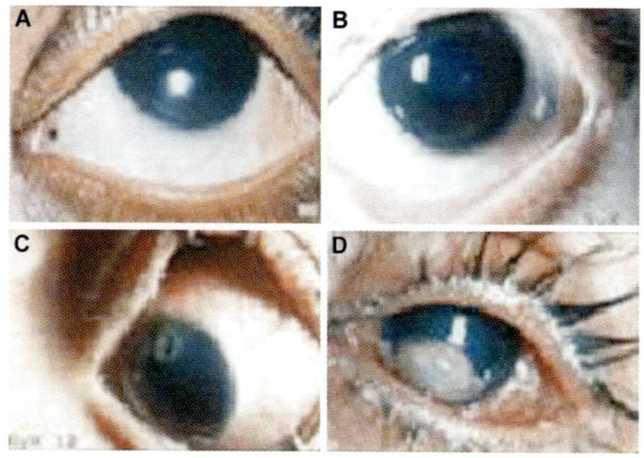

Fig. 9.3: Manifestations of xerophthalmia. (A) Bitot's spot; (B) Corneal xerosis; (C) Keratomalacia; and (D) Corneal scar

- Vitamin A deficiency also results in certain abnormalities of the reproductive system, such as **degeneration of testes, abortions** and production of the **malformed-offspring**.
- Keratinization of epithelium of the seminiferous tubules may also lead to **infertility**.

Hypervitaminosis A

If taken in large quantities for a longer period, vitamin A is toxic, since it is a fat-soluble vitamin and stored in the liver.

Toxicity symptoms include skin abnormalities such as **dry and rough skin, scaly dermatitis, headache, nausea, vomiting** and **loss of appetite, hepatomegaly, painful joints** and several bone abnormalities.

VITAMIN D

Vitamin D is a **sterol (steroid alcohol)**, also called **sunshine vitamin**. Although several forms of vitamin D have been shown to exhibit antirachitic properties, most important of these are:

- Vitamin **D_2 (ergocalciferol)** found in **plant foods**
- Vitamin **D_3 (cholecalciferol)** found in **animal foods**. It is also **synthesized in the skin**.

Vitamin D is, classically, a **prohormone**. It acts as a **precursor to** the hormone, **calcitriol** (1,25-dihydroxy-cholecalciferol).

Provitamin D

A derivative of the cholesterol, called **7-dehydrocholesterol**, is a precursor of vitamin D_3 in animals. It is also called provitamin D. It is synthesized in the human beings from cholesterol and is **converted to vitamin D_3 by UV light, in the skin.** This process is referred to as **photo-biogenesis**.

Active Vitamin D

Vitamin D is activated by two sequential hydroxylation reactions:

- The first step takes place **in the liver**, where it is hydroxylated by cytochrome P450-dependent

25-hydroxylase to **25-hydroxycholecalciferol** [25(OH).D_3].

- From liver, 25-hydroxycholecalciferol is **transported to kidney**, where it is further hydroxylated at position-1, by the mitochondrial enzyme 1-α-hydroxylase, forming **1,25-dihydroxycholecalciferol** [1,25$(OH)_2$.D_3], also called **calcitriol**.

Calcitriol is the physiologically **active form of the vitamin**, which **functions as a hormone** and is **essential for calcium homeostasis**.

Physiological Functions of Vitamin D

- Primary role of vitamin D, in the form of **calcitriol**, is to **regulate blood calcium** level, through its action on **bone, kidneys** and **small intestine**.
- Receptors for calcitriol are also found in a variety of other tissues, hence, vitamin D has also been shown to **inhibit cell proliferation** and **enhance cell differentiation**.

Role of vitamin D in Calcium Metabolism—Calcitriol **induces synthesis of calcium-binding protein, Ca^{2+}-dependent ATPase and alkaline phosphatase**, which are essential for the regulation of serum calcium and phosphorus.

Net result is achieved through its action in the intestine, bone and kidney:

- **In the intestine**, due to stimulation of synthesis of the calcium-binding protein, 1,25$(OH)_2$.D_3 increases **intestinal absorption of calcium** as well as phosphorus.
- **In the bone**, calcitriol **stimulates synthesis of osteocalcin**, which, in turn, mobilizes calcium from bone, i.e. it **causes demineralization of bone**.
- **In the kidney**, active vitamin D **increases tubular reabsorption of calcium and excretion of phosphorus.**

Overall effect of the three processes, thus, is to **increase serum calcium level towards normal**.

Daily Requirement

RDA for vitamin D for normal adults has been suggested as **600 IU** (15 μg) **per day**.

Sources

As vitamin D can be synthesized in the body by the action of the ultraviolet light on the skin, hence, sunshine is the best **source** of vitamin D.

Besides sunshine, rich sources of vitamin D are **milk, butter, egg yolk, fish oil and liver oil.**

Deficiency Symptoms

Deficiency of vitamin D, generally, does not occur, as it can be synthesized in the body. Deficiency however, may occur due to lack of sunshine.

Vitamin D deficiency leads to rickets in children (Fig. 9.4).

In adults vitamin D deficiency results in osteomalacia.

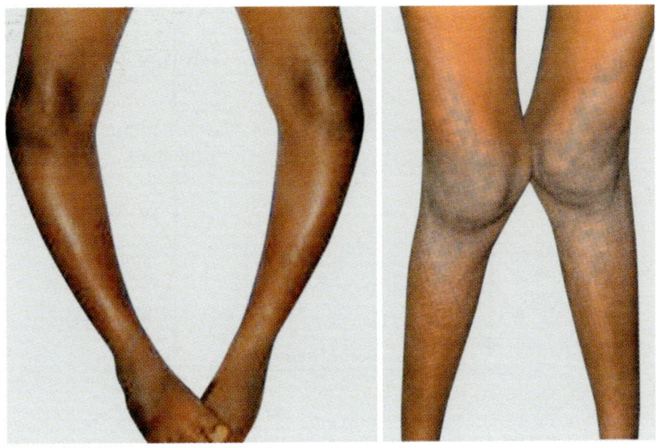

Fig. 9.4: Rickets (bowed-legs and knock-knees)

Hypervitaminosis D

Extremely large doses of vitamin D, over a long period, may lead to **hypercalcemia, hyperphosphatemia, anorexia, nausea, vomiting** and **diarrhea**, besides **bone pain** and metastatic **calcification of the soft tissues** including kidney, myocardium, pancreas and uterus.

VITAMIN E

Several compounds belonging to the group of tocopherols, such as α, **β**, γ **and** δ **tocopherols, exhibit vitamin E activity**.

- The α-tocopherol has highest biological activity as well as widest distribution. It is an alcohol with a **phytol** and **trimethylhydroquinone.**
- Commercially, vitamin E is available, both, as a natural substance as well as a synthetic compound.
- **Natural** vitamin E is **d-α-tocopherol** and is a single stereoisomer.
- Synthetic vitamin E is **dl-α-tocopherol**, which is **produced commercially**.

Physiological Functions of Vitamin E

Vitamin E performs several functions:

- Vitamin E acts as an **antioxidant**.
- It stabilizes cell membrane and **defends cells against oxidative damage** from free radicals. Since cells damaged by free radicals, are prone to mutations, thus, vitamin E **helps to prevent cancer**.
- Vitamin E also **maintains antioxidant status of β-carotene**.

Daily Requirement

RDA for vitamin E for normal adults has been suggested as **8–10 mg/day**.

Its requirement varies depending upon the level and nature of physical activity, diet, psychological stress, exposure to pollutants and intake of polyunsaturated fatty acids. Normally, **0.8 mg of vitamin E** is required **per g of PUFA**.

Sources

Tocopherols are present in small quantities in **green leafy vegetables** such as spinach and lettuce, **milk and milk products**, and **egg yolk**.

Oils, such as **corn oil, cottonseed oil and sunflower oil** are also rich sources of vitamin E.

Deficiency Symptoms

Vitamin E deficiency results in a range of **degenerative diseases**.

- Its **deficiency is seen in patients with abetalipoproteinemia**, who cannot form chylomicrons and VLDL. As a result of abetalipoproteinemia, vitamin E can neither be absorbed nor distributed.
- Deficiency of vitamin E is **also seen in children with fat malabsorption**, where it results in **severe progressive neuropathy and retinopathy**.
- **Hepatic necrosis, muscular dystrophy, defects in vascular system** and certain **reproductive defects** are also known to occur due to deficiency of vitamin E in various animal species.

VITAMIN K

Vitamin K refers to a family of compounds known as **naphthoquinones**. These include:

- Vitamin K_1 (**phylloquinone**, obtained from plant sources). It is the most biologically active form.
- Vitamin K_2 (**menaquinone**, obtained from animal sources and synthesized by intestinal bacteria) and
- Vitamin K_3 (**menadione**, the water-soluble form, available commercially).

Physiological Functions of Vitamin K

- Vitamin K plays a key role in the formation of **blood clot**. It is required for many reactions in the blood-clotting cascade, which involves the **production** of a series of proteins such as **prothrombin, factor VIII, factor IX and factor X, and fibrin**.
- It also helps in **bone formation**, where it is required in the **carboxylation of osteocalcin**, which is required for mineralization and maturation of bone.

Role of Vitamin K in Gamma Carboxylation

Vitamin K is essential for maintenance of the normal levels of various blood clotting factors such as prothrombin, factor VII, factor IX and factor X. These proteins are synthesized in the liver in their inactive forms and get converted to their biologically active forms by γ-carboxylation, with the help of vitamin K (Fig. 9.5).

> ***Note:*** Reduced synthesis of blood clotting factors forms the basis of internal bleeding arising due to vitamin K deficiency.

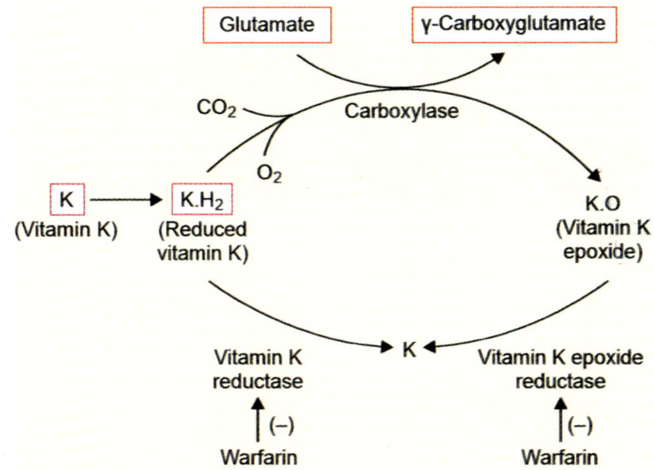

Fig. 9.5: Role of vitamin K in gamma-carboxylation (and synthesis of blood clotting factors)

Daily Requirement

RDA for vitamin K for normal adults has been suggested as **55 μg/day.**

Further, it is advised to administer a **single prophylactic dose of 1 mg of vitamin K_1 to a newborn on the first day of life**.

Sources

Green leafy vegetables such as spinach, lettuce and cabbage, are the rich sources of vitamin K. **Fish, liver and skeletal muscle** are also good sources of this vitamin.

Deficiency Symptoms

Deficiency of vitamin K is seen **in newborns**, due to their sterile intestine, particularly, in **premature infants**, who show **reduced levels of vitamin K, prothrombin and Christmas factor**. This also forms the basis of internal bleeding arising due to vitamin K deficiency.

Common deficiency symptoms include **cutaneous and intramuscular hemorrhages** with **bluish-red discoloration in different parts** of the body.

Vitamin K Antagonists

Anticoagulants such as **dicumarol and warfarin**, due to their **structural similarities** with vitamin K_1, act as antagonists **(anti-vitamins)** of vitamin K.

These compounds act as **competitive inhibitors for the enzymes**, which are concerned with the **activation of** prothrombin and other **coagulation factors**, and require vitamin K for their activation.

Table 9.2 lists various fat-soluble vitamins, their physiological functions, deficiency diseases, sources and daily requirements for adults.

Table 9.2: Fat soluble vitamins, their biological functions, deficiency diseases, sources and recommended daily allowances for adults

Vitamin	*Provitamin*	*Biological functions*	*Deficiency diseases*	*Sources*	*Recommended daily allowances**
Vitamin A (Retinoids)	β-Carotene (Carotenoids)	In vision cycle, growth and maintenance of epithelium	Night blindness; disorders of mucous membrane, bone, nerves; and reproduction	Liver oil, fish oil and vegetable oils	840–1000 μg
Vitamin D (Calciferols)	7-Dehydrocholesterol	Regulation of serum calcium and phosphorus	Rickets and osteomalacia	Fish oil	600 IU
Vitamin E (Tocopherols)	—	As antioxidant	Hemolytic anemia (in infants) and muscular dystrophy	Plant seed oils	8–10 mg
Vitamin K (Napthoquinones)	—	In blood coagulation	Blood clotting failure	Plant seed oils	55 μg

* ICMR-NIN (2020)

Some Important Questions

1. **Name fat-soluble vitamins? Mention their dietary sources, physiological functions and deficiency symptoms.**
2. **Describe physiological functions and deficiency symptoms of vitamin A.**
3. **How is vitamin D activated? Describe its role in calcium metabolism.**
4. **Describe dietary sources, biochemical functions and deficiency symptoms of folate and vitamin B_{12}.**
5. **Given an account of dietary sources, biochemical functions and deficiency symptoms of vitamin C.**
6. **Describe coenzyme forms and biochemical functions of:**
   i. Riboflavin
   ii. Pantothenic acid
   iii. Biotin
   iv. Vitamin B_6
   v. Thiamin
   vi. Niacin
7. **Discuss briefly:**
   i. Role of pyridoxal-5-phosphate in amino acid metabolism
   ii. Physiological functions of vitamin D
   iii. Role of vitamin A in visual process
8. **Write notes on:**
   i. Pellagra
   ii. Beriberi
   iii. Scurvy
   iv. Vitamin B_{12} coenzymes
   v. Calcitriol
   vi. Role of vitamin D in calcium metabolism
   vii. Role of vitamin K in gamma-carboxylation
   viii. Pyridoxine
   ix. Wernicke's encephalopathy
   x. Provitamin A
   xi. Xerophthalmia
   xii. Provitamin D
   xiii. Active vitamin D
   xiv. Rickets
   xv. Vitamin K antagonists
   xvi. Hypervitaminosis A

Chapter 10

Minerals

Minerals are the inorganic substances and represent about 4 to 5% of body weight. These are required by the body in small amounts and perform a variety of functions such as for the formation of bones and teeth, are essential constituents of body fluids and tissues, components of enzyme systems, and are required for normal nerve functions.

CLASSIFICATION OF MINERALS

Based on their daily requirements, minerals are classified into two categories:

- **Major minerals:** These are needed in large amounts, e.g. calcium, phosphorus, sodium, potassium, magnesium, etc.
- **Trace elements:** These are required in, comparatively, small quantities, e.g. iron, zinc, iodine, fluoride, selenium, copper, etc.

CALCIUM

Calcium (Ca) is the most abundant mineral, found in the body. It is found in highest concentration in the body and is needed by all the cells. **Adult human body contains,** nearly, **1.0–1.5 Kg of calcium**, out of which about **99% is found in bones and teeth**, and 1% in the extracellular fluid. Calcium level in the blood is regulated by balancing calcium absorption from the gut, excretion via kidneys, and mobilization and deposition in the bone. These sites are **regulated by** feedback mechanisms, which are controlled by several hormones, including **parathyroid hormone (PTH) and active vitamin D.**

Recommended Daily Allowance

RDA for calcium for normal adults has been suggested as 1000 mg**/day.**

Dietary Sources

Milk, cheese and other dairy products are rich sources of calcium. **Eggs, dry fruits, legumes, green-leafy vegetables** (such as broccoli and cabbage), **fortified soya products and fish** eaten with the bones (such as tinned salmon and whitebait) **are also good sources of calcium**.

Uptake and Excretion of Calcium

- Only about **10–30%** of the dietary calcium is, normally, **absorbed**, mostly in the duodenum.
- **Absorption of calcium depends upon several factors:**
  - In **vitamin D** deficiency, calcium absorption is impaired.
  - Excess of **phosphate** lowers calcium absorption.
  - **Phytic acid** and related substances present in unrefined cereals interfere with the absorption of calcium.
  - Excessive amounts of **fat, fiber and oxalate** in the diet reduce calcium absorption, due to the formation of insoluble salts.
  - Higher amounts of dietary **protein, lactose** and acidic **pH** promote calcium absorption.
- Calcium is excreted in the feces, urine and sweat:
  - Dietary calcium, which is not absorbed in the intestine, is excreted in the feces (nearly 800 mg/d).
  - Amount of calcium excreted in the urine is nearly 200 mg/d.
  - Urinary **excretion is increased** (hypercalciuria) **by ingestion of the excessive** amount of **protein** in the diet, in **acidosis, thyrotoxicosis, hypoparathyroidism** and **restricted physical activity.**
  - **In tropical climate**, calcium **excretion is increased in sweat.**

Physiological Functions

Calcium performs several functions in the body:

- **Formation of bones and teeth:** Bones are the reservoir of Ca in the body.
- **Mediates muscle contraction:** Ca mediates excitation and contraction of muscle fibers.
- **Helps in nerve conduction:** Transmission of nerve impulses from pre-synaptic to post-synaptic region.

- **Mediates secretion of hormones:** Calcium mediates secretion of **insulin, PTH, calcitonin and vasopressin.**
- **Acts as second messenger:** Ca and cAMP act as second messengers of different hormones, such as **glucagon**.
- **Membrane integrity and permeability:** Calcium influences transport of several substances across the membranous barrier.
- **Role in blood coagulation:** Calcium is essential for factor IV in blood coagulation cascade and in the **conversion of prothrombin to thrombin**.
- **Action on heart:** Ca prolongs systole. High Ca concentration also **increases myocardial contractility**.
- **Activation of enzymes: Calmodulin** (Ca-binding regulatory protein) **binds with 4 Ca** ions and leads to **activation of several enzymes**.

Regulation of Serum Calcium (Calcium Homeostasis)

Maintenance of serum calcium level, within the normal limit, is called calcium homeostasis. Serum Ca^{2+} level is regulated in a complex manner by parathyroid hormone (PTH), vitamin D and calcitonin (Fig. 10.1).

Parathyroid hormone: If serum Ca^{2+} concentration falls, secretion of PTH is increased:

- **PTH acts** directly **on osteoclasts** and increases dissolution of bone mineral. This process is called **bone resorption**.
- It also increases the **reabsorption of Ca^{2+} from the kidney tubules**.
- PTH also stimulates 1-α-hydroxylase activity in the kidney which, in turn, **activates vitamin**.
- **Active vitamin D:** It increases serum Ca^{2+} concentration by promoting **intestinal absorption** as well as renal tubular reabsorption of Ca^{2+}.
- **Calcitonin:** It is secreted when serum Ca^{2+} level rises. Its action is to lower serum Ca^{2+} level by promoting deposition of calcium by the osteoblasts. It also promotes renal Ca^{2+} excretion. Thus, PTH and **calcitonin act in opposite directions** in regulating serum calcium.

Deficiency Disorders

- Inadequate intake of calcium, in addition to an inadequate intake of vitamin D, has been demonstrated to contribute to **rickets** in children, and **osteomalacia** in adults.
- **Hypocalcemia may also lead to** osteoporosis, **which is characterized by loss of bone matrix and progressive demineralization. Decreased calcium intake, particularly, during menopause, leads to increased fragility of bones, mainly, of the extremities and pelvis.**
- **Hypocalcemia may also result** in tetany of **skeletal muscles. It is characterized by muscle twitching, spasms and, eventually, convulsions.**

Toxicity

- Very high intake of calcium (2000 mg or more per day) may lead to excessive **calcification of soft tissues,** especially, the kidneys.
- Long term high intakes of calcium may lead to **increased bone fractures in the elderly**, perhaps, due

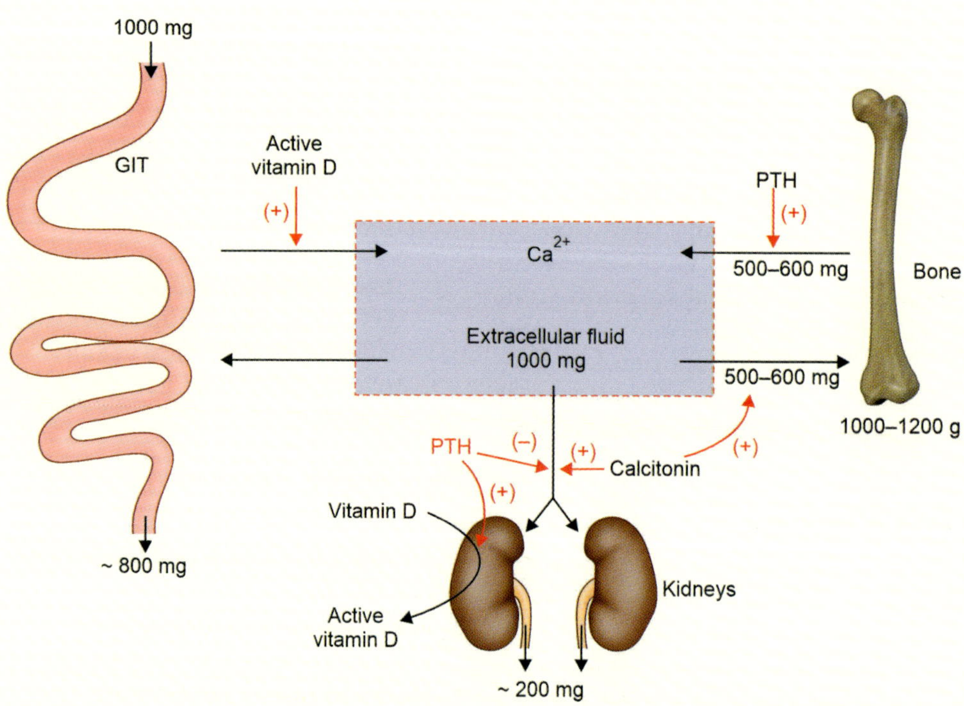

Fig. 10.1: Calcium homeostasis

to high bone remodeling rates that lead to exhaustion of osteoblasts.

- High intakes of calcium may also **interfere with the absorption of other divalent cations,** such as iron, zinc and manganese.
- Another potential adverse effect of excessive calcium intake is constipation.

PHOSPHORUS

A normal **adult body contains** nearly **600–800 g of phosphorus**. About **85%** of it **is present in the skeleton and teeth**, as calcium phosphate crystals. It is **essential for the structure of cell membranes**, as phospholipids. Phosphorus, in the cells, contributes to a number of processes associated with **energy metabolism**.

Recommended Daily Allowance

RDA for phosphorus for normal adults has been suggested as 1000 mg/day.

Dietary Sources

Phosphorus is found in foods containing phosphoproteins, nucleoproteins, phospholipids and glycerophosphates, as well as in the form of inorganic phosphates (chiefly of Ca and Na).

Phosphorus is abundant in **red meat, dairy products, fish, poultry, bread, rice and oats,** and is, usually, found in foods that also contain calcium.

Uptake and Excretion

- Depending upon the presence of other constituents, **about 10–40% of the dietary phosphorus is absorbed as inorganic phosphate in the small intestine**.
- Organic phosphate is hydrolyzed in the intestinal lumen and released as inorganic phosphate, through the action of pancreatic/intestinal phosphatases, e.g. alkaline phosphatase.
- **Absorption** of phosphorus also **depends upon the dietary content of phosphorus** (absorption of phosphorus is increased when its intake is low), as well as **calcium and vitamin D**.
- An increase in dietary magnesium also results in reduction in phosphate absorption.
- About **two-thirds** of the dietary phosphorus are **excreted in the urine**, while the remaining **one-third** is excreted **in feces**.
- PTH increases excretion of phosphate by inhibiting its tubular reabsorption.

Physiological Functions

- As **phosphates**, phosphorus participates in numerous essential functions of the body, e.g. **as a component of DNA and RNA, ATP and other high energy phosphate compounds**, such as creatine phosphate, glucose-6-phosphate, phosphoenolpyruvate, etc.
- **Phosphate with calcium forms hydroxyapatite,** the major inorganic molecule in teeth and bones.
- As part of the phospholipids, phosphorus is present in every cell membrane in the body. Numerous **phospholipid molecules also act as secondary messengers,** within the cytosol.
- As a part of **phosphate buffer**, it is important in intracellular fluid and kidney tubules, where phosphate functions in the **excretion of hydrogen ions.**

Serum Phosphorus Regulation

Absorbed phosphate exists in plasma in two forms, i.e. as phospholipids and in the inorganic form. The inorganic form, like calcium, can be either protein bound or free. In normal adult human beings, **serum phosphorus** (as inorganic phosphorus) varies from **2.5 to 4.5 mg/ 100 ml.** Circulating phosphates are in equilibrium with the skeletal and cellular inorganic phosphates, as well as the organic phosphates. **PTH and serum calcium regulate** the **level of phosphorus in the serum** as well as its reabsorption by the renal tubules.

Deficiency Disorders

- Phosphate deficiency may **result from** long term administration of glucose, or total parenteral nutrition (TPN) without sufficient phosphate, **excessive use of phosphate-binding antacids, hyperparathyroidism,** during treatment of diabetic acidosis, and in those who are **alcoholics.**
- Phosphate deficiency may lead to **neural, muscular, skeletal, hematologic, renal and other abnormalities**.

Toxicity

Persistently high PTH, because of the chronic consumption of low calcium and high phosphorus, may contribute to **increased bone turnover** that, potentially, can result in a reduction of bone mass and density. If this condition is chronic, it could contribute to **fragility fractures** because of excessive resorption and thinning of **trabecular plates at bone sites** throughout the skeleton.

MAGNESIUM

Adult human **body contains** nearly **20–25 g of magnesium** (Mg). About **75% of it is present in bones**, in combination with calcium and phosphorous. Remaining of it is present in soft tissues such as muscle and nervous tissue and in body fluids. Most of the **magnesium in blood is intracellular.**

Recommended Daily Allowance

RDA for magnesium for normal adults has been suggested between **370–440 mg/day**.

Dietary Sources

Whole **grains cereals, potato and seafoods** are good sources of magnesium. Beverages such as **coffee, tea and cocoa** are also rich in magnesium.

Physiological Functions

1. Magnesium is a **component of the bone structure**.
2. It also plays an important role in **nerve impulse transmission**.
3. Magnesium ions (Mg^{2+}) also act as **activator for several enzymes**, particularly those requiring ATP, such as glucokinase, hexokinase, acyl CoA synthetase, alkaline phosphatase, and DNA and RNA polymerases, etc.
4. Mg^{2+} is also required in the synthesis of cAMP and, thus, **mediates the effects of numerous hormones.**
5. Mg^{2+} also **participates in electron transfer** and stabilizes the arrangement of redox centers in cytochrome C oxidase.
6. Mg^{2+} also helps in **contraction of the cardiac and smooth muscles**.

Deficiency Symptoms

Magnesium **deficiency is often observed in alcoholics** and in **patients taking certain types of diuretics,** and those with metabolic acidosis.

Magnesium deficiency may also be observed **in uremic** and children suffering from **kwashiorkor**.

Low serum magnesium levels are also observed **during pregnancy**, particularly during **toxemia of pregnancy, rickets, diarrhea and vomiting**.

Deficiency symptoms include **tremors, depression, hyperirritability, cardiac arrhythmia, muscular weakness** and convulsions.

Low levels of serum magnesium may also result in **tetany**.

Toxicity

Magnesium toxicity may be observed due to increased use of magnesium-containing laxatives and antacids. Chief symptoms include d**rowsiness, lethargy and weakness**.

IRON

Sources, uptake and transport. Heme and nonheme iron functions; deficiency.

Total quantity of iron (Fe), in normal adult human body is about 4 g. Iron may be incorporated in the protoporphyrin ring, both in the Fe^{2+} and Fe^{3+} forms. Fe^{2+}-protoporphyrin complex is called heme, while Fe^{3+}-protoporphyrin complex is designated as hematin.

- **Heme-containing proteins** include **hemoglobin, myoglobin** and several enzymes, such as **catalase and peroxidases**.
- **Nonheme proteins** include **ferritin, transferrin, cytochromes and iron-sulfur proteins**.

Recommended Daily Allowance

Recommended daily allowance (RDA) for iron has been suggested as **19 mg for normal adult males**.

For females the requirement is increased to **29 mg** (due to loss) during menstruation.

During pregnancy RDA is 27 mg while **during lactation it is 23 mg.**

Dietary Sources

Dietary iron is found in two forms, i.e., as heme iron (from animal sources) and nonheme iron (from plant sources).

- Food cooked in **iron cookware** is the best source of iron.
- Animal foods such as **meat, fish and egg**, are good sources of **heme iron**. It is the most bioavailable form of iron.
- **Green-leafy vegetables, cereals, legumes, pulses and beans (whole grains), nuts and fruits**, are good sources of **nonheme iron**, the predominant form of iron found in plant foods.

Uptake and Transport

Absorption of iron, mainly, occurs **in the stomach, duodenum and upper part of the small intestine**. Normally, only about 10% of the dietary iron is absorbed. Efficiency of absorption is increased up to 30% during severe iron deficiency.

Heme iron is **absorbed across the brush border** (mucosa) of the intestinal absorbing cells **(enterocytes)** after it is obtained from the animal sources. After the heme enters cytosol, its **ferrous iron** is enzymatically removed from the ferroporphyrin complex and **combines with apoferritin** to **form ferritin**, similar to free non-heme iron. **Ferritin carries it from brush border to the basolateral membrane** of the absorbing cells. Brush border iron transporter, called **divalent metal transporter 1** (DMT 1), **transports ferrous iron**.

Ferric iron is reduced by the brush border enzyme **ferric reductase**, for its absorption.

Non-heme Iron is transported by transferrin, from intestinal absorbing cells to various tissues.

Unabsorbed iron is **excreted in the feces**.

Physiological Functions

Iron forms a component of several **heme** and **nonheme** proteins:

- **Hemoproteins:**
  - **Hemoglobin** is required for the **transport of O_2** and CO_2.
  - **Myoglobin** is an **oxygen-storage** protein in muscles.

- **Cytochromes** are required in the **electron transport chain** and **oxidative phosphorylation**.
- **Cytochrome P450 system** is responsible for many **biotransformation reactions**.
- Several enzymes contain heme iron, as a part of their prosthetic group, e.g. **catalase, peroxidase, tryptophan pyrrolase, nitric oxide synthases, prostaglandin synthase**, etc.
- As a component of the lysosomal enzyme myeloperoxidase, iron is required for **phagocytosis** and, thus, killing of bacteria by the neutrophils.

- **Nonheme proteins:** Transferrin, ferritin and iron-sulfur proteins (ferridoxins).
  - **Ferridoxins:** These are nonheme iron proteins called **iron-sulfur centers or iron-sulfur proteins.**
    - Due to the presence of iron, Fe-S centers **occur in the oxidized as well as the reduced state.**
    - These are **involved in** various enzymatic oxidation processes, such as in the **mitochondrial electron transport chain**. For example, complex I which passes electrons from NADH to CoQ, contains one molecule of FMN and 6 to 7 Fe-S clusters, that participate in the electron transport.
- **Ferritin:** Ferritin is an iron containing protein **involved in the storage of iron.**
  - The protein component is called **apoferritin,** which consists of 24 subunits of the H chains and the L chains, that are arranged spherically.
  - **Apoferritin,** also called mucosal iron-receptor protein in the upper small intestine, thus, **controls absorption of iron** as it has a very rapid turnover.
  - **Intake of iron** also **regulates the rate of synthesis of apoferritin** so that more protein is available for iron binding when the intake is high.
  - Ferritin, therefore, **acts**, both, **as a sink for iron during its excess intake** as well as **its source during iron deprivation.**
- **Transferrin:** Transferrin is a non-heme iron-**containing serum glycoprotein** (β_1-globulin) synthesized in the liver.
  - Transferrin **transports iron to the sites where it is required**, such as in the bone marrow.
  - The apoprotein part of transferrin is designated as **apotransferrin**. There are two iron-binding sites in an apotransferrin molecule.
  - In a normal healthy adult, nearly one-third of the iron-binding sites is occupied. Thus, total iron-binding capacity **(TIBC) of the serum is directly related to its transferrin concentration.**
  - **In iron overload**, serum **transferrin may be fully saturated.**

Deficiency Disorders

The commonest disorder is iron deficiency **anemia**. It is the commonest disorder of iron metabolism and the commonest form of nutritional anemia.

Causes of anemia: Anemia may be due to several causes, which may include:

- **Inadequate intake:** Malnutrition, pregnancy (increased fetal demand), etc.
- **Poor absorption:** Prolonged gastroenteritis, complete/partial gastrectomy, etc.
- **Increased losses:** Excessive blood loss during menstruation, gastrointestinal hemorrhage, hookworm infections, etc.

Types of anemia: Anemia is a condition, which is characterized by the reduced number of circulating erythrocytes or reduced amount of hemoglobin in them, or both. Based on the RBC size and the hemoglobin content, anemia is of three types:

- **Microcytic hypochromic anemia:** The erythrocytes are much smaller in size and have reduced hemoglobin content. Their number may also be reduced but to a smaller extent. It is caused by iron deficiency (Fig. 10.2).

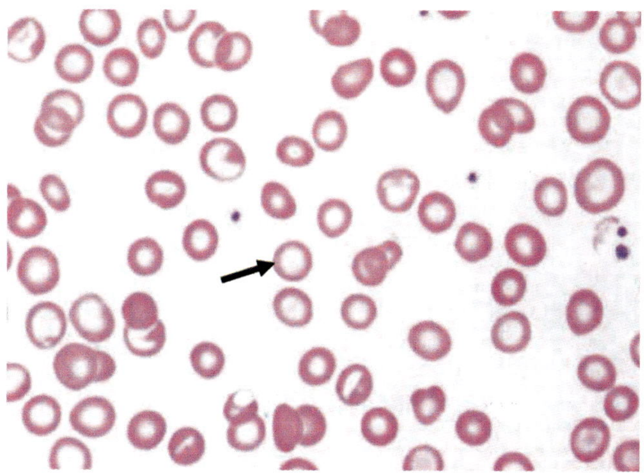

Fig. 10.2: Iron deficiency anemia morphologically characterized by variable degrees of microcytosis and hypochromia which results in widening of the central pallor accounting for greater than one-third of the total RBC diameter (arrow)

- **Macrocytic hyperchromic/normochromic anemia:** The **size of the erythrocytes is increased** while their **number is reduced**, presenting the characteristic blood picture of megaloblastic anemia including pernicious anemia. It is **caused by the deficiency of vitamin B_{12} and/or folic acid.**
- **Normocytic normochromic anemia:** The **size as well as the hemoglobin content of the erythrocytes remains normal** but **number of the circulating erythrocytes is reduced**. It is, usually, a **result of internal or external hemorrhage.**

Symptoms: Anemia is a common feature in children, adolescent girls and females of the childbearing age, particularly, in the developing countries.

- **Children become dull, inactive, lose appetite** and **have poor growth.**

- Deficiency of iron in **females reduce their work capacity**. On exertion, such women get **breathless** and **remain fatigued**.
- Iron deficiency is also associated with **decreased immunocompetence** and **susceptibility to infections**.

Toxicity

Major **cause** of iron overload is **hereditary hemochromatosis**. Frequent blood transfusions and long-term ingestion of large amount of iron can also lead to abnormal accumulation of iron in the liver.

- Consumption of, abnormally, large amount of iron, or in those with a genetic defect resulting in excessive iron absorption, can develop an iron storage condition called **hemosiderosis**. When associated with tissue damage, it is referred to as **hemochromatosis**.
- Increased dietary intake of iron by adult men and postmenopausal women, may contribute to enriched oxidative environment in the body and favors **oxidation of LDL cholesterol, arterial vessel damage** and **other adverse effects, involving the cardiovascular system**.
- Excess iron also **generates excessive amounts of free radicals** that attack cellular molecules, thereby, increasing the number of potentially carcinogenic molecules within cells.

IODINE

Nearly 20–30 mg of iodine is present in adult human body.

Recommended Daily Allowance

RDA for iodine has been suggested as **140 µg/day**.

Dietary Sources

Iodine requirement is, mostly, fulfilled from **drinking water**. Adequate supply of iodine can also be met from **iodized salt**. Besides, **seafoods, fruits, vegetables, cereals and meat** are good sources of iodine.

Physiological Functions

Important function of iodine is the **synthesis of the thyroid hormones** (T_3 and T_4). These hormones perform several functions, which include:

- **Regulation of basal metabolic rate**
- **Growth and development in children.**
- **Synthesis of the thyroid hormones**
  - In the thyroid gland, thyroid hormones are synthesized, as a result of iodination of the tyrosyl residues of the glycoprotein thyroglobulin (Fig. 10.3).
  - For iodination with the tyrosyl residues of thyroglobulin, iodine is first activated by the enzyme peroxidase.

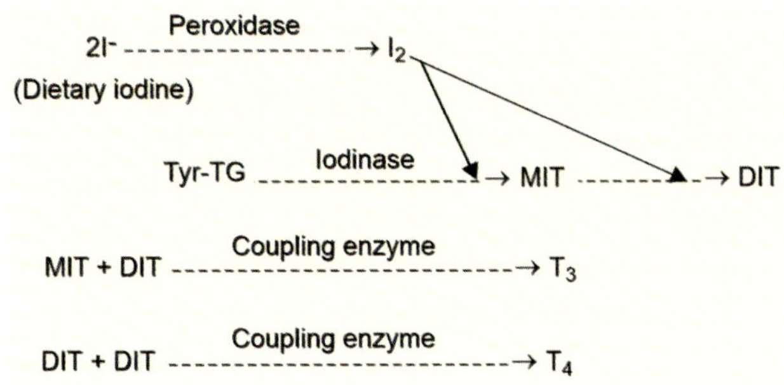

Fig. 10.3: Role of iodine in the synthesis of thyroid hormones

  - Subsequently, iodinase catalyzes iodination of the tyrosyl residues in thyroglobulin, and converts the tyrosine to mono-iodotyrosine (MIT) and di-iodotyrosine (DIT).
  - Thereafter, coupling of either a molecule of MIT with DIT or two molecules of DIT, forms tri-iodothyronine (T_3), or tetra-iodothyronine (called thyroxine or T_4), respectively. This is an intramolecular process and these hormones are synthesized within the protein chain (thyroglobulin).

Thyroid Hormones (T_3 and T_4) Perform various Functions

- **Development of the central nervous system:** Thyroid hormones **stimulate growth of the nerve cell bodies, branching of dendrites and rate of myelination of axons**.
- **Regulation of normal body growth:** Thyroid hormones **promote general growth and calcification of bones**.
- **Regulation of basal energy economy:** Thyroid hormones stimulate **synthesis of various cytochromes, cytochrome oxidase and Na^+/K^+-ATPase enzymes, uncoupling protein-1** (UCP-1, in brown adipose tissue) as well as **other uncoupling proteins (UCP-2 and UCP-3)** in many tissues, and, thus, **regulate** basal metabolic rate **(BMR)**. This is also called **thermogenic action of thyroid hormones**.
- **Regulation of fuel metabolism:** In addition to their ability to regulate BMR, thyroid hormones also **promote** a **positive nitrogen balance** and **synthesis of structural proteins**. The effects of these hormones on carbohydrate metabolism are opposite to that of insulin, hence, they tend to **increase blood glucose levels**. They also upregulate hepatic LDL receptors, thereby **favoring uptake of LDL-cholesterol**.

Deficiency Disorders

Iodine deficiency causes **abnormal enlargement of the thyroid gland**, which is situated in the neck region. In childhood, iodine deficiency causes reduced thyroid functioning, which results in retarded physical and mental growth. It may result in **goiter** (also called endemic goiter) as well as **cretinism**, which results in developmental delays and other health problems.

Iodine deficiency is associated with the development of **endemic goiter**, enlargement of the thyroid gland, **commonly observed in mountainous areas and in regions of high goitrogens intake** (Fig. 10.4).

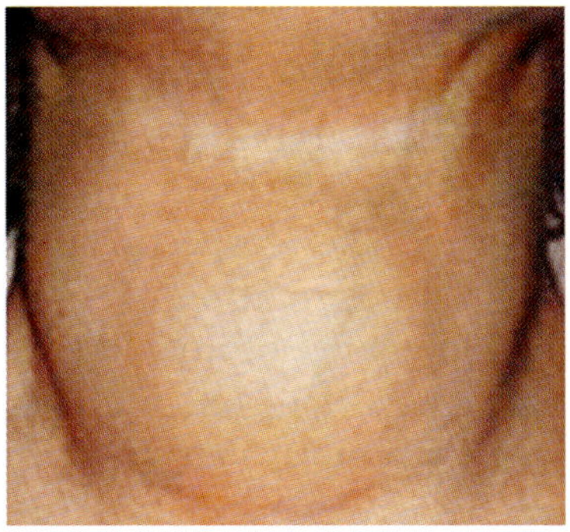

Fig. 10.4: Goiter

Goitrogens are the substances that **exist, naturally, in foods**. They can cause goiter by blocking uptake of iodine, from blood, by the thyroid cells. Foods, containing goitrogens, include **cabbage, turnips, rapeseeds, peanuts, cassava, sweet potatoes and soybeans**. Goitrogens can be inactivated by heating or cooking.

Severe iodine deficiency during gestation and early postnatal growth, results in cretinism in infants, a syndrome **characterized by mental deficiency, spastic diplegia or quadriplegia, deaf mutism, dysarthria, a characteristic shuffling gait, short stature and hypothyroidism** (Fig. 10.5).

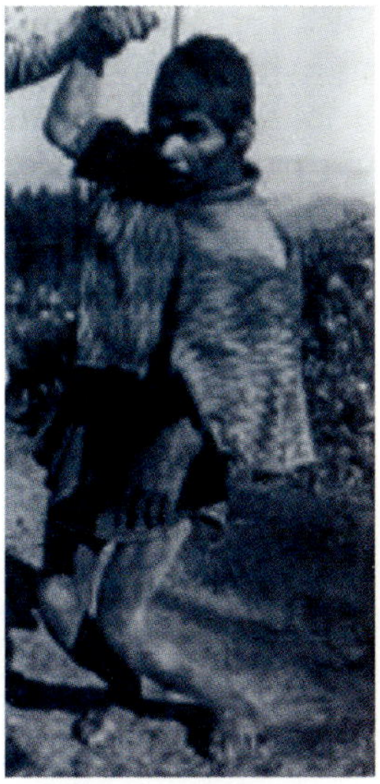

Fig. 10.5: Cretinism

Toxicity

Long term iodine intake, much higher than the physiologic requirement, may result in **hypothyroidism**, goiter formation or **hyperthyroidism**.

FLUORIDE

Fluoride is present in traces, in several tissues, mainly, bones, teeth, thyroid gland and skin.

Recommended Daily Allowance

RDA for fluoride has been suggested between **2 and 3 mg/day**.

Dietary Sources

Drinking water is an important source of fluoride, in a human diet. Besides, fluoride can also be obtained from **tea and fish**.

Functions of Fluoride

- The main function of fluoride is in the **mineralization of bones and teeth**.
- Fluoride also acts as an **antibacterial agent**, in the oral cavity and **protects teeth from dental caries**.

Deficiency Disorders

Deficiency of fluoride promotes development of **dental caries** in children, and **osteoporosis** in adults, particularly, in the postmenopausal women.

Dental caries: Dental caries is characterized by destruction of the tooth enamel due to the action of microorganisms on sugars. Breakdown of the enamel, in turn, exposes the dentine and leads to cavity formation (Fig. 10.6).

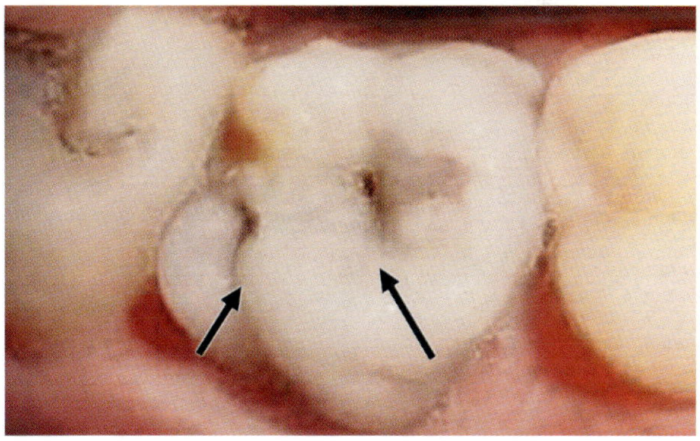

Fig. 10.6: Dental caries (formation of cavities)

Toxicity

Large doses of fluoride may be toxic. It may lead to **fluorosis**, which is an important public health problem in many parts of the world. It is due to the reason that high content of fluoride in rocks results in increased levels of fluoride in the groundwater. Fluoride toxicity may manifest in two major forms, i.e. as **dental fluorosis and skeletal fluorosis**, which **together** constitute **endemic fluorosis**:

- **Dental fluorosis:** It occurs, mainly, in children, who are exposed to high fluoride intake, before the completion of mineralization of the tooth enamel.

Their teeth exhibit mottled enamel. **Mottling** is confined to the permanent teeth and **is characterized by multiple, minute white flecks and yellow/brown spots**, which are **scattered irregularly over the tooth surface** (Fig. 10.7).

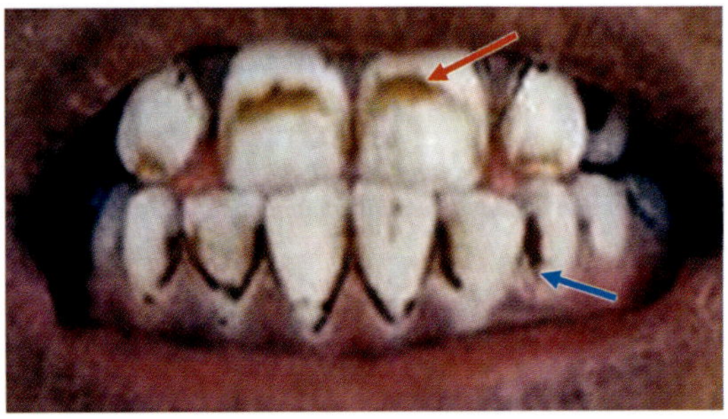

Fig. 10.7: Dental fluorosis. The teeth of the upper jaw (the two central incisors) show mottling and discoloration (red arrow) horizontally aligned on the enamel surface, away from the gums. It cannot be cleaned by a dentist. However, the teeth of the lower jaw show discoloration along the gums (blue arrow) due to dirty teeth (not fluorosis), which can be cleaned by a dentist

- **Skeletal fluorosis:** Its clinical features include **pain, inflammation and restricted movement of the joints** and **stiffness of the spine**. Further, significantly higher intake of fluoride (more than 3 mg/L, in drinking water) results in a variant of severe form of the skeletal fluorosis called **genu valgum** (knock-knee; Fig. 10.8).

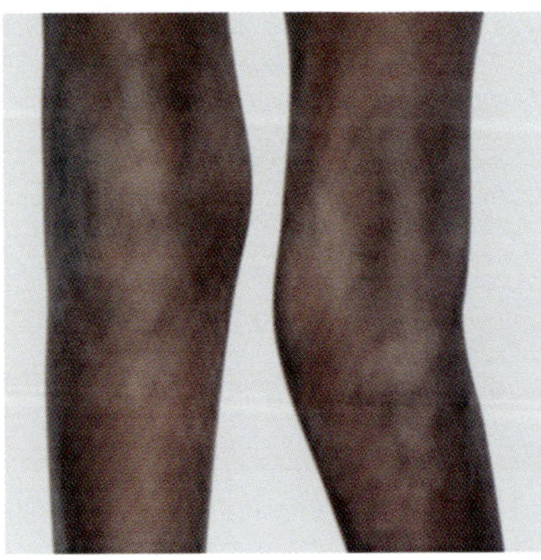

Fig. 10.8: Skeletal fluorosis. Deformed but mobile joints

COPPER

Adult **human body contains 100–150 mg** of copper, out of which, nearly, 50% is found in muscles and 25% in bones.

Recommended Daily Allowance

RDA for copper has been suggested as **1.5–1.7 mg/day.**

Dietary Sources

Nuts, leafy vegetables, dried legumes, egg yolk, and fish and liver meat, are good sources of copper.

Physiological Functions

- Copper is a **component of many enzymes**, particularly, those which require vitamin C, such as **cytochrome oxidase, ferroxidase (ceruloplasmin), tyrosinase, ascorbic acid oxidase, superoxide dismutase**, etc.
- It is also a constituent of α-aminolevulinate synthase and ferroxidase I, and thus, **helps in the metabolism of iron and biosynthesis of hemoglobin.**
- Copper is also an important **constituent of** several other proteins, such as **erythrocuprein, cerebrocuprein and hepatocuprein**, which are present in the bone marrow, brain and liver, respectively.
- It also helps in the **formation of bone and elastin fibers**, and **maintenance of myelin sheath.**
- Copper is also important for **infant growth, brain development, immune system and strong bones.**

Deficiency Disorders

- Some of the symptoms of copper deficiency include **hypercholesterolemia, demineralization of bones, leukopenia, demyelination of the neural tissue and alopecia** (loss of hair).
- There is also **microcytic normochromic anemia**, which cannot be cured by iron supplementation alone, since copper (as ferroxidase) is essential for the intestinal absorption of iron and in its metabolism.
- Copper deficiency in infants has been found to be associated with a condition described as Menkes disease.

Menkes disease is an X-linked hereditary disease due to **failure of copper absorption** across the serosal membrane of intestinal mucosal cells. This, in turn, leads to **low concentrations of copper** in the plasma and the liver. It also results in **deficiency of various copper containing oxidases** (tyrosinase, lysyl oxidase, etc.), leading to various systemic manifestations such as **skeletal malformation, mental retardation, defective thermoregulation and immunodeficiency**. Menkes disease is also called **kinky hair syndrome**, due to the failure to keratinize **hair which become kinky and steel grey** (Fig. 10.9).

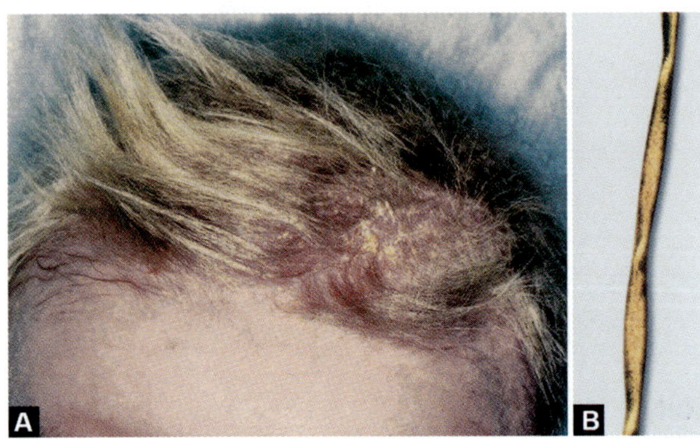

Fig. 10.9: Copper deficiency results in defective keratinization: (A) Menkes kinky hair which feels like steel wool (steely hair syndrome); (B) Pili torti: Twisting of the hair shaft on its own axis

Copper Toxicity

Copper toxicity may manifest as **diarrhea, blue-green discoloration of the saliva, hemolysis, proteinuria and renal failure**. Increased amount of copper is deposited in the liver and brain in Wilson's disease.

Wilson's disease (also known as **hepatolenticular degeneration)** is an **autosomal recessive inherited disorder** in which there is a **positive copper balance** due to **deficient synthesis of ceruloplasmin in the liver.** The net result is the **accumulation of Cu^{2+}** to highly toxic levels, mainly, in the liver and the basal nuclei of the brain. This, in turn, promotes the **generation of free radicals** leading to **extensive cell damage**. There may be **liver failure, neurological disturbances and characteristic Kayser-Fleischer rings in the cornea** (Fig. 10.10).

ZINC

Total **body content** of zinc in an adult man **is about 2.0 g.** Choroid of the eye, liver, prostate gland and prostate fluid contain high concentration of zinc.

Recommended Daily Allowance

RDA for zinc has been suggested as **13–17 mg/day**.

Dietary Sources

Zinc is present in many foods, but is most readily absorbed from **meat. Colostrum** is a rich source of zinc. It is also present in **milk, cheese, eggs, shellfish, wholegrain cereals, nuts and pulses**.

Physiological Functions

- Zinc, primarily, an intracellular ion, **functions with more than 300 enzymes**. It also **participates in the metabolism of carbohydrates, lipids, proteins and nucleic acids**.
- In the nucleus, zinc **stabilizes RNA and DNA structure**, and is required for the activity of **RNA polymerases**.
- Zinc also functions in **chromatin proteins, involved in transcription and replication**.
- It is also involved in the **integrity of subcellular organelles, in transport processes, immune functions and expression of genetic information**.

Deficiency Disorders

Since body stores of zinc are small, dietary deficiency can therefore produce symptoms promptly, particularly, when the soil content is low.

- Severe zinc deficiency is **seen in alcoholics, chronic renal disease, severe gastroenteritis and malabsorption, and protein-energy malnutrition**.
- There is **poor wound healing, loss of appetite, poor growth and alopecia** (loss of hair).
- **Impairment of sexual development in children**.
- **Impairment in brain functions**.
- Certain **fetal abnormalities during pregnancy** besides hypogonadism, dwarfism (stunted growth) and gross skin lesions with severe acrodermatitis.
- **Delayed recovery from diarrhea**.

Zinc Toxicity

- Zinc, when consumed in excessive amounts, produces toxic effects, such as **acute gastrointestinal irritation, gastric ulcers, nausea and vomiting**.
- It also interferes with the utilization and functions of copper, and may cause anemia.

ROLE OF OTHER MINERALS

Recommended daily allowances, dietary sources, physiological functions and deficiency disorders of several minerals are described in Table 10.1.

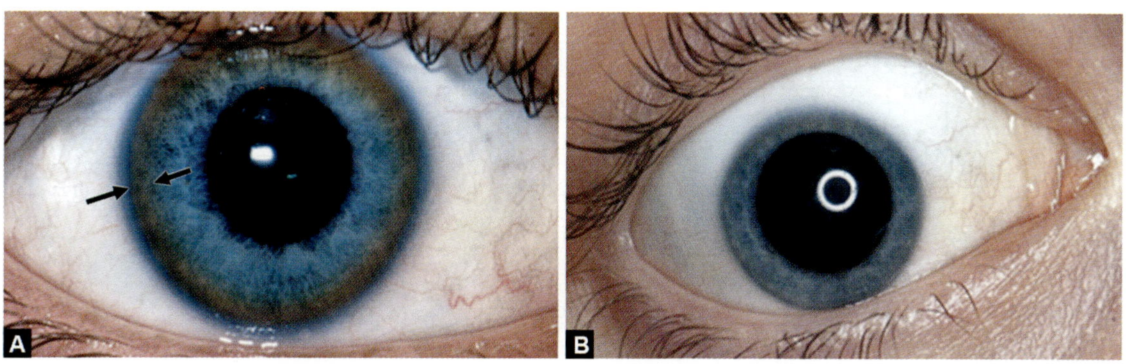

Fig. 10.10: Wilson's disease. (A) Kayser-Fleischer ring (arrows); (B) Complete resolution following copper-chelating (penicillamine) treatment

Table 10.1: Recommended daily allowances for adults, dietary sources, physiological functions and deficiency disorders of some of the minerals

Minerals	*Recommended daily allowances**	*Dietary sources*	*Physiological functions*	*Deficiency disorders*
Sodium	2000 mg	Common salt	Water and electrolyte balance	
Potassium	3500 mg	Fruits, vegetables and dairy products	Acid base balance	Cardiac arrhythmia
Calcium	1000 mg	Milk and milk products, eggs, dry fruits, legumes, cabbage and cauliflower	Calcification of bones and teeth, blood coagulation, cofactor for adenylate cyclase. Ca^{2+}-ATPase, and protein kinases	Rickets in children and osteomalacia in adults
Phosphorus	1000 mg	Milk and milk products, eggs, meat, legumes and cereals	Calcification of bones and teeth, component of nucleic acids, regulation of blood pH and activator for enzymes involved in phosphorylation/ dephosphorylation	Neural, muscular, skeletal, hematological and renal abnormalities
Magnesium	370–440 mg	Whole grain cereals, potatoes and seafoods	Cofactor for various ATP-dependent enzymes required in the synthesis of fatty acids and proteins, phosphorylation of glucose and its derivatives in the glycolytic pathways and transketolase reactions	Tremors, muscle spasms, personality changes, anorexia, nausea and vomiting, tetany, convulsions and coma
Iron	19 mg	Meat, fish, eggs, green-leafy vegetables, cereals and legumes	Component of heme and nonheme proteins, such as hemoglobin, catalase and cytochromes	Iron deficiency anemia, reduced work capacity and immunocompetence
Zinc	13–17 mg	Meat, seafoods, eggs legumes and milk	Cofactor for various enzymes that participate in reactions involving either synthesis or degradation of carbohydrates, lipids, proteins and nucleic acids	Short stature, hypogonadism, mild anemia and reduced immune functions
Copper	1.5–1.7 mg	Nuts, leafy vegetables, dried legumes, egg-yolk, fish and liver meat	Component of several enzymes, such as cytochrome oxidase, ferroxidase (ceruloplasmin), tyrosinase, ascorbic acid oxidase and superoxide dismutase	Anemia, neutropenia, skeletal abnormalities and Menke's syndrome
Iodine	140 µg	Drinking water, iodized salt, sea-foods, fruits, vegetables, cereals and meat	Synthesis of iodine-containing hormones (T3 and T4), regulation of BMR in adults, growth and development in children	Endemic goiter and cretinism
Fluoride	2–3 mg	Drinking water and tea	Development of tooth enamel and as antibacterial agent	Dental caries and osteoporosis
Selenium	40 µg	Plant-foods, cereals, fish and meat	Component of selenoproteins, such as glutathione peroxidase and selenoprotein-P	Liver necrosis
Manganese	4 mg	Nuts, whole grain cereals, legumes and leafy-vegetables	Component of many enzymes, such as glutamine synthetase, pyruvate carboxylase and superoxide dismutase	Sterility, skeletal abnormalities and ataxia in offspring
Chromium	50 µg	Brewer's yeast, mushroom, black pepper, liver, whole grains, nuts and cheese	Potentiates insulin action and influences carbohydrate, lipid and protein metabolism	Insulin resistance and lipid abnormalities
Molybdenum	100–200 µg	Pulses, cereals, green-leafy vegetables and meat	Component of enzymes, such as xanthine oxidase, aldehyde oxidase and sulfite oxidase	Mental changes, abnormalities of sulfur and purine metabolism
Cobalt	1–2 µg	Food from the animal origin	Component of vitamin B_1	Macrocytic anemia and pernicious anemia

* ICMR-NIN (2020)

Some Important Questions

1. **Describe dietary sources, recommended daily allowance and physiological functions of calcium.**
2. **Describe role of parathyroid hormone, vitamin D and calcitonin in calcium metabolism.**
3. **Name iron-containing proteins found in the body and describe their functions. Describe disorders related to iron metabolism.**
4. **Describe:**
   i. Regulation of calcium metabolism
   ii. Fluoride toxicity
   iii. Role of copper in iron metabolism
   iv. Physiological functions of zinc
   v. Factors affecting absorption of iron
   vi. Physiological functions of phosphorus
5. **Write notes on:**
   i. Copper
   ii. Wilson's disease
   iii. Physiological functions of calcium
   iv. Ferritin
   v. Transferrin
   vi. Anemia
   vii. Menke's disease
   viii. Kinky-hair syndrome
6. **Discuss:**
   i. Hepatolenticular degeneration
   ii. Goiter
   iii. Factors affecting absorption of calcium

Unit IV

Energy Generation and Metabolism of Macronutrients

Chapter 11

Biological Oxidation

As discussed in Chapter 7, dietary carbohydrates, lipids and proteins are the sources of energy for the cells, which is stored within the chemical bonds that hold them together. Eukaryotic cells use these **three major processes to transform this energy held in the chemical bonds of food** molecules into more readily usable forms, often energy-rich carrier molecules.

- The first process in the eukaryotic energy pathway is **glycolysis**, which, literally, means sugar splitting. During glycolysis, each molecule of **glucose is split** and, ultimately, **converted into two molecules of pyruvate in the cytoplasm**.

  Glycolysis is actually a series of ten chemical reactions that requires the input of two molecules of ATP. This input is used to generate four new ATP molecules, which means that **glycolysis results in a net gain of two ATP**. Besides, **two NADH molecules are also produced**, which serve as electron carriers for other biochemical reactions in the cell.
- When oxygen is available, pyruvate produced by glycolysis becomes the input for the next portion of the eukaryotic energy pathway. During this stage:
  - Each **pyruvate** molecule, from the cytoplasm, **enters the mitochondrion**, where it is **converted into acetyl CoA** (two-carbon energy carrier). The third carbon of pyruvate combines with oxygen and is released as carbon dioxide. At the same time, **an NADH** carrier is also generated (*see* Fig. 3.14).
  - **Acetyl CoA** then **enters** a pathway **called citric acid cycle**, which is the second major energy process used by cells. In eight steps, **citric acid cycle generates three NADH, one $FADH_2$ and one GTP.**
- The **third** major **process** in the eukaryotic energy pathway involves an **electron transport chain** (described below), catalyzed by several protein complexes located in the mitochondrional inner membrane.

This process, called **oxidative phosphorylation, transfers electrons from NADH and $FADH_2$ through the membrane protein complexes**, and ultimately to oxygen, where they combine to form water. As electrons travel through the protein complexes in the chain, a gradient of hydrogen ions, or protons, is formed across the mitochondrial membrane. Cells harness the energy of this proton gradient to create **2.5 ATP molecules for every electron that travels from NADH**, along the chain.

Together, **these processes that occur inside the mitochondrion, the citric acid cycle and oxidative phosphorylation, are referred to as respiration**, a term used for processes that couple the uptake of oxygen and the production of carbon dioxide.

TRANSFER OF ELECTRONS THROUGH MEMBRANE PROTEIN COMPLEXES

Electrons from NADH and $FADH_2$ (generated during the processes of glycolysis and citric acid cycle) **are transferred into the inner mitochondrial membrane through membrane protein complexes**, which comprise **malate-aspartate shuttle and glycerol phosphate shuttle**.

- **Malate-aspartate Shuttle**
  - Firstly, **pyruvate**, formed in the cytosol during glycolysis, **is converted to oxaloacetate**.
  - Thereafter, **with** the help of **NADH, oxaloacetate is reduced** and converted **to malate**.
  - Malate is **transported into the inner mitochondrial membrane.**
  - **In the matrix**, malate is **reconverted back to oxaloacetate with** the help of **NAD^+**, within the mitochondria. During this reaction, **NAD^+ is converted to NADH**, which **enters the electron transport chain**.
  - Since **oxaloacetate** cannot be transferred from the matrix back to the cytosol, it **is converted to aspartate**.
  - Aspartate is **transferred to the cytosol and is reconverted back to oxaloacetate**, to re-enter the shuttle.
  - Thus, the malate-aspartate shuttle **transfers electrons from NADH into the inner mitochondrial membrane**, for their use in the electron transport chain (Fig. 11.1).

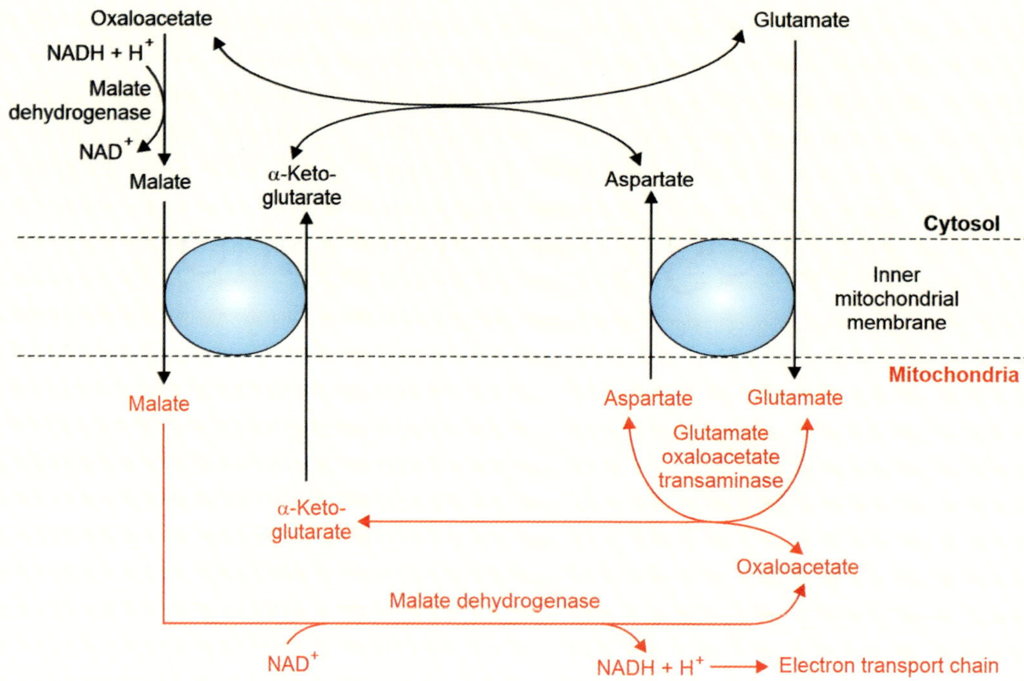

Fig. 11.1: Malate-aspartate shuttle

- **Glycerol phosphate shuttle:** It helps in the transfer of electrons from $FADH_2$ into the inner mitochondrial membrane, for their use in the electron transport chain (Fig. 11.2).

ELECTRON TRANSPORT CHAIN

Electron transport chain (ETC) is also referred to as mitochondrial electron transport chain. Various components of **the ETC** include NAD^+-linked dehydrogenase, flavin-linked dehydrogenase, iron-sulphur proteins, coenzyme Q and various cytochromes.

NAD^+-linked Dehydrogenase

NAD-linked dehydrogenase reaction reduces NAD to NADH, and, in turn, converts a reduced member of the oxidation reduction reaction to the oxidized form, such as malate to oxaloacetate.

In this process, two electrons and two protons are removed, out of which, both the electrons and one of the protons are transferred to NAD^+. Since only one of the protons (as an anhydride ion, i.e. H^-, one hydrogen atom containing an additional electron) is accepted by NAD^+, the second proton (H^+) is released free into the aqueous environment. Some of the NAD-linked dehydrogenases include malate dehydrogenase, lactate dehydrogenase, etc.

Flavin-linked Dehydrogenase

NADH, which is produced as a result of the NAD-linked dehydrogenase reaction, is oxidized by the FMN-linked NADH dehydrogenase. In this process, isoalloxazine ring of FMN accepts two electrons and one proton from NADH plus one proton from the aqueous environment, and pass them onto the coenzyme Q. This type of reaction employs a flavin nucleotide as an electron acceptor, which forms a part of the flavin-

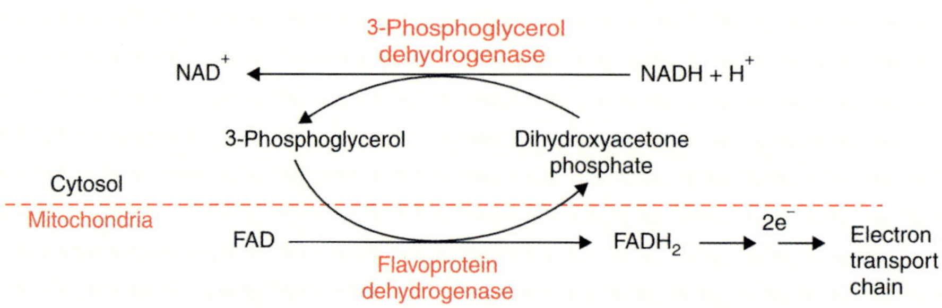

Fig. 11.2: Glycerol phosphate shuttle

linked dehydrogenase. Either FMN or FAD can be utilized in the oxidation reduction reaction. FMN-linked NADH dehydrogenase is a complex enzyme, having a flavoprotein and at least four iron-sulfur centers. Some of the flavin-linked dehydrogenases include NADH dehydrogenase, succinate dehydrogenase, etc.

Iron-sulfur Centers

Iron-sulfur centers, also called iron-sulfur clusters, form prosthetic group of the iron-sulfur protein, a non-heme iron protein. Iron component of the iron-sulfur center is bound to cysteine residue of the protein as well as to the acid labile sulfur. Iron-sulfur clusters undergo one electron oxidation-reduction. During the transfer of reducing equivalents, iron is converted from ferric (Fe^{3+}) to ferrous (Fe^{2+}), on and off the flavin moiety. Iron-sulfur centers function in the transfer of electrons from $FMN.H_2$ to coenzyme Q and from cytochrome b to cytochrome c_1.

Coenzyme Q

Acceptor of the electrons and protons from NADH dehydrogenase is coenzyme Q (CoQ), also called ubiquinone. It is neither a protein nor a nucleotide, but is a lipophilic electron carrier. It serves as a mobile electron transporter within the mitochondrial membrane and operates between the flavin-linked dehydrogenase and cytochrome b. With the addition of two reducing equivalents ($2H^+ + 2e^-$), CoQ is reduced to $CoQ.H_2$. Hydrogen atoms collected by CoQ are released into the mitochondrial matrix and, ultimately, form water with the molecular oxygen.

Cytochromes

Cytochromes are a class of proteins containing heme as a prosthetic group, and are called hemoproteins. Various cytochromes of the mammalian mitochondria are designated as cytochrome a **(cyt a), cyt b, cyt c,** etc. They carry electron from CoQ to molecular oxygen, sequentially, and thus, act as transelectronases. Each cytochrome accepts a pair of electrons from its predecessor, thereby, converting Fe^{3+} to Fe^{2+}. Transfer of electrons from one cytochrome to another, and eventually to cytochrome oxidase, accomplishes regeneration of Fe^{3+}. No hydrogen transfer takes place in this segment of the electron transport chain.

Cytochrome $a.a_3$, also called **cytochrome oxidase**, is the terminal unit of the electron transport chain. This component functions in the transport of electrons by the reversible oxidation and reduction of its iron. Copper ions are involved in the transfer of electrons from cyt a to a_3. The a_3 component, finally, reacts with oxygen.

NAD-linked dehydrogenase, flavin-linked dehydrogenase and CoQ are involved in the transfer of both, hydrogen and electrons. Electron transfer reactions from NADH through CoQ involves transport of two e^-, whereas reactions between CoQ and O_2, involving various cytochromes, are one e^- transfer reactions.

ORGANIZATION OF ELECTRON TRANSPORT CHAIN

Above components of the electron transport chain are arranged in the inner mitochondrial membrane. These components participate in a sequential manner, in four complexes, which contain redox centers with progressively increasing affinity for electrons, i.e. with the increasing standard redox potential. Electrons travel through this chain from lower to higher standard redox potential and are carried from complex II to complex III by CoQ, and from complex III to complex IV by cyt *c* (Fig. 11.3).

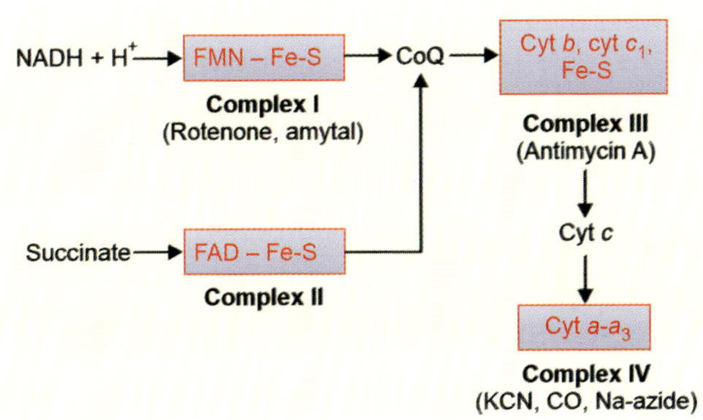

Fig. 11.3: Four complexes of the electron transport chain and their inhibitors (shown in parentheses)

Complex I

Complex I, also called NADH dehydrogenase complex, catalyzes the first reaction, in which protons and electrons are accepted from NADH + H^+ and are transferred to CoQ. Complex I, thus, catalyzes the oxidation of NADH by the reduction of CoQ.

- Complex I contains a flavoprotein (Fp), consisting of one molecule of FMN as the prosthetic group and an iron-sulfur protein (Fe.s). NADH transfers electrons to FMN, which, in turn, gets reduced to $FMN.H_2$.

$$\mathbf{NADH + H^+ + FMN \rightarrow NAD^+ + FMN.H_2}$$

- Electrons from $FMN.H_2$ are then transferred, via Fe.s, to CoQ.
- Thus, complex I accepts the pair of electrons from NADH and transfers them to CoQ. As a result of it, NADH is oxidized to NAD^+, while CoQ is reduced to $CoQ.H_2$.

$$\mathbf{NADH + H^+ + CoQ \rightarrow NAD^+ + CoQ.H_2}$$

- This, in turn, results in large negative free energy change, which is utilized to translocate four protons out of mitochondria.

Complex II

Complex II, also called succinate. CoQ reductase, accepts reducing equivalents from succinate, via FAD.

- FAD is reduced to $FAD.H_2$ and the electrons enter electron transport chain at the level of CoQ.

$$FAD.H_2 + CoQ \rightarrow FAD + CoQ.H_2$$

- Thus, CoQ facilitates the transfer of electrons from NADH or $FADH_2$ through complex I or complex II, respectively, to complex III.

Complex III

Complex III, also called cytochrome reductase, consists of Fe.s protein, cyt b and cyt c_1. It catalyzes oxidation of the reduced CoQ, i.e. Converts $CoQ.H_2$ to CoQ.

- In this process, cyt c receives electrons from complex III and delivers them to complex IV.
- During the process of the transfer of electrons, iron in the heme group, shuttles between Fe^{3+} and Fe^{2+}.

$$CoQ.H_2 + cyt\ c\ (Fe^{3+}) \rightarrow CoQ + cyt\ c\ (Fe^{2+})$$

- This, in turn, also results in large negative free energy change, which is utilized to translocate four protons, which are pumped out of mitochondria.

Complex IV

Complex IV, also called cytochrome oxidase, catalyzes oxidation of the reduced cyt c by the molecular oxygen (½O_2). It is the terminal accepter of the electrons, which is tightly bound to the mitochondrial membrane. The functional unit is referred to as cytochrome $a.a_3$, which contains two heme groups and two copper ions.

- In this complex, two electrons are accepted from cyt c and pass on to molecular oxygen.

$$Cyt\ c\ (Fe^{2+}) + ½O_2 \rightarrow Cyt\ c\ (Fe^{3+}) + H_2O$$

- In addition, two protons are pumped out to the inter membrane space.

Inhibitors of the Electron Transport Chain

Inhibition of the mitochondrial electron transport chain results in impairment of its energy-generating function and may cause death of the organism. Several compounds are known to inhibit electron transport chain at the specific site. They block transport of electrons; inhibit oxygen consumption and synthesis of ATP. These include:

- **Rotenone** (a fish poison), **barbiturates** (such as amytal) and **certain antibiotics**, like piericidin A which **inhibit** flow of electrons through **complex I**.
- Antibiotics, such as **British antilewisite** (BAL) and **antimycin A, inhibit complex III.**
- **Cyanide, azide, carbon monoxide (CO) and hydrogen sulfide (H_2S)** act at **complex IV**. Cyanide and azide bind to Fe^{3+}, whereas CO binds to Fe^{2+}.

Cyanide poisoning: Ingestion of **potassium cyanide**, or inhalation of **hydrogen cyanide** gas, **causes rapid and extensive inhibition of the mitochondrial electron transport chain**, at the cytochrome oxidase step.

Cyanide binds to Fe^{3+} in the heme of the cytochrome $a.a_3$ component, at the terminal step in the electron transport chain and **prevents oxygen from reacting with the cyt $a.a_3$** as the final electron acceptor. As a result of it, **mitochondrial respiration and energy production is stopped**, and **cell death occurs**, rapidly, from tissue hypoxia, particularly, of the central nervous system.

OXIDATIVE PHOSPHORYLATION

Generation of ATP from ADP and Pi is termed as **phosphorylation. Phosphorylation coupled with biological oxidation**; the process **is called oxidative phosphorylation.**

As discussed above, **during electron transfer, protons are also expelled from mitochondria**, thereby, **producing a proton gradient** across the mitochondrial membrane. The **free energy stored in this electrochemical gradient is used for the synthesis of ATP.**

- Oxidative phosphorylation, thus, is a descriptive blend of the two processes operating simultaneously, i.e. the **oxidation of a metabolite by oxygen via electron transport chain** and the **phosphorylation of ADP.**
- Within this sequential process, there are **three different sites** for the phosphorylation of ADP (to form ATP).
- **Efficiency of the oxidative phosphorylation system is expressed in terms of the P/O ratio.**

P/O ratio: It is the **ratio of the number of moles of ATP generated to the number of atoms of oxygen reduced** by the electron transport chain. Since, there **are 3 sites of generation of ATP** in the electron transport system, thus, the **P/O ratio is 2.5**, if **reducing equivalents enter the chain through NADH.** On the other hand, **for the FAD. H_2 requiring reactions P/O ratio is only 1.5**, because electrons and protons enter through complex II only.

> ***Note:*** As per old concept, the values for ATP generation (P/O ratios) were described as 3.0 and 2.0, respectively. However, recent research has described these values as 2.5 and 1.5, respectively.

Most accepted theory of oxidative phosphorylation is referred to as **chemiosmotic theory**. According to this theory:

- Electrons and protons are sequentially transferred, via different components of the electron transport chain, from complex I and complex II to complex III and complex IV and finally to oxygen.
- **During the flow of electrons** from NADH or FAD. H_2 to ½O_2, **protons (H^+) are transported across the membrane**, into the intermembrane space, thereby creating H^+-gradient across the membrane.
- **Once the gradient is established, H^+ flow back**, spontaneously, downhill across the membrane. The **potential energy stored in this gradient is harvested by** a fifth protein complex, referred to as **complex V** (Fig. 11.4).

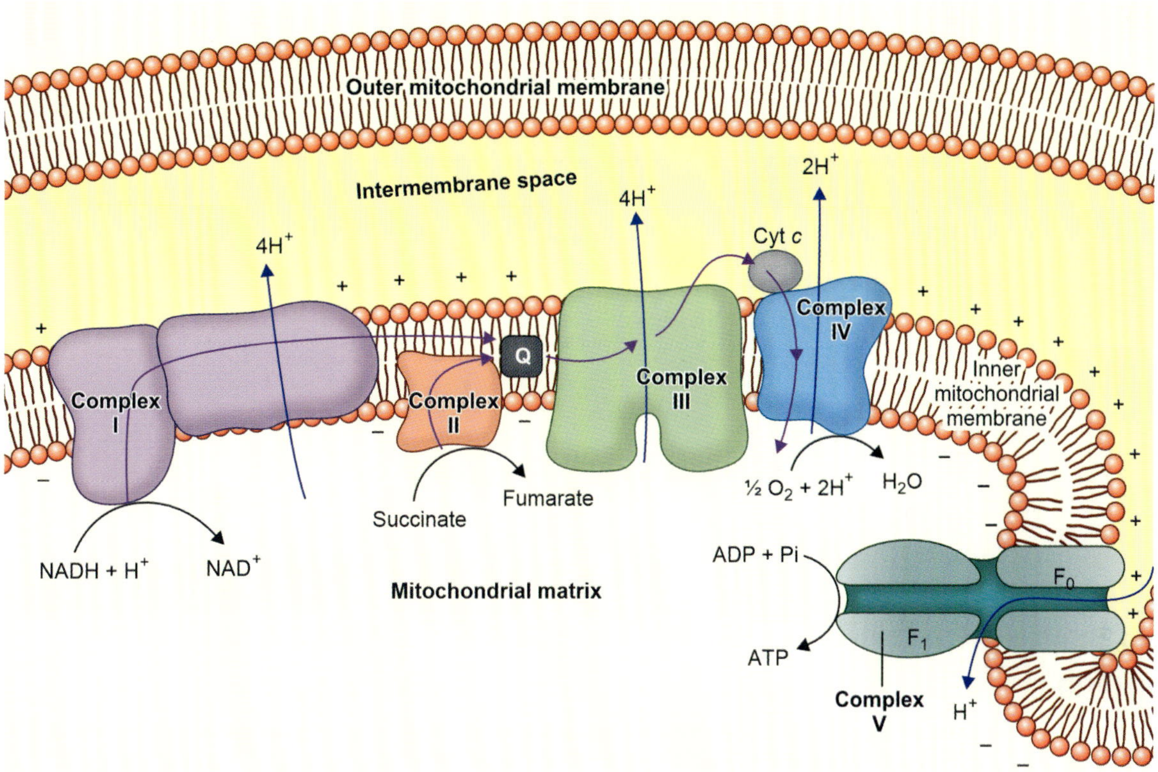

Fig. 11.4: Chemiosmotic theory of oxidative phosphorylation

- In complex V, **protons traverse the membrane at** certain sites, designated as **F_0** protein of the **F_1–F_0 complex.**
- The **energy of proton gradient** and also the **membrane potential, promote a reaction of two protons with oxygen of the phosphate.** Water is eliminated and the resulting highly reactive phosphate group (Pi) joins ADP, **to generate ATP.**

A large amount of ATP (more that 90% of the total ATP synthesized in the body) is produced in oxidative phosphorylation.

Inhibitors and Uncouplers of Oxidative Phosphorylation

Inhibitors and uncouplers of oxidative phosphorylation stop ATP synthesis:

- **Inhibitors:** Oligomycin **binds to the F_0 subunit of the mitochondrial F_1-F_0-ATPase, suppresses oxygen consumption** and, thus, the phosphorylation of **ADP** to ATP.
- **Synthetic uncouplers:** 2,4-Dinitrophenol is a proton ionophore which **uncouples phosphorylation from electron transport**, resulting in the accumulation of ADP. The **energy**, normally, conserved as ATP, **is lost as heat**. In this situation, electron transport may continue, but **without the generation of ATP**.
- **Physiological uncouplers:** They dissipate the chemical energy of ATP in the form of heat and are one of the mechanisms for **thermoregulation** (Table 11.1).

Table 11.1: Physiological uncouplers
• Uncoupling protein 1 (thermogenin)
• Unconjugated bilirubin
• Free fatty acids
• Thyroxine
• Estrogen

SUBSTRATE LEVEL PHOSPHORYLATION

Besides oxidative phosphorylation, a small amount **of ATP (only about 10%) is also generated in the cytosol, within certain individual steps of a metabolic pathway.** It is referred to as substrate level phosphorylation.

In substrate level phosphorylation there is **transfer of a phosphate group from a very high energy phosphate donor to ADP**. For example, **two reactions of the glycolytic process**, which are **catalyzed by phosphoglycerokinase and pyruvate kinase**.

Phosphorylation of ADP by creatine phosphate, catalyzed by creatine kinase, also represents an important mode of ATP generation in the muscle. Besides, **succinate thiokinase catalyzed reaction in Krebs cycle** is also an example of substrate level phosphorylation (Fig. 11.5).

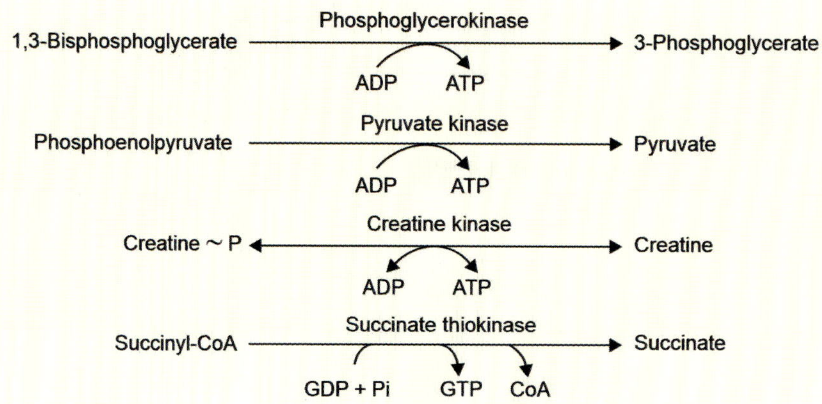

Fig. 11.5: Substrate level phosphorylation

Some Important Questions

1. Explain the process of oxidative phosphorylation and its inhibitors and uncouplers.

2. Discuss briefly:

i. Respiratory chain and sites of ATP production
ii. Oxidative phosphorylation and uncouplers
iii. Mitochondrial respiratory chain
iv. Diagrammatic representation of the electron transport chain
v. Malate aspartate shuttle
vi. Glycerolphosphate shuttle
vii. Inhibitors of oxidative phosphorylation

3. Write notes on:

i. Respiratory chain
ii. Oxidative phosphorylation
iii. Substrate level phosphorylation
iv. Coenzyme Q
v. Iron-sulphur centers
vi. Cytochromes
vii. P/O ratio

Chapter 12

Metabolism of Carbohydrates

As discussed in Chapter 8, all **dietary carbohydrates are digested and absorbed** as glucose, which enters the liver.

METABOLIC FATES OF GLUCOSE

In the liver, glucose is utilized in various metabolic pathways which include **glycolysis** (oxidized to produce energy), **glycogenesis** (stored as glycogen in the liver and muscle) and **pentose phosphate pathway** (to produce pentoses and NADPH). During starvation, when blood glucose is low, glucose is released from glycogen **(glycogenolysis)** or produced via **gluconeogenesis** (Fig. 12.1)

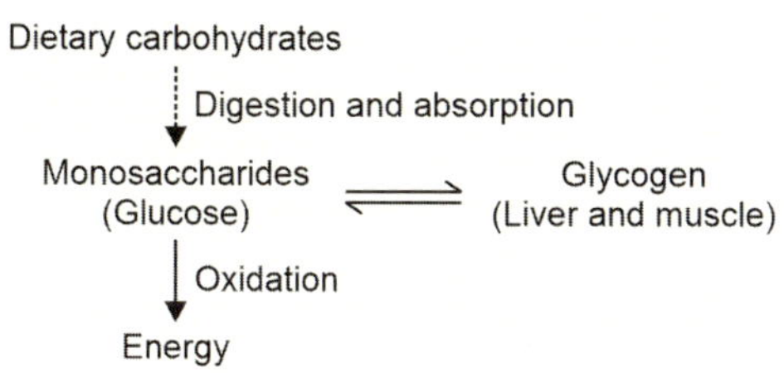

Fig. 12.1: Metabolic fates of glucose

GLYCOLYSIS

Glycolysis, also called Embden Meyerhof (or **Embden Meyerhof Parnas**) pathway, is a process of utilization (catabolism) of glucose, mainly, in the **liver (aerobic glycolysis) and skeletal muscle (anaerobic glycolysis)**.

Glycolytic enzymes are present in the extramitochondrial compartment of the cell to produce energy.

Outline of Glycolysis

Various reactions of the glycolytic pathway are outlined in Fig. 12.2.

1. **Glucose is** first **converted to glucose-6-phosphate.** This reaction is catalyzed by the **enzyme hexokinase**, which requires ATP and Mg. Hexokinase is present in all the tissues.

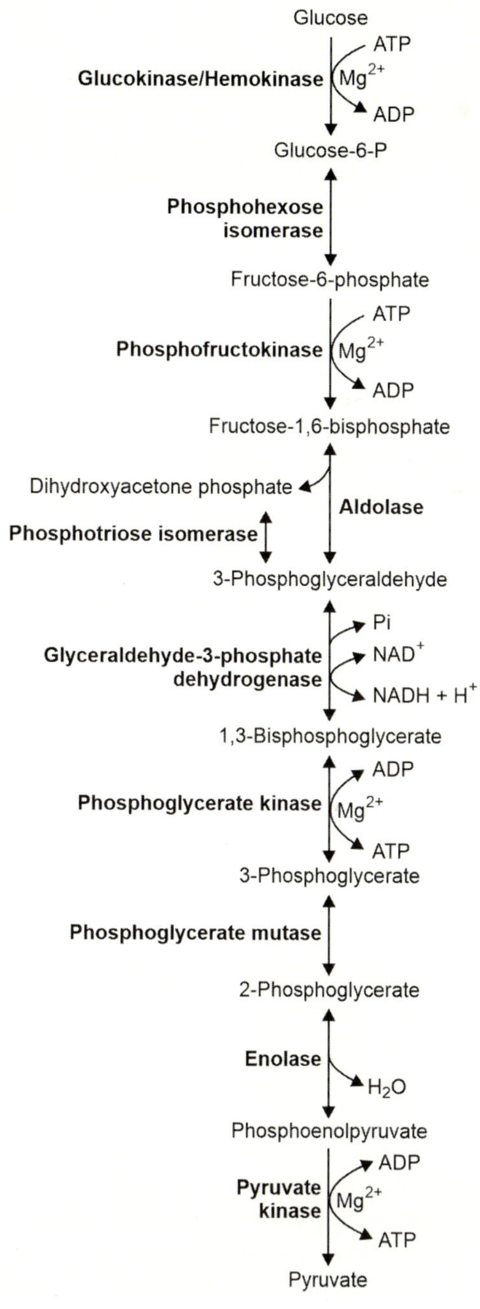

Fig. 12.2: Outline of glycolysis

In the fed state, this reaction is catalyzed by another enzyme, called **glucokinase**. This enzyme is found in the liver, where it is induced by high glucose concentration after meals.

2. In the next reaction, **glucose-6-phosphate is isomerized**, in a freely reversible reaction, **to fructose-6-phosphate**, by the enzyme **phosphohexose isomerase.**
3. **Fructose-6-phosphate** is then **phosphorylated by** an allosteric enzyme **phosphofructokinase to** form **fructose-1,6-bisphosphate**.

   This is an irreversible reaction and requires ATP.
4. Thereafter, **fructose-1,6-bisphosphate** (a hexose) is **cleaved by aldolase to** 3-phosphoglyceraldehyde **(glyceraldehyde-3-phosphate)** and **dihydroxyacetone phosphate**, two trioses.
5. Subsequently, **only 3-phosphoglyceraldehyde enters the pathway**.

   So, **dihydroxyacetone phosphate** also gets **converted to 3-phosphoglyceraldehyde**. This reaction is catalyzed **by** the enzyme **phospho-triose isomerase**.

   Glycerol also enters glycolytic pathway at this point.
6. In the next step, in presence of NAD^+ and inorganic phosphate (Pi), **glyceraldehyde-3-phosphate dehydrogenase oxidizes 3-phosphoglyceraldehyde to 1,3-bisphosphoglycerate**.
7. In the next step, **1,3-bisphosphoglycerate is converted to 3-phosphoglycerate.** This reaction is catalyzed **by** the enzyme **phosphoglycerate kinase**.

   In this reaction, there is a **generation of ATP**. It is called substrate-level production of ATP (i.e. **substrate-level phosphorylation**).

   Arsenate inhibits phosphorylation at **this step** and, thus, ATP production.
8. Thereafter, **3-phosphoglycerate** is **converted to 2-phosphoglycerate by** the enzyme **phosphoglycerate mutase.**
9. In the next step, **enolase converts 2-phosphoglycerate to** a high-energy compound, called **phospho-enolpyruvate**.

   Enolase requires Mg^{2+} for its activity but **is inhibited by fluoride.**

   Since fluoride inhibits this reaction, therefore, **fluoride is added to the blood, as a preservative, in glucose estimation.**
10. Subsequently, **phosphoenolpyruvate is converted to pyruvate,** irreversibly. This reaction is catalyzed **by** the enzyme **pyruvate kinase**, which, in turn, phosphorylates ADP to ATP.

    Deficiency of pyruvate kinase leads to hemolytic anemia.

OXIDATION OF PYRUVIC ACID

Pyruvic acid is reduced to lactic acid under anaerobic conditions or is oxidized to acetyl CoA under aerobic conditions.

Outline of Pyruvate Oxidation

- **Under anaerobic conditions: Pyruvate is reduced to lactate**. This reaction is catalyzed **by** the enzyme **lactate dehydrogenase**, which requires NADH.

  Tissues such as skeletal muscle, when function under hypoxic conditions, produce large amount of lactic acid.
- **Under aerobic conditions: Pyruvate is** transported into mitochondria, where it is **oxidatively decarboxylated to acetyl CoA by** the enzyme **pyruvate dehydrogenase complex** (Fig. 12.3).

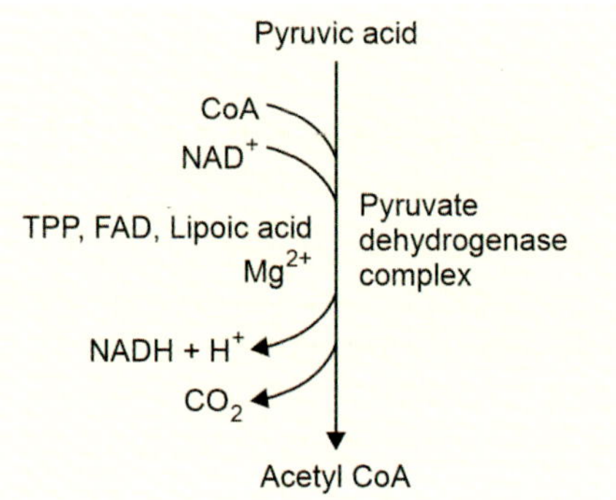

Fig. 12.3: Oxidation of pyruvic acid to acetyl CoA

Pyruvate dehydrogenase complex requires five coenzymes, i.e. TPP, CoA, NAD, FAD and lipoic acid. Insulin stimulates its activity, whereas acetyl CoA, NADH and increased ATP/ADP ratio inhibit it.

Bioenergetics (ATP production) of Glycolysis

Number of ATP produced during glycolysis vary, depending upon the condition:

- **Under anaerobic condition**, conversion of 1,3-bisphosphoglycerate to 3-phosphoglycerate and phosphoenolpyruvate to pyruvate, each produces one ATP. Thus, a total of 2 ATP are produced per molecule of a triose, or **4 molecules of ATP per molecule of hexose** (Fig. 12.4).

  As 2 ATPs are used in the initial two reactions of the process, i.e. in the conversion of glucose to glucose-6-

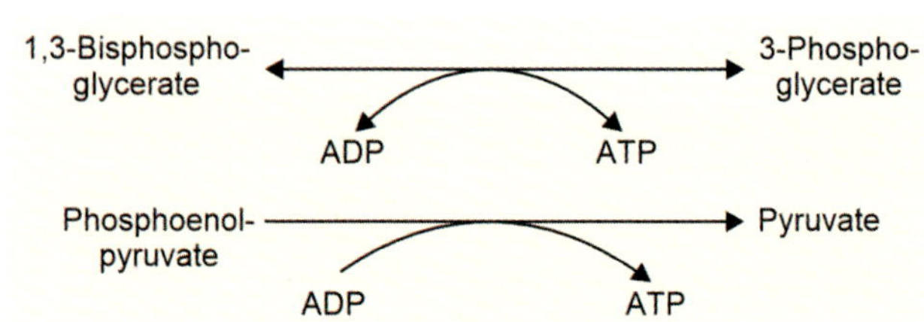

Fig. 12.4: ATP producing steps in anaerobic glycolysis

phosphate and fructose-6-phosphate to fructose-1,6-bisphosphate, the **net energy yield** per molecule of glucose is only **2 ATP**.

- **Under aerobic conditions** NADH, which is produced during the conversion of 3-phosphoglycerte to 1,3-bisphosphoglycerate, can enter the electron transport chain and release 2.5 ATP, thus, additionally, 5 more ATP are produced per molecule of glucose. Therefore, a **total yield** under aerobic conditions **is 9 ATP** while the **net yield is 7 ATP**.

Biomedical Importance of Glycolysis

In the liver and other tissues, **aerobic glycolysis is the main source of ATP. In the muscle, anaerobic glycolysis** provides energy **during exercise**.

Regulation of Glycolysis

There are three irreversible steps which are catalyzed by **hexokinase, phosphofructokinase and pyruvate kinase**. These are also the sites of the regulation of glycolysis.

Insulin stimulates these enzymes and increases utilization of glucose by glycolysis. On the other hand, glucagon inhibits this process.

CITRIC ACID CYCLE

Citric acid cycle or Krebs cycle, also called **tricarboxylic acid cycle (TCA cycle)** is a process of the **oxidation of acetyl CoA** (active acetate, produced under aerobic glycolysis) to **CO_2 and H_2O**.

During the course of oxidation of acetyl CoA reducing equivalents are produced, which enter respiratory chain and generate large amount of ATP.

Outline of Citric Acid Cycle

Reactions of the TCA cycle are outlined in Fig. 12.5.

1. In the first step, **acetyl CoA** (formed from pyruvate under aerobic condition) **combines with oxaloacetate and forms citric acid** (a tricarboxylic acid).

   This reaction is catalyzed **by** the enzyme **citrate synthase**, also called the condensing enzyme.
2. **Citrate is** then rearranged to cis-aconitate, which is subsequently **changed to isocitrate**. Both of these steps are catalyzed **by aconitase.**

   Conversion of citrate to isocitrate is **inhibited by fluoroacetate.**
3. In the next step, in the presence of **isocitrate dehydrogenase, isocitrate is converted to oxalo-**

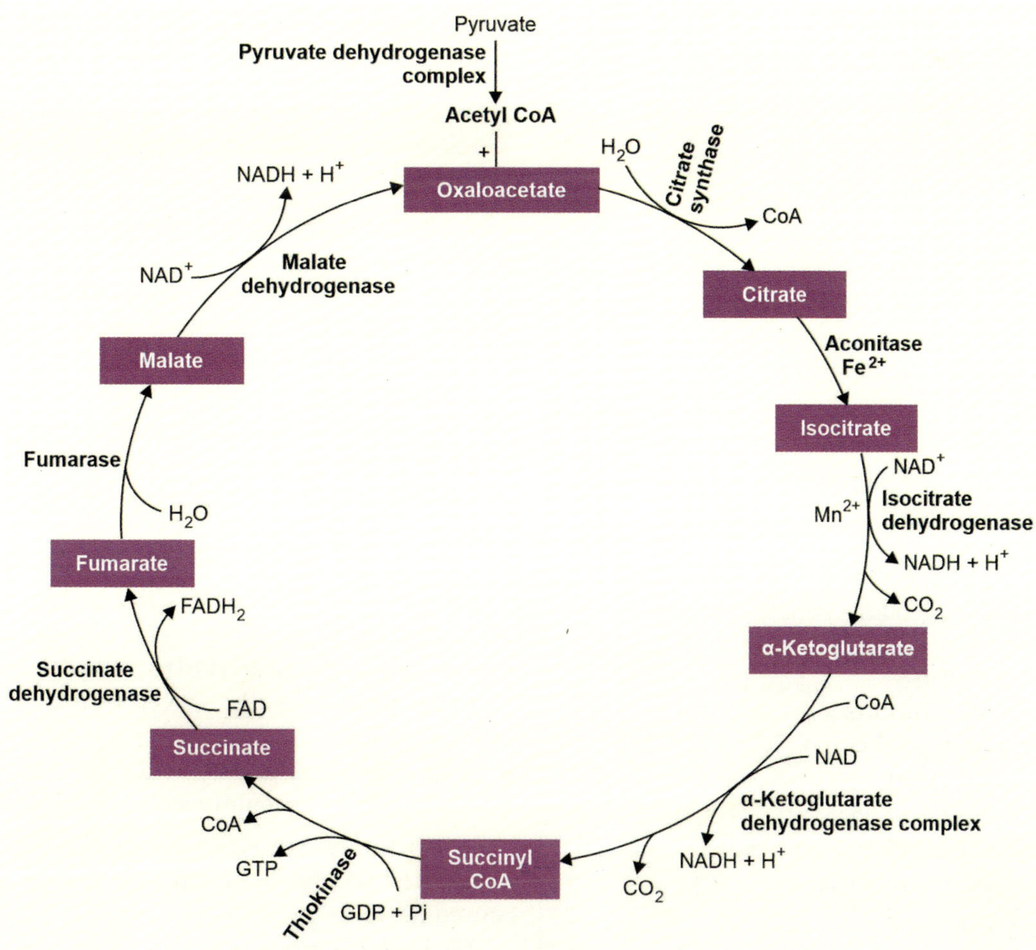

Fig. 12.5: Outline of citric acid cycle

succinate, which is subsequently **decarboxylated to α-ketoglutarate**.

4. Thereafter, **α-ketoglutarate** undergoes **oxidative decarboxylation** and gets converted **to succinyl CoA**.

   This reaction is similar to the conversion of pyruvate to acetyl CoA. α-Ketoglutarate dehydrogenase complex, which also requires five coenzymes, i.e. TPP, NAD^+, FAD, coenzyme A and lipoic acid, catalyzes this reaction.

5. In the next step, **succinyl CoA is converted to succinate, by** the enzyme **succinate thio-kinase**.

   During this reaction, a molecule of GTP is formed. This is known as **substrate level phosphorylation**, as a high-energy molecule is formed at the substrate level.

6. Thereafter, **succinate is converted to fumarate, by** the enzyme **succinate dehydrogenase**.

   Due to structural similarities between malonate and succinate, **malonate inhibits** succinate dehydrogenase, **competitively**.

7. In the next step, with the addition of a molecule of water, **by** the enzyme **fumarase** (fumarate hydratase), **fumarate is converted to L-malate**.

8. Finally, **malate dehydrogenase**, in the presence of NAD^+, **converts malate to oxaloacetate**.

Bioenergetics (ATP Production) of Citric Acid Cycle

As a result of oxidation of one molecule of acetyl CoA in the Krebs cycle, three molecules of NAD^+ and one molecule of FAD are reduced.

Reducing equivalents (from NADH + H^+) enter respiratory chain and result in the production of 2.5 molecules of ATP. Similarly, FADH2 yields 1.5 ATP. Besides, there is also a substrate level production of GTP.

Thus, **total ATP yield**, per molecule of acetyl CoA, is 10 ATP (Table 12.1).

As mentioned above, conversion of pyruvate to acetyl CoA also generates NADH + H^+ and gives 2.5 ATP. Thus, total number of ATP produced from oxidation of pyruvate is **12.5**.

Table 12.1: Energy producing steps in citric acid cycle

Reaction	*Reducing equivalents produced as*	*Number of ATP produced*
Isocitrate → α-Ketoglutarate	NADH + H^+	2.5
α-Ketoglutarate → Succinyl CoA	NADH + H^+	2.5
Succinyl CoA → Succinate	—	1 (As GTP)
Succinate → Fumarate	$FADH_2$	1.5
Malate → Oxaloacetate	NADH + H^+	2.5
	Total	**10**

Since 2 molecules of pyruvate are formed from one molecule of glucose, therefore, in addition to energy yield during aerobic glycolysis (5 ATP) a molecule of glucose also produces 25 ATP via the Krebs cycle. Thus, a total of **30 molecules of ATP are obtained, when a molecule of glucose is completely oxidized to CO_2 and H_2O under aerobic conditions**, i.e. via glycolysis and Krebs cycle.

Biomedical Importance of Citric Acid Cycle

Citric acid cycle has a dual role, i.e. it is important in oxidation as well as synthetic processes. It is, thus, **amphibolic** in nature.

- It is **catabolic** for the **oxidation of carbohydrates, lipids and proteins**, as they are completely oxidized to CO_2 and H_2O, and **release energy**.
- It is also important in the **anabolic** reactions, as various **intermediates** of the cycle can be **used for the biosynthesis of the nonessential amino acids.**
- Various **intermediates** of the cycle are also potentially glucogenic and thus, can give rise to glucose in liver and kidney.

Regulation of Citric Acid Cycle

TCA cycle is regulated by the availability of acetyl CoA, oxaloacetate and NADH. **Citrate synthase, isocitrate dehydrogenase and α-ketoglutarate dehydrogenase** are the rate limiting enzymes of the TCA cycle.

METABOLISM OF GLYCOGEN

GLYCOGENESIS

Glycogenesis **(glycogen synthesis)** is the process of the synthesis of glycogen, wherein glucose is used and forms glycogen. Although, it is operative in several tissues, liver and muscle are the main organs for the synthesis of glycogen. Glycogenesis is **stimulated by insulin.**

Though glycogen is synthesized from glucose, **excess intake of carbohydrate will not increase glycogen level in liver or muscle** due to the reason that:

- **Glycogen concentration is tightly regulated by hormones.**
- All the **dietary carbohydrates are digested and absorbed as glucose** (*see* Chapter 8).
- Furthermore, as mentioned above, **glucose is mainly catabolized via glycolysis and is converted to pyruvate and finally to acetyl CoA.**
- **Acetyl CoA** has various metabolic fates, but **is primarily used in fatty acid synthesis and is finally converted to triacylglycerols** (*see* Chapter 13).

Accordingly, excess of dietary carbohydrate is not converted to glycogen but to triacylglycerols and is stored as fat.

Various reactions of glycogenesis are described in Fig. 12.6.

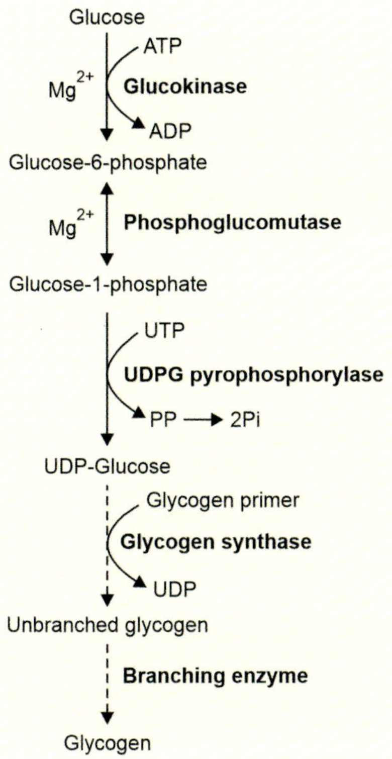

Fig. 12.6: Outline of glycogenesis

1. Firstly, **glucose is activated** (phosphorylated) **to form glucose-6-phosphate.**
2. **Glucose-6-phosphate is isomerized to glucose-1-phosphate, by** the enzyme **phosphoglucomutase**.
3. **Glucose-1-phosphate** reacts with UTP and gets **converted to** uridinediphosphate glucose (**UDP-Glu** or UDPG). This reaction is catalyzed **by UDPG pyro-phosphorylase** (glucose-1-phosphate uridyl-transferase).
4. **From UDP-Glu, glucose is transferred to the glycogen** primer (i.e. the preformed oligosaccharide). This reaction is catalyzed by the enzyme **glycogen synthase**.

   The incoming glucose is linked to the primer at the non-reducing end by 1,4-α-glycosidic linkage and results in elongation of the pre-existing branch. This results in the formation of an unbranched glycogen.
5. Once the straight chain containing nearly 11 glucose residues is formed, branching enzyme removes a block of 7–8 glycosyl residues from the growing chain and transfers it to the neighboring chain.

   The branch point again grows with the addition of the glucose molecules at the 1 → 4 linkage. This, in turn, results in the formation of a highly branched glycogen structure.

GLYCOGENOLYSIS

Glycogenolysis (glycogen breakdown) is the process of the conversion of glycogen to either glucose-6- phosphate in muscle or free glucose in liver and kidney (Fig. 12.7).

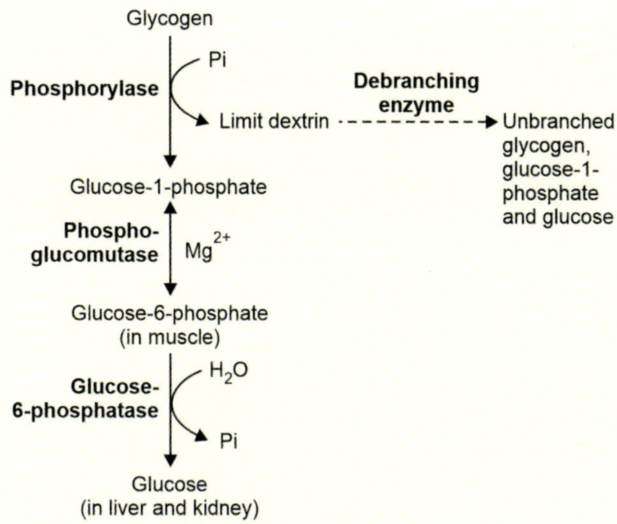

Fig. 12.7: Outline of glycogenolysis

1. In the first step, glucose molecules are sequentially removed from glycogen as glucose-1-phosphate. This reaction is catalyzed by the enzyme phosphorylase. It is the rate limiting step of this pathway.

   Phosphorylase hydrolyzes the α-1,4-glycosidic bonds and removes glucose units as glucose-1-phosphate, until nearly four glucose residues are left. After the action of phosphorylase, glycogen is partially hydrolyzed, leaving limit dextrin.
2. Limit dextrin is further hydrolyzed by the debranching enzyme to glucose-1-phosphate and free glucose. Debranching enzyme is a bifunctional enzyme. Its first unit has glycosyltransferase activity, which removes a strand of three glucosyl residues from the four glucosyl-residues of the branch and attaches the same to the nonreducing end of another branch. This reaction forms a new α-(1 → 4) linkage and thus, three more glucose units become available for the phosphorylase reaction (Fig. 12. 8).

   The α-(1 → 6) bond, which is linking the remaining glucosyl residue on the branch point to the main chain, is hydrolyzed by the second unit of the debranching enzyme that is referred to as amylo-(α-1,6-) glucosidase. This glucosyl-residue is released as free glucose, rather than as glucose-1-phosphate, leaving the unbranched glycogen molecule.

   Cooperative and repetitive actions of phosphorylase and debranching enzyme result in complete hydrolysis of glycogen.
3. Glucose-1-phosphate, produced as a result of the action of phosphorylase, is converted to glucose-6-phosphate by the enzyme phosphoglucomutase.

   Glucose-6-phosphate is the end product of glycogen breakdown in muscle, where it is used in the glycolytic pathway to liberate energy that is required during exercise. Thus, glycogenolysis is

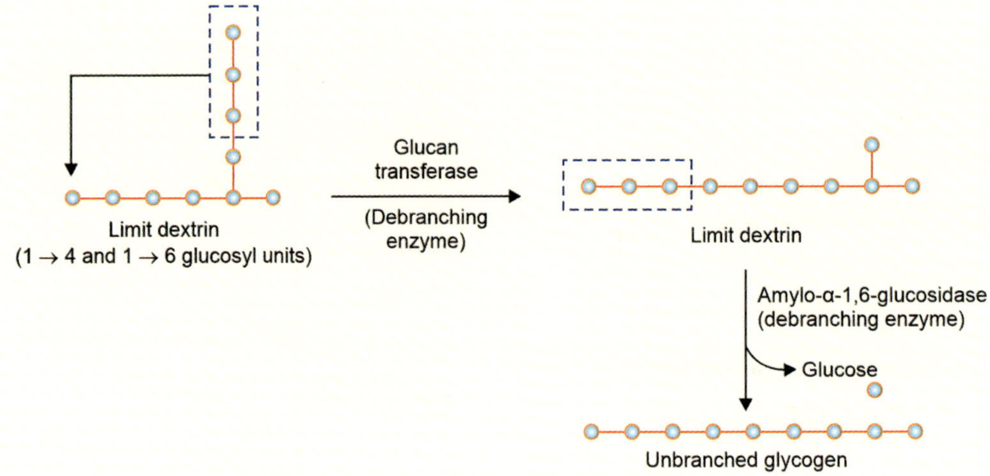

Fig. 12.8: Removal of a branch point by the debranching enzyme during glycogenolysis

followed by glycolysis, due to the absence of the enzyme glucose-6-phosphatase **in the muscle**.

4. **In the liver and kidney**, glucose-6-phosphate is further hydrolyzed to glucose. This reaction is catalyzed by glucose-6-phosphatase.

Biomedical Importance of Glycogen Metabolism

Glycogen, which is stored in the liver, is converted to free glucose and is used to maintain blood glucose level in a hypoglycemic state. On the other hand, in the muscle, glycogen is used for providing energy during exercise.

Regulation of Glycogen Metabolism

Glycogen metabolism in the liver is controlled by glucagon while in the muscle and other tissues, it is controlled by insulin and norepinephrine/epinephrine.

Glycogenesis is regulated by glycogen synthase, whereas glycogenolysis is regulated by glycogen phosphorylase. Both the enzymes are under allosteric control and are regulated by the availability of ATP and glucose-6-phosphate, reversibly.

Glycogen Storage Disorders

This is a group of inherited disorders that are associated with glycogen metabolism, where an abnormal type or quantity of the glycogen is deposited in different tissues. According to the deficiency of the enzyme involved, more than 15 types of glycogen storage diseases are known to occur. Some of these are described in Table 12.2.

Three of these (type I, type II and type III) are most common in children.

Table 12.2: Some of the glycogen storage diseases

Type	*Glycogen storage disease*	*Deficient enzyme*	*Features*
I	von Gierke disease	Glucose-6-phosphatase	Liver, renal and intestinal epithelial cells are loaded with glycogen. There also occurs hypoglycemia, lactic acidosis, ketosis, hyperlipidemia and hyperuricemia
II	Pompe's disease	Lysosomal acid maltase	Accumulation of glycogen in the lysosomes. It is fatal and may result in heart failure
III	Cori disease or Forbes disease	Debranching enzyme	Accumulation of the branched polysaccharide in liver, muscle, heart and leucocytes.
IV	Andersen disease	Branching enzyme	Accumulation of amylopectin, hence also referred to as amylopectinosis. Death may occur due to liver or cardiac failure within first year of life.
V	McArdle's syndrome	Muscle phosphorylase	Muscle has abnormally high glycogen content. There is diminished exercise tolerance with little or no lactate in blood after exercise
VI	Her's disease	Liver phosphorylase	High glycogen content in liver. There is also a tendency towards hypoglycemia

GLUCONEOGENESIS

Gluconeogenesis (neo-glucogenesis) is the process of the formation of glucose from various non-carbohydrate sources such as the glucogenic amino acids, lactate, glycerol, or propionate.

- Gluconeogenesis takes place in the fasting state or on a low carbohydrate diet, particularly, in the liver and some other tissues, which are solely dependent on glucose for their energy demand. It does not take place in muscle.
- Gluconeogenesis thus, enables maintenance of blood glucose when all the dietary glucose has been absorbed and oxidized. This process is essential since blood glucose level has to be maintained, to support metabolism of the tissues that use glucose as the primary substrate such as the brain, red blood cells and lens.

Gluconeogenesis is said to be the reversal of glycolysis but truly it is not a reversal of glycolysis, since there are three irreversible reactions in the glycolytic pathway (Fig. 12.9).

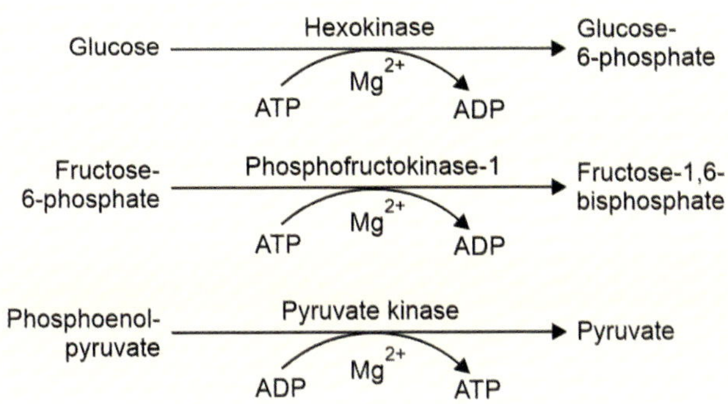

Fig. 12.9: Irreversible steps in glycolysis

A. Reversal of Glycolysis

It includes the following set of reactions:

1. Conversion of pyruvate to phosphoenolpyruvate:

- In the reversal of the pyruvate to phosphoenolpyruvate, pyruvate is first converted to oxaloacetate by the enzyme pyruvate carboxylase, in mitochondria.
- Thereafter, malate dehydrogenase converts oxaloacetate to malate, which is freely transported across the mitochondrial membrane. Malate thus, comes out from the mitochondria to the cytosol where it is reconverted back to oxaloacetate by the same enzyme. This also reduces NAD^+ to $NADH + H^+$. This enzyme, thus, not only transports oxaloacetate (via malate) but also reducing equivalents from mitochondria into cytosol. Reactions of gluconeogenesis, thus, occur in the cytosol as well as mitochondria.
- In the next step, oxaloacetate is converted to phosphoenolpyruvate, by the enzyme phosphoenolpyruvate carboxy-kinase (PEP-carboxy-kinase).

2. Conversion of fructose-1,6-bisphosphate to fructose-6-phosphate: Fructose-1,6-bisphosphate is converted to fructose-6-phosphate by the enzyme fructose-1,6-bisphosphatase.

3. Conversion of glucose-6-phosphate to glucose: Glucose-6-phosphate is converted to glucose by the enzyme glucose-6-phosphatase. This enzyme is not found in the muscle and adipose tissue.

B. Conversion of Lactate to Glucose

Lactate is produced during the process of anaerobic glycolysis. For its conversion to glucose, firstly, lactate is oxidized to pyruvate. This reaction is catalyzed by the enzyme lactate dehydrogenase, which requires NAD^+. Subsequently, pyruvate is converted to glucose by the reversal of the glycolytic reactions.

C. Conversion of Glucogenic Amino Acids to Glucose

Various glucogenic amino acids transfer their α-amino group by transamination and release carbon skeletons which form intermediates of the citric acid cycle (Table 12.3).

Table 12.3: Conversion of glucogenic amino acids to the citric acid cycle intermediates

Amino acid	*Citric acid cycle intermediate formed*
Gly, Ala, Ser, Thr, Cys, Trp and HO-Pro	Pyruvate
Arg, His, Glu, Gln and Pro	α-Ketoglutarate
Phe and Tyr	Fumarate
Val, Ile and Met	Succinyl CoA

These citric acid cycle intermediates, in turn, can form glucose by the reversal of the glycolytic reactions, via pyruvate.

D. Conversion of Glycerol to Glucose

Glycerol is produced as a result of lipolysis in the adipose tissue. Glycerol kinase converts it to α-glycerol-phosphate in the liver, which is later reduced by a dehydrogenase to dihydroxyacetone phosphate and can enter glycolysis at this point (Fig. 12.10).

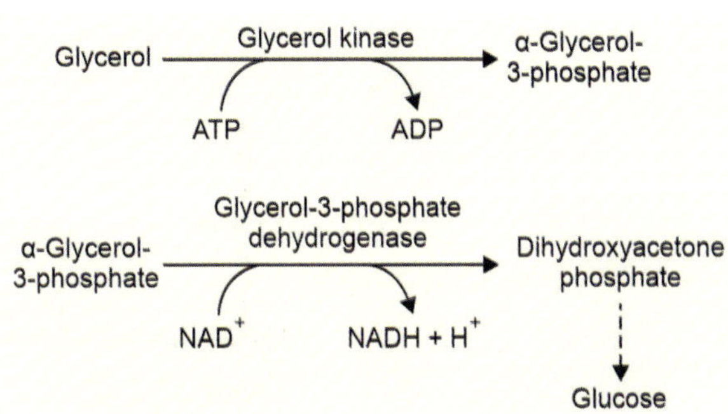

Fig. 12.10: Conversion of glycerol to glucose

E. Conversion of Propionyl CoA to Glucose

Oxidation of fatty acids containing odd number of carbon atoms, in addition to acetyl CoA, also produces a molecule of propionyl CoA, particularly, in ruminants. In human beings, propionyl CoA is obtained from Ile, Val and Thr. It is converted to D-methyl-malonyl CoA by propionyl CoA carboxylase. D-Methyl-malonyl CoA is then converted to L-methyl-malonyl CoA and finally by an isomerase to succinyl CoA which is an intermediate of the citric acid cycle. Succinyl CoA, in turn, can be converted to glucose via pyruvate (Fig. 12.11).

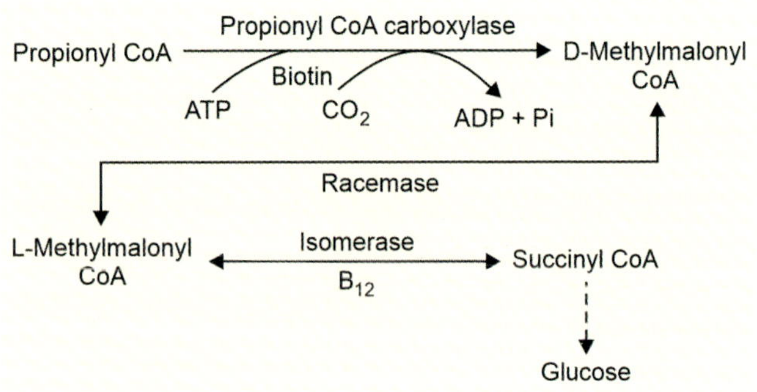

Fig. 12.11: Conversion of propionyl CoA to glucose

Biomedical Importance of Gluconeogenesis

Gluconeogenesis occurs in the fasting state or on a low carbohydrate diet in the liver and other tissues, which are solely dependent on glucose for their energy demand. Thus, it enables the maintenance of blood glucose, when it is in short supply.

Regulation of Gluconeogenesis

Gluconeogenesis is regulated by pyruvate carboxylase, phosphoenolpyruvate carboxy-kinase, fructose-1,6-bisphosphatase and glucose-6-phosphatase, which catalyze reversal of the irreversible steps of glycolysis.

METABOLISM OF LACTATE

Tissues, such as skeletal muscle, when function under hypoxic conditions, produce large amount of lactic acid. The direction of the reaction depends upon the relative intracellular concentrations of pyruvate and lactate.

A large amount of lactate is produced in tissues such as red blood cells, lens and cornea, etc. Elevated concentration of lactate in the blood is termed as **lactic acidosis.** Lactic acidosis occurs when there is reduced supply of oxygen, such as in myocardial infarction, pulmonary embolism, or during shock.

Lactic acid is transported to the liver and reforms glucose by the process of gluconeogenesis and becomes available for the muscle and other tissues. This process is called **Cori cycle**.

CORI CYCLE

The end product of glycogen breakdown in the muscle is glucose-6-phosphate, and not free glucose, due to the absence of glucose-6-phosphatase. Glucose-6-phosphate, so produced, is used for energy production, particularly, during exercise (anaerobic glycolysis) and results in the production of lactic acid. Lactic acid is transported to the liver and reforms glucose by the process of gluconeogenesis. Glucose via circulation again becomes available for its oxidation in the muscle and other tissues. This is called lactic acid cycle or Cori cycle. It results in the net exchange of glycogen (via glucose-6-phosphate) and lactic acid in the two tissues, i.e. the muscle and the liver (Fig. 12.12).

PENTOSE PHOSPHATE PATHWAY

Pentose phosphate pathway, also called hexose monophosphate shunt **(HMP shunt)**, is the second major pathway for the metabolism of glucose. Enzymes for this pathway are localized in the cytosol, while reducing equivalents are accepted by $NADP^+$ instead of NAD^+. This pathway is operative in many tissues such as liver, erythrocytes, lactating mammary glands, testes and adipose tissue. Rate of the HMP shunt reactions is increased by insulin.

In the overall process, six molecules of glucose are utilized to give six molecules of CO_2 and six molecules

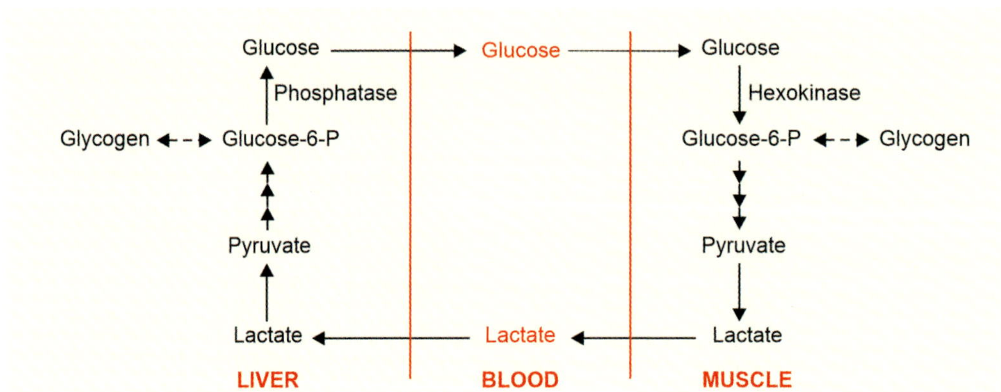

Fig. 12.12: Glucose-lactate cycle (Cori cycle)

of pentoses. The pentoses are subsequently, rearranged to give four molecules of fructose-6-phosphate and two molecules of glyceraldehyde-3-phosphate. Two trioses also form a hexose by the reversal of glycolysis thus, **regenerating five molecules of hexoses** (Fig. 12.13).

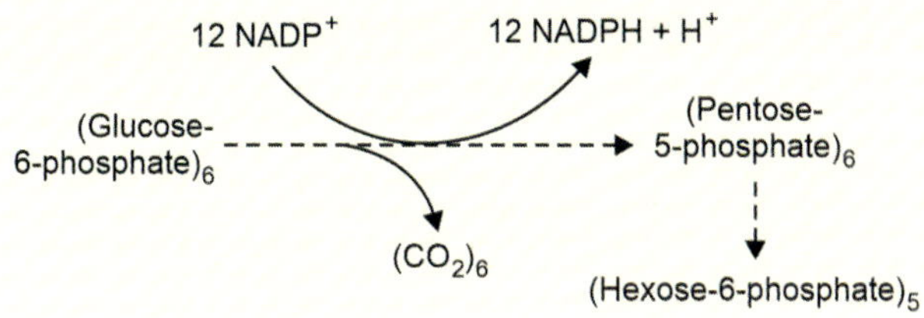

Fig. 12.13: HMP shunt: Overall process

Reactions of the pentose phosphate pathway are outlined in Fig. 12.14:

1. Firstly, **glucose is activated to glucose-6-phosphate by** the enzyme **hexokinase**.
2. Thereafter, **glucose-6-phosphate is changed to 6-phosphogluconolactone** and, subsequently, to **6-phospho-gluconate by** the enzyme **glucose-6-phosphate dehydrogenase**. This enzyme is induced by insulin. During this process $NADP^+$ is reduced to NADPH + H^+.

Glucose-6-Phosphate Dehydrogenase Deficiency

G6PD deficiency is an X-linked inherited disease characterized by hemolytic anemia due to inability to detoxify oxidizing agents. The molecular defect is a point mutation in the G6PD gene. Highest prevalence is seen in the Middle East, tropical Africa and Asia, and parts of Mediterranean. Babies with G6PD deficiency suffer from neonatal jaundice appearing 1–4 days after birth due to increased bilirubin production resulting from hemolysis.

G6PD deficiency impairs the ability of RBC to form NADPH which is essential for the maintenance of reduced glutathione (GSH), a potent intracellular antioxidant. This results in reduced detoxification of reactive oxygen species (free radicals such as superoxide anion as well as nonradicals like hydrogen peroxide) which damage the RBC membrane with consequent hemolysis. Extreme caution should be taken when prescribing antibiotics (sulfamethoxazole, chloramphenicol, etc.), antimalarials (primaquine) and antipyretics (acetanilide), to these patients since these drugs readily trigger hemolysis.

3. In the next reaction, a hexose is converted to a pentose, i.e. **6-phosphogluconate is oxidized by** the enzyme **6-phosphogluconate dehydrogenase, to** form an intermediate called **3-keto-6-phosphogluconate**. This reaction also generates NADPH + H^+.
4. Subsequently, **by** the enzyme **6-phosphogluconate decarboxylase**, a carbon is removed from 3-**keto-6-phospho-gluconate** as CO_2, leaving a pentose called **ribulose-5-phosphate**.

   These two enzymes, i.e. glucose-6-phosphate dehydrogenase and 6-phosphogluconate dehydrogenase, are the regulatory enzymes of this shunt.
5. In the second stage of the shunt, **ribulose-5-phosphate changes to other pentoses:**
   - Ribulose-5-phosphate is changed **to ribose-5-phosphate by** the enzyme **ribose-5-phosphate keto-isomerase.**

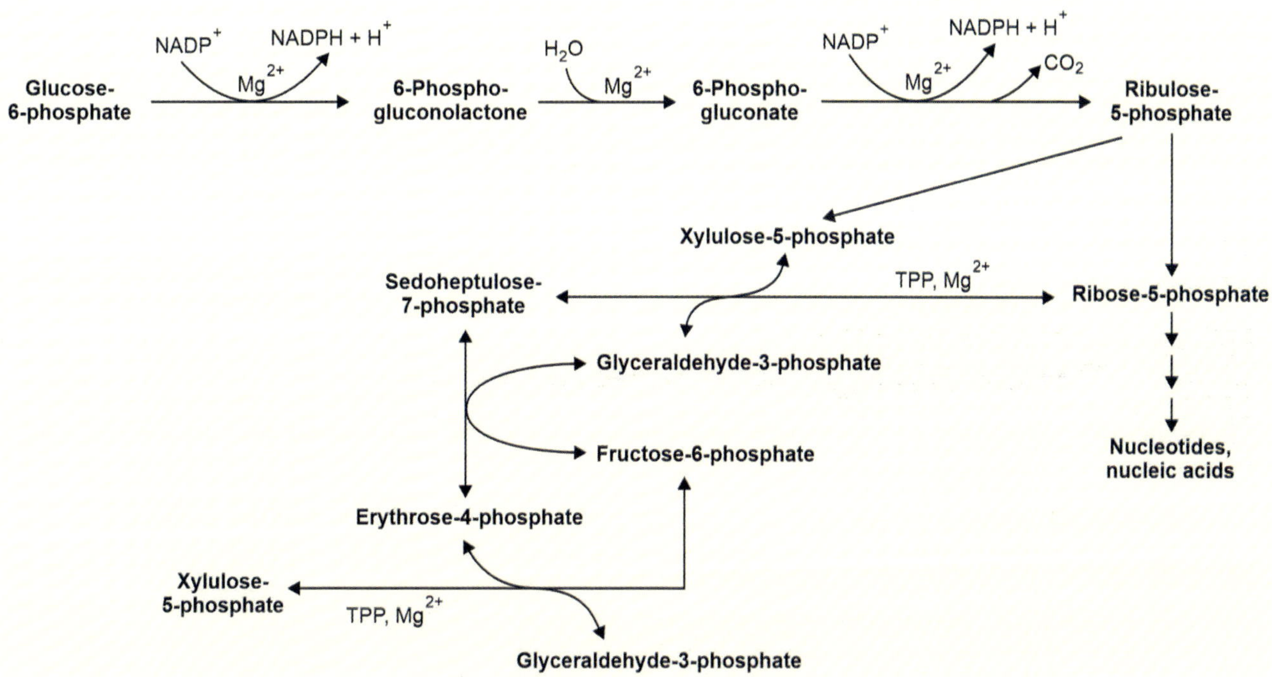

Fig. 12.14: Outline of HMP shunt

- It is also converted **to xylulose-5-phosphate by** the enzyme **ribulose-5-phosphate epimerase.**

6. In the next reaction, **carbon skeletons of the two pentoses are rearranged:**
   - Firstly, **transketolase transfers a ketol group** (the first 2 carbon atoms) from xylulose-5-phosphate to ribose-5-phosphate, **forming sedoheptulose-7-phosphate and glyceraldehyde-3-phosphate.** Transketolase requires TPP as a coenzyme.
   - Subsequently, **an aldol group** (3 carbons moiety) is transferred by the enzyme **trans-aldolase, from sedoheptulose-7-phosphate to glyceraldehyde-3-phosphate, forming fructose-6-phosphate and erythrose-4-phosphate.**
7. Thereafter, **transketolase** further **transfers a ketol group** (2 carbons moiety) **from xylulose-5-phosphate to erythrose-4-phosphate, forming fructose-6-phosphate and glyceraldehyde-3-phosphate.**

Biomedical Importance of HMP Shunt

- **In the liver:** In the liver HMP shunt serves as a source of NADPH and pentoses.
  - **Generation of NADPH:** Two molecules of $NADP^+$ are reduced to NADPH per molecule of glucose-6-phosphate, in the pentose phosphate pathway. NADPH, so produced, is used for the various anabolic reactions such as synthesis of fatty acids and cholesterol.
  - **Source of pentoses:** Pentose phosphate pathway is also important source of pentoses which are required for the synthesis of nucleic acids.
- **In the erythrocytes:** NADPH is utilized by glutathione reductase in the erythrocytes to maintain the reduced state of glutathione and prevent their hemolysis. This reaction is important for the detoxification of H_2O_2, which is produced in erythrocytes. If accumulates, H_2O_2 decreases their life span and causes hemolysis.

FORMATION OF GLUCURONIC ACID

Glucuronic acid can be obtained in small amounts from the diet. It can also be obtained from the intracellular lysosomal degradation of glycosaminoglycans (proteoglycans) or via the uronic acid pathway (Fig. 12.15).

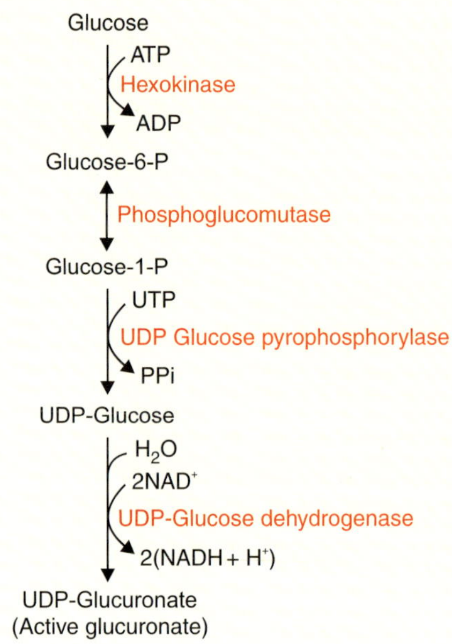

Fig. 12.15: Uronic acid pathway

The active form of glucuronic acid is UDP-glucuronic acid, which is produced by oxidation of UDP-glucose, by UDP-glucose dehydrogenase.

UDP-Glucuronic acid is the donor of glucuronic acid, both for the formation of proteoglycans and for conjugation and detoxification reactions that occur in the liver. In the liver, glucuronic acid is conjugated to steroid hormones, bilirubin, and many drugs, which in turn increases the water solubility of these hydrophobic compounds, facilitating their excretion in urine.

Some Important Questions

1. **Outline reactions of the citric acid cycle. Give energetic of the cycle and explain the amphibolic role of this cycle.**
2. **Outline pentose phosphate pathway reactions. Discuss significance of the pathway in the liver and the erythrocytes.**
3. **Give outline of glycolysis. What are its regulatory steps? What is the energy yield of this pathway?**
4. **Define glycogenolysis. Outline reactions of this pathway.**
5. **What is glycogenesis? Give reactions of glycogenesis.**

6. Explain:

i. Why aerobic glycolysis releases more energy than anaerobic glycolysis?
ii. How glycolysis can be reversed?
iii. Citric acid cycle and its energetics

7. Write notes on:

i. Glycogenolysis
ii. Glycogenesis
iii. Gluconeogenesis
iv. Glycogen storage diseases
v. Energetics of the citric acid cycle
vi. Oxidation of pyruvate to acetyl CoA
vii. Cori cycle
viii. Lactate metabolism
ix. Glucose-6-phosphate dehydrogenase deficiency

Chapter 13

Metabolism of Lipids

As discussed in Chapter 8, digestion of dietary lipids results in the formation and release of chylomicrons, which transport triacylglycerols to the liver and adipose tissue. Triacylglycerols are subsequently hydrolyzed to release fatty acids which are oxidized to produce energy.

OXIDATION OF FATTY ACIDS

Major pathway for the oxidation of fatty acids occurs **in mitochondria.** This pathway is called as β-oxidation of fatty acids and was proposed by Knoop.

In this process, **oxidation** of fatty acids **occurs at the β-carbon atom** (carbon-3) and **two-carbon fragments are successively removed** from the carboxyl end of fatty acyl CoA. This, in turn, results in the elimination of two terminal carbon atoms **as acetyl CoA**, thereby leaving fatty acyl CoA that has two carbon atoms less than the original fatty acid.

Outline of β-Oxidation of Fatty Acids

The process of β-oxidation of a fatty acid is outlined in Fig. 13.1.

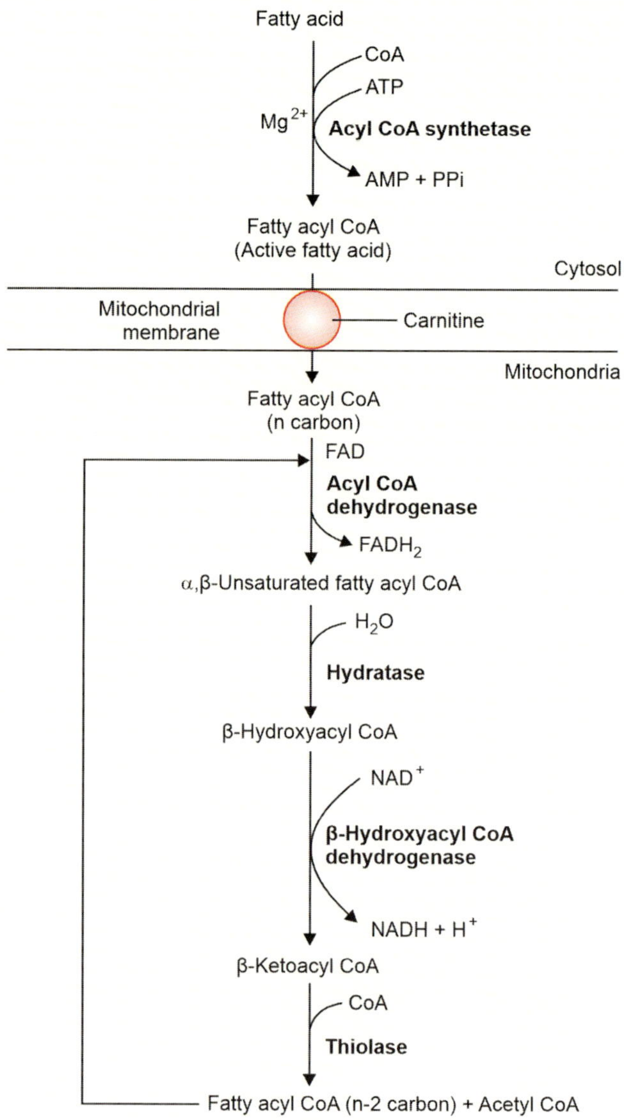

Fig. 13.1: Outline of β-oxidation of fatty acid

β-Oxidation of a fatty acid involves activation of fatty acid, its transport into mitochondria and oxidation of the fatty acid within the mitochondria.

- **Activation of fatty acids:** A **long chain fatty acid** (fatty acid containing >12 carbons) enters the cell, where it is **converted to its CoA derivative** by the enzyme **long chain fatty acyl CoA synthetase (thiokinase) in the cytosol**.
- **Transport of fatty acids from cytoplasm into mitochondria:** The process of **β-oxidation occurs in the mitochondrial matrix;** thus, **fatty acid must be transported** across the mitochondrial membrane.

  Whereas, the **short chain fatty acids can cross the inner mitochondrial membrane,** it is, however, impermeable to **long chain fatty acids**. So, long chain fatty acids are to be transported from cytosol to the mitochondrial matrix. **Long chain fatty acids are transported with the help of** a carrier referred to as **carnitine**. This process is called **carnitine shuttle.**
  - During this process, firstly, an **acyl group is transferred from the cytosolic CoA to carnitine,**

by the enzyme **carnitine palmitoyl transferase-I** (CPT-I. This enzyme is associated with the outer mitochondrial membrane and is also referred as carnitine acyl transferase-I or CAT-I). As a result of it, acyl CoA is **converted to acylcarnitine** and CoA is released.
- Thereafter, acylcarnitine is **transported into the mitochondrial matrix by** a protein called **carnitine acyl-translocase.**
- Finally, **CPT-II** (also called CAT-II, which is present in the inner mitochondrial membrane) catalyzes the **transfer** of the acyl group from **acylcarnitine** which is converted to acyl CoA in the mitochondrial matrix and carnitine is released.

Carnitine can be obtained from the dietary meat. A small amount of it can also be synthesized in the liver and kidney from lysine and methionine. Carnitine deficiency can be observed in patients with a liver disease, malnutrition or in strict vegetarians.

- **The process of β-Oxidation of Fatty Acids in Mitochondria:** Thereafter, the process of β-oxidation of the fatty acid (acyl CoA) occurs in mitochondria, in four steps, which results in reducing the chain length of the fatty acid by two carbon atoms. This includes:
  - **Oxidation** of the fatty acid: After activation of the fatty acid, such as palmitic acid, and its entry into the mitochondrial matrix, flavoprotein containing acyl CoA dehydrogenase removes two hydrogen atoms from the α- and β-positions of the fatty acyl CoA, reduces FAD to $FADH_2$ and the fatty acyl CoA to α,β-unsaturated fatty acyl CoA or enoyl CoA.
  - **Hydration** of the α,β-unsaturated fatty acyl CoA: In the next reaction, **enoyl CoA hydratase** adds a molecule of water at the double bond and converts **α,β-unsaturated fatty acyl CoA** (enoyl CoA) to **β-hydroxy-acyl CoA**.
  - **Oxidation** of β-hydroxy-acyl CoA: Thereafter, **β-hydroxy-acyl CoA dehydrogenase** oxidizes **β-hydroxy-acyl CoA and converts it to β-ketoacyl CoA.**
    - **Cleavage** of β-ketoacyl CoA: In the last step, acyl CoA: Acyl-transferase, also called **thiolase**, in the presence of CoA, results in thiolytic cleavage of the **β-ketoacyl CoA** and **converts** it **to acetyl CoA and fatty acyl CoA which has two carbon atoms less** than the original fatty acyl CoA.

These four steps are repeated, i.e. the fatty acyl CoA again undergoes above four set of reactions, starting with acyl CoA dehydrogenase, and in each cycle a molecule of acetyl CoA, $FADH_2$ and NADH are produced.

Thus, a fatty acid is sequentially degraded to acetyl CoA.

Deficiency of medium chain fatty acyl CoA dehydrogenase results in a clinical condition referred to as **sudden infant death syndrome (SIDS)**, also called **Reye's syndrome**. It is an autosomal recessive disorder, which, in turn, **reduces fatty acid oxidation**. Features of the disease include **vomiting, lethargy and coma,** accompanied with the **hypoketotic hypoglycemia and dicarboxylic aciduria**. Symptoms appear after more than 12 hours of fast and are more complicated on prolonged starvation, usually, within two years of life. Treatment includes a carbohydrate-rich diet.

ATP Production During β-Oxidation of Fatty Acids

A molecule of **palmitic acid** ($C_{15}H_{31}COOH$), when undergoes β-oxidation, **releases 8 molecules of acetyl CoA** in seven rounds. As mentioned above, in every round, one molecule each of **$FADH_2$ and NADH + H^+ are** also **produced**, which, in turn, generate 1.5 and 2.5 ATP, respectively. Thus, a total of 28 ATP molecules are produced during this process. In addition, each molecule of acetyl CoA, when oxidizes via the citric acid cycle, produces 10 ATP. Therefore, additionally, 80 ATP are produced from 8 molecules of acetyl CoA. Hence, **a total of 108 ATP molecules are produced from one molecule of palmitic acid.** As two high-energy phosphate bonds are hydrolyzed from one molecule of ATP, which is changed to AMP, thus, a total of 2 ATP are used during activation of the fatty acid. Therefore, there is a **net yield of 106 ATP** when one molecule of palmitic acid (fatty acid with 16 carbons) is completely oxidized.

Oxidation of Fatty Acids Containing Odd Number of Carbon Atoms

Oxidation of a saturated **fatty acid with odd number of carbon atoms proceeds in the same way** as a saturated fatty acid with even number of carbons, until final three carbons are reached. Thus, **in addition to acetyl CoA,** a fatty acid with odd number of carbon atoms **also produces a molecule of propionyl CoA** (containing 3 carbon atoms).

Propionyl CoA is **converted to succinyl CoA** and is **used in the TCA cycle.**

Oxidation of Unsaturated Fatty Acids

Unsaturated fatty acids are also **activated, transported across the inner mitochondrial membrane and undergo β-oxidation**, by the process similar to that of a saturated fatty acid. However, since double bonds in the naturally occurring unsaturated fatty acids are found in *cis*-configuration (compared to those produced during β-oxidation, which have *trans*-configuration) hence, **three additional enzymes are required** for their oxidation. These include:

- Enoyl CoA isomerase,
- Dienoyl CoA reductase, and
- 3,2-Enoyl CoA isomerase.

Thus, in addition to the other enzymes of β oxidation, these three enzymes are also required for the oxidation of the unsaturated fatty acids.

METABOLIC FATES OF ACETYL CoA

Acetyl CoA is, mainly, used in the **Krebs cycle**. Besides Krebs cycle, acetyl CoA can also be used for the **synthesis of fatty acids** and **cholesterol**. A small quantity of it is also converted to **ketone bodies** in the liver (Fig. 13.2).

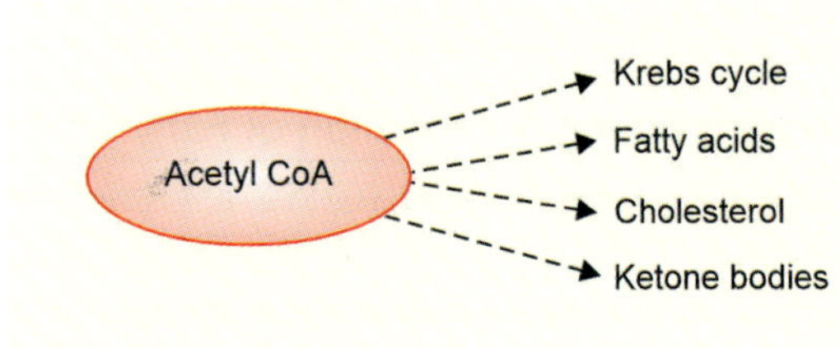

Fig. 13.2: Metabolic fates of acetyl CoA

METABOLISM OF KETONE BODIES

Three compounds, namely, **acetoacetate, β-hydroxybutyrate and acetone** are collectively referred to as ketone bodies (acetone bodies).

- The process of **synthesis of ketone bodies** is called **ketogenesis**.
- The process of **degradation** (oxidation) of ketone bodies is called **ketolysis.**
- Clinical condition resulting from the increased synthesis of ketone bodies is called **ketosis**. Ketosis occurs in **severe diabetes, starvation** or on **high-fat low-carbohydrate diet**.
- Ketone bodies are diffused into the blood. In a normal man, concentration of ketone bodies is, usually, less than 3 mg/100 mL of blood.
- Their **increased concentration in blood** is called **ketonemia**. In conditions, such as during prolonged starvation or impaired glucose oxidation, like **diabetes mellitus**, when fat becomes the source of energy and lipolysis is accelerated, there is increased production of acetyl CoA, which cannot be utilized in the Krebs cycle (due to lack of oxaloacetate) and forms ketone bodies.
- Ketonemia results in **increased excretion of ketone bodies** in urine. It is referred to as **ketonuria.**

SYNTHESIS OF KETONE BODIES

Synthesis of ketone bodies (ketogenesis) occurs in mitochondria, in the liver, since liver has a highly active system for the production of acetoacetate, which is also referred to as the principal ketone body. Synthesis of acetoacetate is outlined in Fig. 13.3.

- Firstly, **2 molecules of acetyl CoA condense** and **form aceto-acetyl CoA.**
- **Aceto-acetyl CoA** further reacts with one more molecule of **acetyl CoA** and **forms HMG CoA** (β-hydroxy-β-methyl-glutaryl CoA).
- Thereafter, HMG CoA lyase splits HMG CoA and converts it to acetyl CoA and acetoacetate (the parent ketone body).

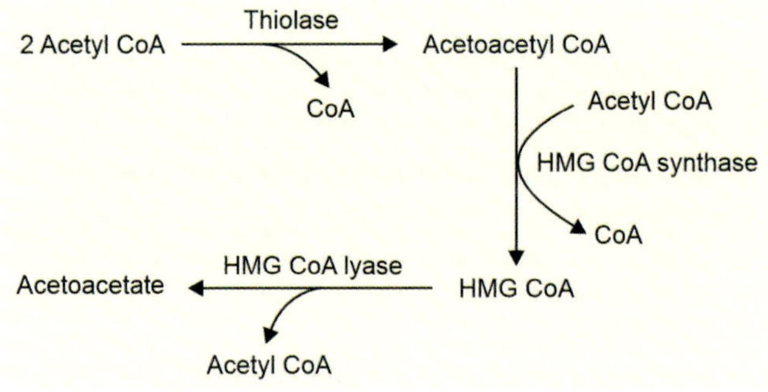

Fig. 13.3: Synthesis of acetoacetate

- In the mitochondria, a part of **aceto-acetyl CoA is reduced** by NADH-dependent β-hydroxybutyrate dehydrogenase **to β-hydroxybutyrate.**
- Some of the acetoacetate is **also** decarboxylated spontaneously by a non-enzymatic reaction and is **converted to acetone**.

Under normal conditions, acetone formation is negligible, but when acetoacetate accumulates, such as **in severe diabetic ketoacidosis**, amount of **acetone in blood is increased** to the extent that it is **detectable in breath** of the patient. **Acetoacetate and β-hydroxybutyrate**, both, are strong acids. They slowly **deplete alkali reserve** of the body. This, in turn, results in **metabolic acidosis,** also called **ketoacidosis**. These are also used as a source of energy in the peripheral tissues such as kidney and muscle during starvation. During starvation even brain starts utilizing ketone bodies.

Degradation of Ketone Bodies

Degradation of ketone bodies is also referred to as ketolysis.

- **Oxidation of β-hydroxybutyrate:** A mitochondrial enzyme **β-hydroxybutyrate dehydrogenase,** oxidizes **β-hydroxybutyrate** and **converts** it **to acetoacetate**.
- **Oxidation of acetoacetate:** Acetoacetate is oxidized after its activation to aceto-acetyl CoA. Since liver does not contain the concerned enzyme, ketone bodies cannot be utilized in the liver.
  - In the first reaction, **acetoacetate** reacts **with succinyl CoA,** in the presence of the enzyme ***trans-acylase*** (acetoacetate-succinyl CoA transferase, also called thiophorase), and is **converted to aceto-acetyl CoA.**
  - Thereafter, **aceto-acetyl CoA is hydrolyzed to** two molecules of **acetyl CoA by** the enzyme thiolase (β-keto-thiolase).
  - **Acetone is oxidized** very slowly, mainly, **through lungs.**

SYNTHESIS OF FATTY ACIDS

Mammals can synthesize a major portion of the saturated as well as monounsaturated fatty acids by the process called *De novo* synthesis. In human beings, fatty acid synthesis occurs, primarily, in the cytosol, in the liver and lactating mammary glands.

The process of *De novo* **synthesis of fatty acid synthesis** includes **transport of acetyl CoA** from mitochondria **to cytosol,** its **conversion to malonyl CoA** and **synthesis of palmitic acid** (a saturated, straight chain, 16-carbon-containing fatty acid), which is synthesized first, and is, subsequently, changed to other fatty acids.

- **Transport of Acetyl CoA from Mitochondria to Cytosol:** First step in fatty acid synthesis is the transfer of the acetate units from mitochondria to the cytosol. For this purpose:
  - **Acetyl CoA condenses with oxaloacetate and forms citrate.**
  - **Citrate is then translocated from mitochondria** to the **cytosol**, where it is **cleaved by the enzyme ATP-citrate lyase** and is converted back to acetyl CoA and oxaloacetate in the cytosol (Fig. 13.4).

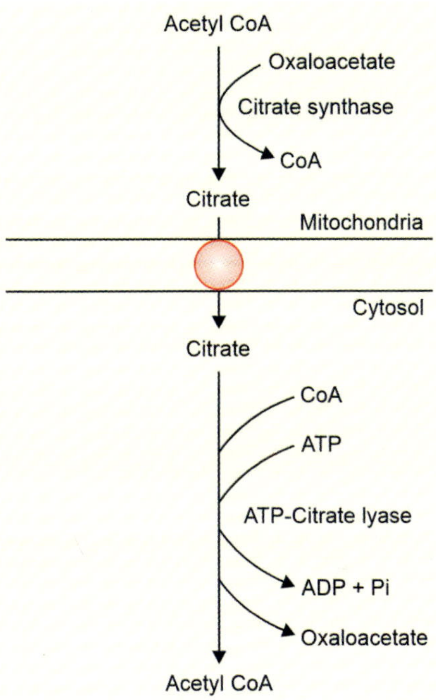

Fig. 13.4: Transport of acetyl CoA from mitochondria to cytosol

- **Conversion of Acetyl CoA to Malonyl CoA:** In the cytosol, **acetyl CoA** is carboxylated, and **converted to malonyl CoA** by a biotin-containing enzyme, referred to as **acetyl CoA carboxylase.**
- **Synthesis of Palmitic Acid: In eukaryotes, synthesis of palmitic acid** occurs in the cytosol by the enzyme referred to as **fatty acid synthase.**

Fatty acid synthase: Fatty acid synthase is a **multifunctional,** dimeric **enzyme, composed of the two identical subunits.** Its **each monomer** is a multicatalytic polypeptide **with seven different enzyme** activities plus a domain that covalently binds a molecule of 4′-phosphopantotheine. During fatty acid synthesis, 4′-phosphopantotheine carries acetyl and acyl units on its terminal **thiol (–SH) groups.**

Individually, these **enzyme activities** of the fatty acid synthase complex **are** designated as:

- Acetyl CoA-ACP acetyl *trans*-acylase,
- Malonyl CoA-ACP *trans*-acylase,
- Condensing enzyme (β-Ketoacyl-ACP synthase),
- β-Ketoacyl ACP reductase,
- β-Hydroxy-acyl ACP dehydratase, and
- Enoyl-ACP reductase.

In addition, it has **two –SH groups,** called pantotheinyl-SH group, which is referred to as the **ACP-SH**, and the thiol-SH group that is designated as the **CYS-SH**.

In prokaryotes, fatty acid synthase is a multienzyme complex and the 4′-phosphopantotheine domain is present on a separate protein, referred to as **acyl carrier protein** (ACP).

Outline of fatty acid synthesis is shown in Fig. 13.5.

1. Fatty acid synthesis starts with the **transfer of** a molecule of **acetate,** from acetyl CoA **to the ACP-SH.** This reaction is catalyzed **by the** acetyl CoA-ACP-**acetyl-*trans*-acylase** domain of the fatty acid synthase complex and the two-carbon fragment is transferred to the CYS-SH, which is a temporary holding site.

   At the same time, malonyl CoA-ACP *trans*-acylase domain of the fatty acid synthase transfers three-carbon malonate unit from **malonyl** CoA to the vacant –SH group of ACP.
2. In the next step, malonyl group loses CO_2 and transfers the acetyl group, by β-ketoacyl-ACP-**synthase** domain of the fatty acid synthase, which, in turn, **causes condensation of the two acetyl groups** on the CYS–SH **and forms** a four-carbon **aceto-acetyl unit** that is attached to the ACP domain.
3. Thereafter, β-ketoacyl ACP **reductase** domain of the fatty acid synthase **reduces** keto group of the **aceto-acetyl-S-ACP to β-hydroxy-butyryl-S-ACP** (β-hydroxy-acyl-S-ACP).
4. In the next step, β-hydroxy-acyl-ACP **dehydratase** domain of the fatty acid synthase removes a molecule of H_2O from **β-hydroxy-acyl-S-ACP** and introduces a double bond in it, **to** form **crotonyl-S-ACP** (α, β-***trans***-butenyl-ACP or α,β-unsaturated acyl-S-ACP).
5. In the next step, **crotonyl-S-ACP is reduced by** the enoyl-ACP **reductase** domain of the fatty acid synthase, and is **converted to butyryl-S-ACP** (acyl-S-ACP).

   As a result of these reactions, a four-carbon compound is formed whose three terminal carbons are fully saturated and remain attached to ACP.

   The above steps are again repeated, beginning with the transfer of the butyryl-chain to the cys-SH, repeated five more times (each time incorporating two-carbon units, which are derived from malonyl CoA, and are attached to the growing fatty acid chain, at the carboxyl end). After the chain length reaches 16 carbons, process is terminated with the formation of palmitoyl-S-ACP.

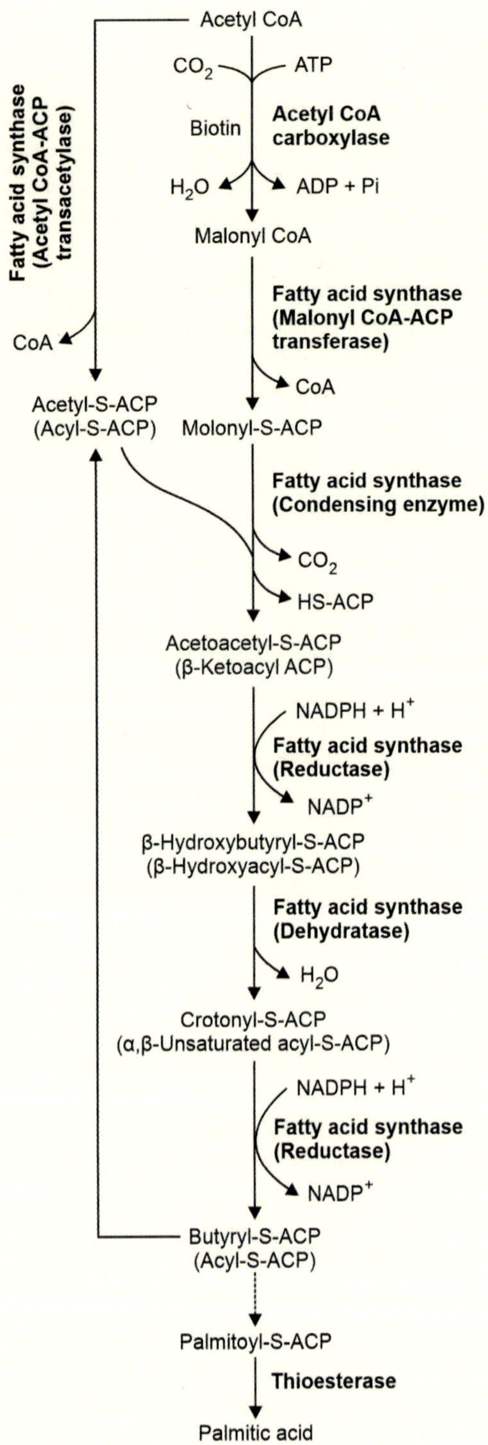

Fig. 13.5: Outline of fatty acid synthesis

6. Thereafter, palmitoyl **thio-esterase cleaves** the thioester bond with the release of **palmitate**.

Reducing equivalents **(NADPH + H+)**, which are **used in the biosynthesis of fatty acids, are derived from the pentose phosphate pathway**.

Synthesis of Other Fatty Acids

Palmitate, produced by fatty acid synthase catalyzed reactions is modified by chain elongation and desaturation.

METABOLISM OF TRIACYLGLYCEROLS

As discussed above, products of the lipid digestion, primarily, free fatty acids (≈70%) and β-monoacylglycerols, are used for the resynthesis of triacylglycerols, which are incorporated into and released as chylomicrons. It is the way dietary triacylglycerols reach peripheral tissues and are either stored in the adipose tissue (for use at the time of necessity) or are oxidized in the liver and muscle.

In a homeostatic situation, there is continuous synthesis and breakdown of triacylglycerols in the adipose tissue.

LIPOGENESIS

Triacylglycerols, as mentioned above, are the principle dietary lipids as well as lipids of the fat depot in the body. Excessive amounts of dietary carbohydrates are also stored as triacylglycerols in the adipose tissue. The process of biosynthesis of triacylglycerols is referred to as lipogenesis, which, though, mainly, occurs in the liver and adipose tissue; lactating mammary glands, kidneys and epithelial cells of the intestinal mucosa are also active in this respect.

Lipogenesis involves **activation of free fatty acids** and **α-glycerol phosphate** (Fig. 13.6).

- **Synthesis of L-α-glycerol phosphate:** L-α-glycerol phosphate, required for the esterification of fatty acids, can be synthesized in two ways:
  - **In most of the tissues** which contain glycerol kinase, glycerol is directly converted to **L-α-glycerol phosphate**.
  - Alternatively, **in muscle and adipose tissue**, which lack glycerol kinase, L-α-glycerol phosphate is formed by the **reduction of dihydroxyacetone phosphate**, an intermediate of glycolysis. The reaction is catalyzed by glycerol-3-phosphate dehydrogenase.
- **Activation of fatty acids:** Free **fatty acids**, in the presence of ATP and CoA, are activated **to acyl-CoA, by thio-kinase** (fatty acyl-CoA synthetase).
- **Re-esterification of glycerol phosphate:** After the synthesis of L-α-glycerol phosphate and activation of fatty acids, triacylglycerols are synthesized by re-esterification. In this process:
  - A molecule of **acyl-CoA combines with α-glycerol phosphate** and **forms 1-acylglycerol-3-phosphate** (lysophosphatidic acid). The reaction is catalyzed **by glycerol-3-phosphate acyltransferase**.
  - L-Acylglycerol-3-phosphate **acyltransferase** (lyso-phosphatidyl-acyltransferase) **converts 1-acylglycerol-3-phosphate to 1,2-diacylglycerol phosphate** (**DAG** or phosphatidic acid).

    DAG is a common intermediate for the biosynthesis of, both triacylglycerols as well as phospholipids.
  - **Phosphatase** (phosphatidic acid phosphohydrolase) **hydrolyzes phosphatidic acid and forms 1,2-diacylglycerol**.

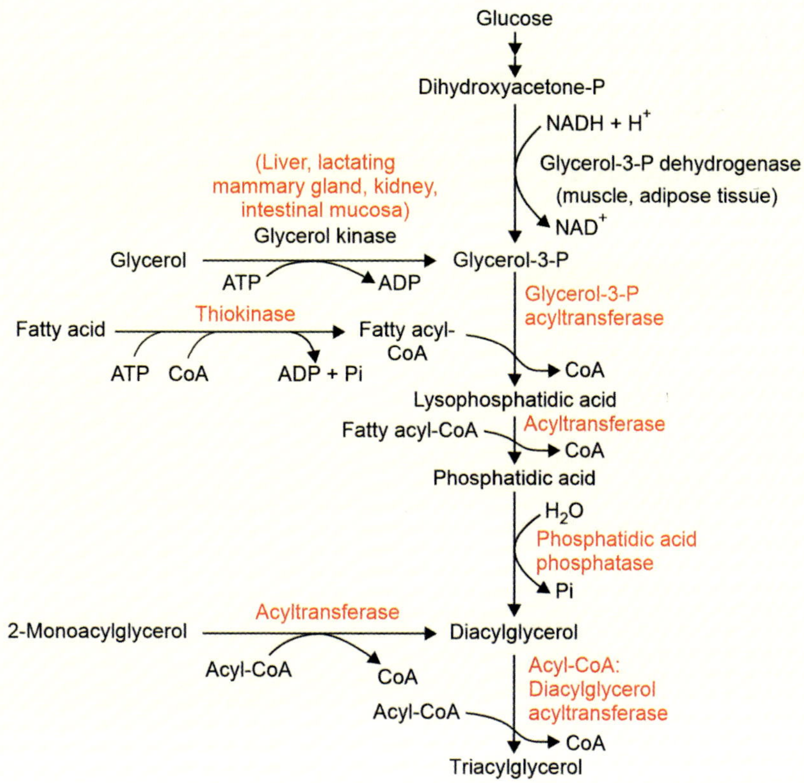

Fig. 13.6: Biosynthesis of a triacylglycerol

In many tissues, especially, in the intestinal mucosa, 1,2-diacylglycerol is also formed from 2-monoacylglycerols, since monoacylglycerols are directly absorbed in the intestinal mucosa. The reaction involves the transfer of an acyl group by the enzyme monoacylglycerol acyltransferase.

- Diacylglycerol **acyltransferase** esterifies diacylglycerol and **forms triacylglycerol**.

Generally, palmitic acid is mainly present in position 1 while oleic acid at positions 2 and 3 of a triacylglycerol in the human adipose tissue.

LIPOLYSIS

The process of the **breakdown of triacylglycerols** is called lipolysis. **Key enzymes** for the release of energy from these stores are called lipases.

There are two types of lipases involved in the hydrolysis of triacylglycerols:

- **Lipoprotein lipase:** It is located on the surface of the endothelial cells of capillaries and, possibly, of the adjoining tissues. Lipoprotein lipases remove fatty acids from 1 and/or 3 positions of a triacylglycerol, and/or diacylglycerol, when they are present in lipoproteins (VLDL and chylomicrons). The enzyme requires apoprotein C-II for its activity. Insulin also activates the enzyme. Fatty acids that are released are either bound to serum albumin or are taken up by the tissues. Monoglycerides, which are produced, may either pass into the cells or are further hydrolyzed by the serum monoacylglycerol hydrolase.
- **Hormone sensitive lipase:** This is a distinct type of lipase which hydrolyzes fatty acids from triacylglycerols that are stored in the adipose tissue. It is regulated by lipolytic hormones such as epinephrine, glucagon and ACTH. These hormones stimulate cAMP-mediated phosphorylation of the inactive enzyme. Insulin and prostaglandins inhibit enzyme activity.

Process of lipolysis: Sequence of hydrolysis of fatty acids from different positions of triacylglycerol depends upon specificities of the particular lipase (Fig. 13.7).

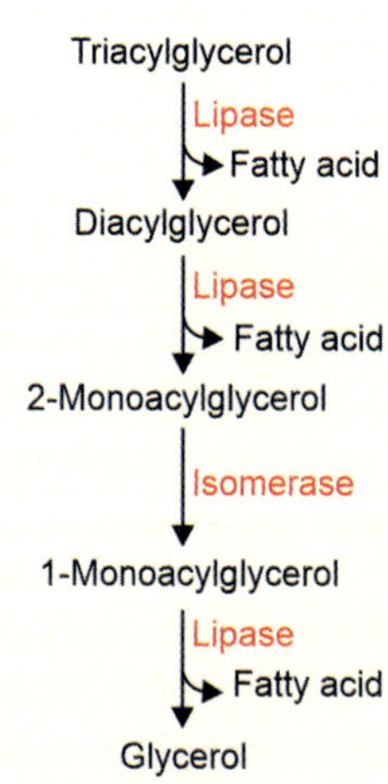

Fig. 13.7: Lipolysis

Fatty acids and glycerol, so produced, are released into circulation in blood. Fatty acids are bound to serum albumin, transported to different tissues, and are oxidized to CO_2 and H_2O, with the liberation of energy. Glycerol returns to the liver, where it is converted to dihydroxyacetone phosphate and enters the glycolytic pathway, or is converted to glucose via gluconeogenesis.

METABOLISM OF CHOLESTEROL

An adult man contains about 1 g cholesterol/kg body weight. Cholesterol content in **normal** human **blood varies between 130 to 220 mg/100 mL**, which is equally distributed between plasma and erythrocytes. About 30% of the circulating cholesterol occurs free, while the remaining of it exists in the form of cholesterol esters.

SYNTHESIS OF CHOLESTEROL

Important sites for cholesterol biosynthesis include **liver, skin, intestine, adrenal cortex and reproductive tissues**, including ovaries, testes and placenta. All the carbon atoms of cholesterol are derived from acetate (acetyl CoA), which is obtained from several sources such as oxidation of long chain fatty acids, ketogenic amino acids and glucose (via pyruvate). Synthesis of cholesterol is called *de novo* synthesis.

De novo synthesis of cholesterol is outlined in Fig. 13.8.

- Firstly, **two** molecules of **acetyl CoA** condense to **form aceto-acetyl CoA**. This reaction is catalyzed **by** the enzyme **aceto-acetyl CoA thiolase**.
- Thereafter, in the presence of the enzyme β-hydroxy-β-methyl-glutaryl CoA synthase **(HMG CoA synthase)**, **aceto-acetyl CoA** further condenses **with** another molecule of **acetyl CoA** and **forms** β-hydroxy-β-methyl-glutaryl CoA **(HMG CoA)**.

  HMG CoA, however, **does not lead to increased cholesterol synthesis in starvation**. This is due to the reason that during starvation there is decreased oxidation of glucose and the available amounts of acetyl CoA and oxaloacetate are used in the citric acid cycle. Thereafter, when the oxidation of fatty acids is increased, acetyl CoA (due to the limited supply of oxaloacetate) is used for the synthesis of ketone bodies and fatty acids, which are used as a source of energy during starvation.
- In the next step, an NADPH-dependent enzyme, **HMG CoA reductase, converts HMG CoA to mevalonic acid.**

  This is the **regulatory step in cholesterol biosynthesis.**
- Thereafter, there occur **stepwise transfer of the two γ-phosphate** groups **from two molecules of ATP**. These reactions are catalyzed **by two kinases**, called mevalonate kinase (enzyme I) and phosphomevalonate kinase (enzyme II).
- Subsequently, **decarboxylation** takes place **by** the enzyme **decarboxylase** (pyro-phospho-mevalonate decarboxylase).

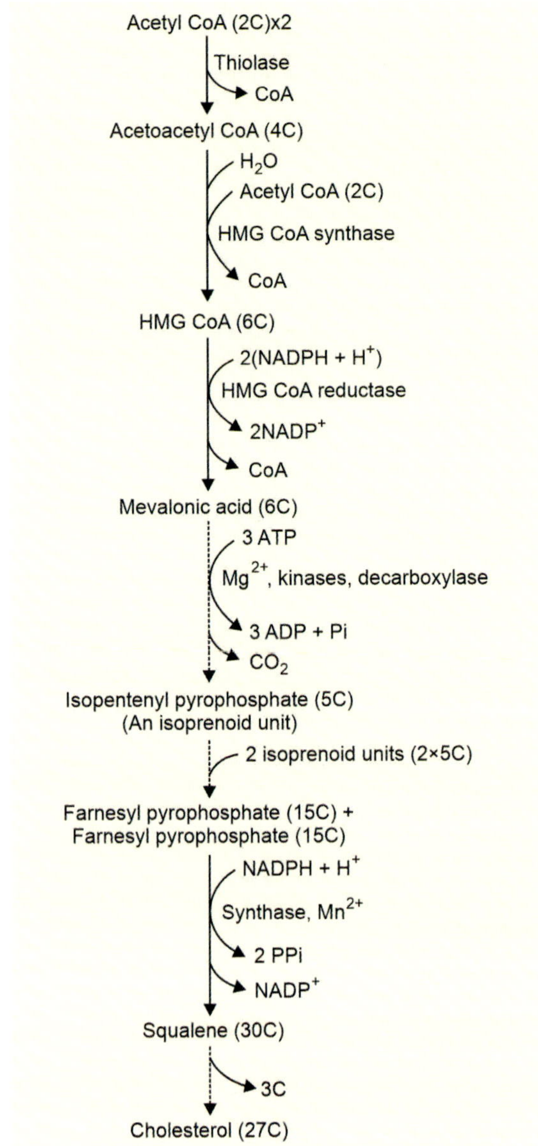

Fig. 13.8: Outline of cholesterol synthesis

Thus, **phosphorylation and decarboxylation of mevalonic acid forms** isopentenyl-pyrophosphate, which is also called **active isoprenoid unit.**

- In the next step, the **isoprenoid unit** (isopentenyl-pyrophosphate) is **isomerized to another isoprenoid unit**, designated as 3,3-dimethylallylpyrophosphate, **by** the enzyme isopentenyl-pyrophosphate **isomerase.**
- Thereafter, stepwise **condensation of the three isoprenoid units** (5C units) leads to the formation of a 15-carbon unit called **farnesyl-pyrophosphate** (15C).

  In this process, **first two isoprenoid units** (a molecule each of isopentenyl-pyrophosphate and 3,3-dimethylallylpyrophosphate) **condense** together and **forms** a 10-carbon unit, called **geranyl-pyrophosphate** (10C). The 10C unit **further condenses with another isoprenoid unit** (a molecule of isopentenyl-pyrophosphate) and forms farnesyl-pyrophosphate (15C). This reaction is catalyzed by the enzyme **geranyl-transferase.**

- In the next step, fusion of the **two molecules of farnesyl-pyrophosphate forms** a 30-carbon compound, called **squalene (30C)**.
- Subsequently, by **ring closure and removal of the three methyl groups, squalene is converted to cholesterol** (which has 27 carbon atoms).

TRANSPORT AND REGULATION

Cholesterol is a hydrophilic molecule, so it is minimally soluble in water. For its transport in blood, cholesterol is packaged in lipoproteins, where it is present in two forms. Nearly, thirty percent of the total cholesterol is present in free form while the remaining is present in the esterified form.

Regulation of Cholesterol Metabolism

Cholesterol synthesis is regulated by dietary cholesterol, feedback inhibition and its disposal by the liver.

- **By dietary cholesterol:** Rate of ***de novo*** **synthesis** of cholesterol is **inversely related to** the amount of **dietary cholesterol.** When dietary cholesterol intake is reduced, cholesterol synthesis is increased in the liver and the intestine, to meet needs of the other tissues. On the other hand, when dietary cholesterol intake is increased, its synthesis is reduced.
- **By feedback inhibition:** Cholesterol **inhibits its own synthesis by feedback inhibition.** HMG CoA reductase regulates cholesterol synthesis. **Cholesterol inhibits** activity of **HMG CoA reductase** by **suppressing its synthesis and promoting inactivation.**
- **By disposal from the liver:** Liver removes cholesterol by several processes:
  - **By esterification: Lecithin:** cholesterol acyltransferase (LCAT) and HDL are important for the esterification of cholesterol. **LCAT is** a plasma enzyme which is **produced**, mainly, **by the liver.** It **transfers one fatty acid from carbon-2 of lecithin to the 3-hydroxyl group of cholesterol.** This reaction is freely reversible and **utilizes cholesterol, which is present in HDL**.

    Cholesterol esters, so formed, diffuse into core of the HDL particle, where they are transported from the tissues and plasma to the liver, which further metabolizes and excretes it. This is referred to as the **reverse transport of cholesterol**, since HDL provides the vehicle for the transport of cholesterol from the peripheral tissues to the liver. In a normal healthy adult, on a low cholesterol diet, about 1300 mg of cholesterol is returned to the liver, each day.
  - **By excretion:** Free cholesterol as well as **bile acids/salts are excreted in bile.**
  - **By incorporation into VLDL:** In the liver, cholesterol is also **incorporated into VLDL and is secreted into circulation.**

CATABOLISM (METABOLIC FATES) OF CHOLESTEROL

Free cholesterol is **present** in abundance, **in bile**. It is also present in large amount in the **myelin structure of the brain and in biological membranes**.

Cholesterol is also used in the biosynthesis of **bile acids, steroid hormones and vitamin D** (Fig. 13.9).

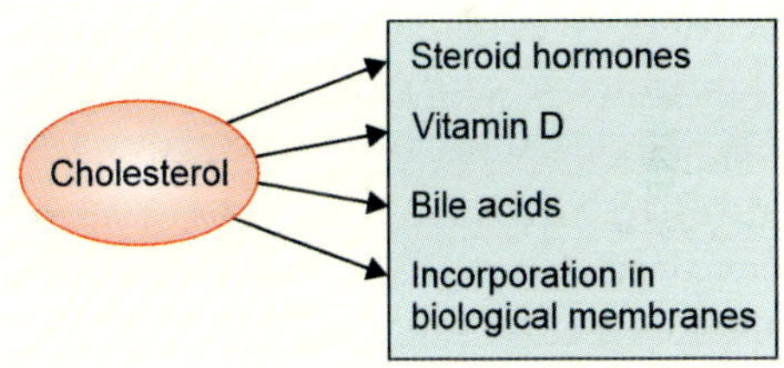

Fig. 13.9: Metabolic fates of cholesterol

Some Important Questions

1. **Outline β-oxidation of fatty acids. How much energy is produced when a molecule of palmitic acid is oxidized to acetyl CoA?**
2. **Outline *de novo* synthesis of fatty acid. What is the source of reducing equivalents?**
3. **Outline cholesterol synthesis. How its synthesis is regulated?**
4. **Describe briefly:**
   i. Role of carnitine in fatty acid oxidation
   ii. Metabolic fates of cholesterol
   iii. Process of β-oxidation of fatty acid
   iv. Synthesis of cholesterol and its regulation
   v. Oxidation of fatty acids containing odd number of carbon atoms
5. **Write notes on:**
   i. Ketone bodies
   ii. Lipolysis
   iii. *De novo* synthesis of fatty acids
   iv. Sudden infant death syndrome
   v. Rey's syndrome
   vi. Metabolic fates of acetyl CoA
   vii. Lipogenesis

Chapter

14

Metabolism of Proteins

As discussed in Chapter 8, digestion of proteins releases amino acids, which are absorbed by the liver.

In the liver, **amino acids are** either **used for protein synthesis** or are catabolized to release ammonia (which is converted to urea) while the remaining molecule (the carbon skeleton) is either converted to glucose or to ketone bodies.

UTILIZATION OF PROTEINS FOR ENERGY

Excess of the dietary **amino acids are** degraded to common metabolites and are **used as a source of energy (metabolic fuel)**. According to the formation of the end product, i.e. glucose and/or ketone bodies, various amino acids are classified into three groups, as follows:

1. **Glucogenic amino acids:** These amino acids serve as precursors of glucose, which are used in gluconeogenesis, for glucose formation. For example, alanine, glutamate and valine forms pyruvate, α-ketoglutarate and succinyl CoA, respectively. As these are the intermediates of the citric acid cycle and can be converted to glucose by gluconeogenesis, these amino acids are called glucogenic amino acids. Glucogenic amino acids include **glycine, alanine, serine, aspartic acid, asparagine, glutamic acid, glutamine, proline, valine, methionine, cysteine, histidine and arginine**.
2. **Ketogenic amino acids:** These amino acids are degraded to form ketone bodies. These include **leucine and lysine**. End products of the catabolism of leucine are acetyl CoA and aceto-acetyl CoA, whereas the end product of the catabolism of lysine is aceto-acetyl CoA.
3. **Both glucogenic and ketogenic amino acids:** Catabolic products of these amino acids are used in the formation of, both, ketone bodies as well as glucose. For example, catabolism of phenylalanine, in addition to an intermediate of the citric acid cycle (i.e. formate) also forms acetyl CoA or aceto-acetyl CoA, the precursors of ketone bodies. Therefore, these amino acids are referred as glucogenic as well as ketogenic. These include **isoleucine, phenylalanine, tryptophan and tyrosine**.

Classification of amino acids based on metabolic fate, as a source of energy, is shown in Table 14.1.

Table 14.1: Classification of amino acids based on metabolic fate

Metabolic fate of amino acids	*End products of their catabolism*
Glucogenic	
Gly, Ala, Ser, Cys, HO-Pro	Pyruvate
Glu, Gln, Pro, Arg, His	α-Ketoglutarate
Val, Met	Succinyl CoA
Asp, Asn	Oxaloacetate
Glucogenic and Ketogenic	
Ile	Succinyl CoA and acetyl CoA
Phe and Tyr	Fumarate and acetoacetyl CoA
Trp	Pyruvate and acetoacetyl CoA
Thr	Pyruvate and acetyl CoA
Ketogenic	
Leu	Acetyl CoA and acetoacetyl CoA
Lys	Acetoacetyl CoA

REMOVAL OF THE AMINO GROUP AS AMMONIA FROM AMINO ACIDS

There are two processes by which the α-amino group can be removed from amino acids. These are referred to as **deamination** and **transamination**.

DEAMINATION

Process of the removal of α-amino group from amino acids is referred to as deamination. Liver and kidney are the main organs which are responsible for the deamination of amino acids. Deamination may take place either by **oxidative** or **nonoxidative** process.

Oxidative Deamination

Liver and kidney contain several enzymes which catalyze deamination of amino acids, such as amino acid oxidases. There are two types of amino acid oxidases, called L-amino acid oxidases and D-amino acid oxidases:

- **L-Amino Acid Oxidases:** L-amino acid oxidase is linked to FMN (the prosthetic group) and catalyzes the oxidation of L-amino acids, producing α-keto acids, ammonia and water as the final products (Fig. 14.1).

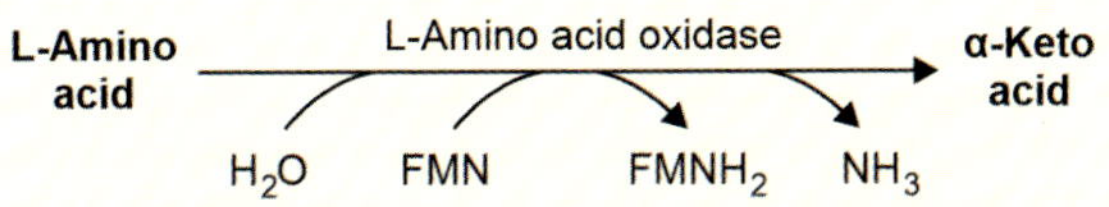

Fig. 14.1: L-Amino acid oxidase reaction

- **D-Amino Acid Oxidases:** Some of the tissues also contain FAD-linked D-amino acid oxidases which catalyze oxidation of glycine and the D-amino acids.

Nonoxidative Deamination

Dehydratase, sulf-hydrase and histidase catalyze deamination of serine, cysteine and histidine, respectively. They catalyze dehydration followed by nonoxidative deamination of the amino acid, spontaneously (Fig. 14.2).

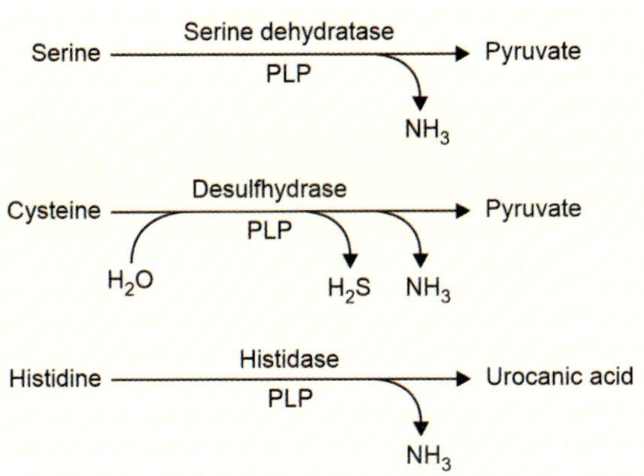

Fig. 14.2: Nonoxidative deamination reactions

TRANSAMINATION

Transamination is a process of the transfer of α-amino group from amino acid to keto acid. As a result of it, the amino acid is converted to keto acid while the keto acid is converted to amino acid (Fig. 14.3).

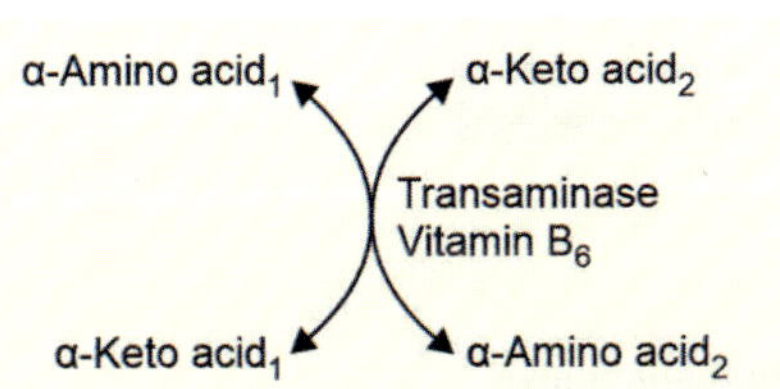

Fig. 14.3: Transamination reaction

Enzymes, which catalyze transamination, are called transaminases (aminotransferases). Although, liver contains several transaminases, most important of these are glutamate pyruvate transaminase (GPT, also called alanine aminotransferase or ALT) and glutamate oxaloacetate transaminase (GOT, also called aspartate aminotransferase or AST). Transaminases catalyzed reactions are shown in Fig. 14.4.

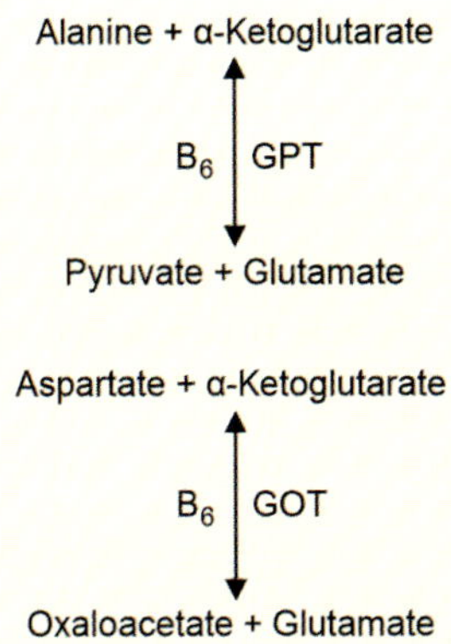

Fig. 14.4: GPT and GOT catalysed reactions

Diagnostic Significance of Transaminases

Serum GOT and GPT have diagnostic significance. They are present in large amount in cardiac muscle and liver, respectively. Although, serum levels of both the enzymes are raised in heart as well as liver diseases, SGOT is markedly raised in myocardial infarction while SGPT is more increased in liver disorders such as viral hepatitis or toxic liver necrosis (Table 14.2).

Table 14.2: Diagnostic significance of transaminases

Enzyme	*Comparatively more raised in*
SGOT	Cardiac disorders, e.g. myocardial infarction
SGPT	Liver disorders, e.g. viral hepatitis

AMMONIA METABOLISM (REMOVAL OF AMMONIA FROM BODY)

- **In the liver,** ammonia is released from different amino acids by trans-amidation and is used for the synthesis of urea, which is excreted in urine.

Trans-amidation

Trans-amidation **(trans-deamination)** refers to the process where transamination is coupled with oxidative deamination.

In the process of transamination, as mentioned above, α-amino group (ammonia) is either transferred from glutamate (which is converted to α-ketoglutarate) or transferred to α-ketoglutarate (which is converted to glutamate). Thus, an obligate amino acid or the α-keto acid which participate in these reactions is either glutamate or α-ketoglutarate. Since there are several transaminases, most of the amino acids transfer α-amino group to α-ketoglutarate and convert it to glutamate. As a result of it, glutamate pool is increased.

Glutamate, formed as above, is oxidatively deaminated by a specific enzyme, referred to as glutamate dehydrogenase (GDH). It is present in most of the tissues, both in cytoplasm and mitochondria. It is an anaerobic dehydrogenase and can use both NAD and NADP as a coenzyme. It catalyzes degradation as well as synthesis of glutamate. Though GDH catalyze synthesis as well as degradation of glutamate, it is important in the deamination of glutamate, which is produced as a result of transamination of most of the amino acids with α-ketoglutaric acid (Fig. 14.5).

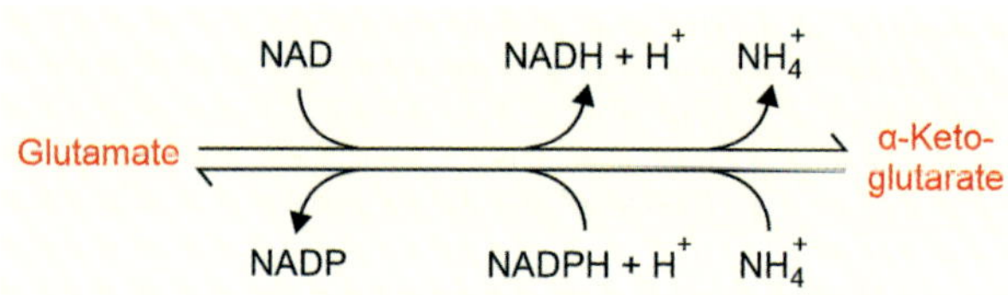

Fig. 14.5: Reactions catalyzed by glutamate dehydrogenase

- **In the brain,** since ammonia cannot cross blood–brain barrier, it reacts with glutamate and forms glutamine. This reaction is catalyzed by the enzyme glutamine synthetase. Glutamine is transported to the kidney where glutaminase removes amide group from glutamine as ammonia and forms glutamate.

Thus, ammonia from brain is transported to the kidney and is excreted as ammonium ions (NH_4^+). This is called glutamine cycle (Fig. 14.6).

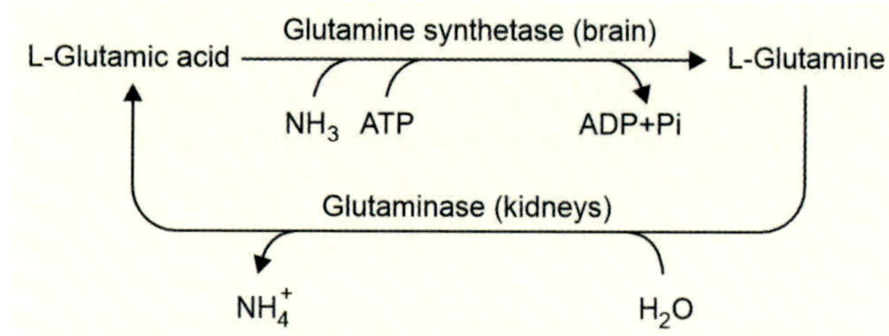

Fig. 14.6: Synthesis and degradation of glutamine

UREA FORMATION

Urea cycle is the process by which ammonia, a highly toxic water insoluble substance, is converted to urea, which is less toxic, water soluble, excretory waste product. Urea cycle occurs in the liver.

Outline of urea cycle is given in Fig. 14.7.

1. In the first step, ammonia reacts with carbon dioxide and forms carbamoyl-phosphate, in the mitochondria. This reaction is catalyzed by the enzyme carbamoyl-phosphate synthetase (CPS), which requires N-acetyl-glutamate as coenzyme.
2. Thereafter, ornithine trans-carbamoylase transfers carbamoyl group from carbamoyl-phosphate to ornithine and forms citrulline.
3. In the next step, in the presence of the enzyme arginine-succinate synthetase, citrulline combines with L-aspartate and forms arginine-succinate.

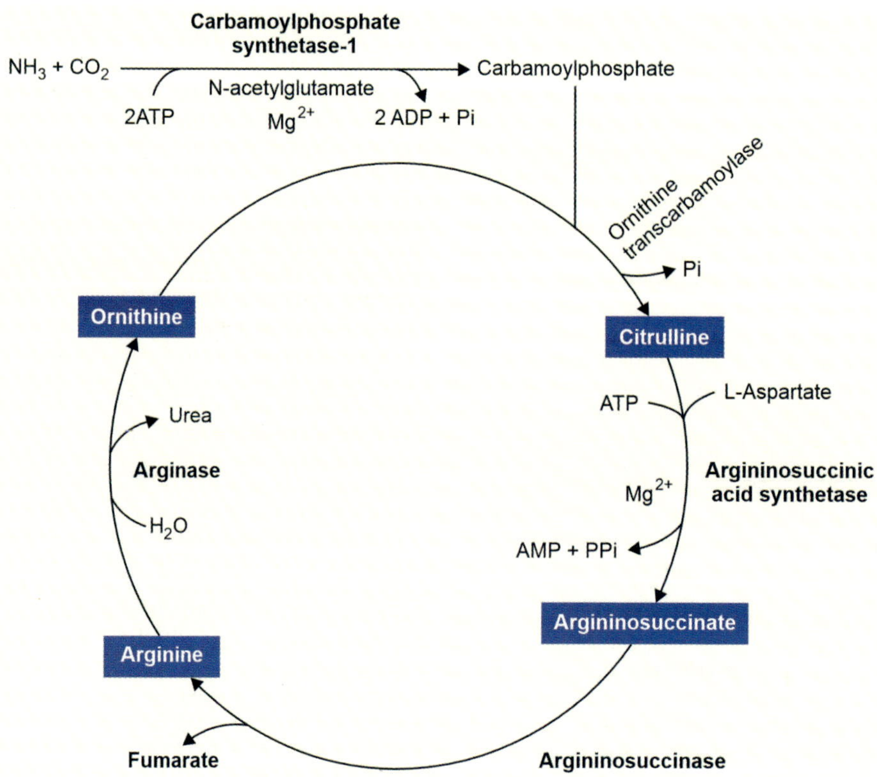

Fig. 14.7: Urea cycle

4. Subsequently, arginine-succinase hydrolyzes arginine-succinate to arginine and fumarate. Fumarate, which is released in this reaction, enters mitochondria where it is converted to oxaloacetate via citric acid cycle. Hence, urea cycle is coupled with the Krebs cycle, both of which were discovered by Sir Hans Krebs and his coworkers. Thus, urea cycle is also called urea bicycle (Krebs-Henseleit cycle).
5. In the last reaction, arginine is hydrolyzed by the enzyme arginase, to ornithine and urea. Ornithine is transported to mitochondria and re-enters the cycle. Urea cycle is the mechanism for the excretion of nitrogen in humans and other primates. In the synthesis of urea, two atoms of nitrogen are derived from two different sources, i.e. from NH_3 and the amino group of aspartic acid.

Inborn Errors of Urea Formation

A defect in any enzyme of the urea cycle may result in an inborn error. In general, since ammonia is very toxic, a metabolic disorder of urea cycle may result in coma and may be potentially fatal (Table 14.3).

Table 14.3: Inborn errors of metabolism of urea cycle

Enzyme	*Disorder*
Carbamoylphosphate synthetase	Hyperammonemia type I
Ornithine trans-carbamoylase	Hyperammonemia type II
Argininosuccinate synthetase	Citrullinemia
Argininosuccinase	Argininosuccinic aciduria
Arginase	Hyperargininemia

AMINO ACIDS FUNCTIONS

PHOSPHOCREATINE FORMATION

Creatine is present in the muscle, liver, kidney and brain. It is stored in the muscle as phosphocreatine (creatine-phosphate). Three amino acids, i.e. glycine, arginine and methionine are used for the synthesis of creatine (Fig. 14.8).

- First, the guanidino group of arginine is transferred to glycine and forms guanido-acetate. This reaction is catalyzed by the enzyme arginine-glycine trans-aminidase, in the kidney.
- Subsequently, guanido-acetate methyl-transferase transfers methyl group from S-adenosylmethionine, in the liver and forms creatine.
- Creatine is stored in muscle as phosphocreatine.

Conversion of Creatine to Phosphocreatine

Phosphocreatine is the form in which high energy phosphate is stored in the muscle. It is **synthesized from creatine by the transfer of a high energy phosphate group from ATP**. This reaction is catalyzed **by creatine-phosphokinase** (CPK), also called creatine kinase (CK).

- During resting condition creatine phosphate is utilized to phosphorylate ADP and creatine is released as creatinine.
- During exercise ATP is used as a source of energy and is converted to ADP.

Creatinine is the **anhydride form of creatine**. As mentioned above, it is **formed in the muscle from creatine phosphate by a nonenzymatic reaction**, irreversibly.

- Creatinine is one of the major nonprotein nitrogenous excretory products. Nearly 1.0–1.5 g of creatinine is excreted in the urine, in 24 hours.
- Its total excretion is independent of the amount of dietary protein but is related to muscle mass.
- Serum creatinine as well as amount of creatinine excreted by an individual remains constant from day to day and by calculating creatinine clearance, one can determine renal function, in terms of glomerular filtration rate.
- Only traces of creatine are normally present in the urine. Large quantities may be excreted in muscular dystrophies, during starvation and pregnancy.

TRANSMETHYLATION

Methionine is an **essential amino acid** and cannot be formed in the body. It is a **glycogenic amino acid**, as the end product of its catabolism is succinyl CoA. Methionine also acts as a **lipotropic factor**.

Metabolism of methionine is outlined in Fig. 14.9.

- The first and the most important step in the metabolism of methionine is catalyzed by adenosyl-transferase, which converts methionine to S-adenosyl-methionine (SAM), also called active methionine.
- Active methionine acts as a methyl carrier and donor, and helps in transmethylation and formation of several methylated products.
- Transmethylation reactions are catalyzed by specific methyltransferases, which transfer a methyl group from SAM to an acceptor molecule.
- Transmethylation reactions are important in the formation of several methylated products of biological significance (Table 14.4).

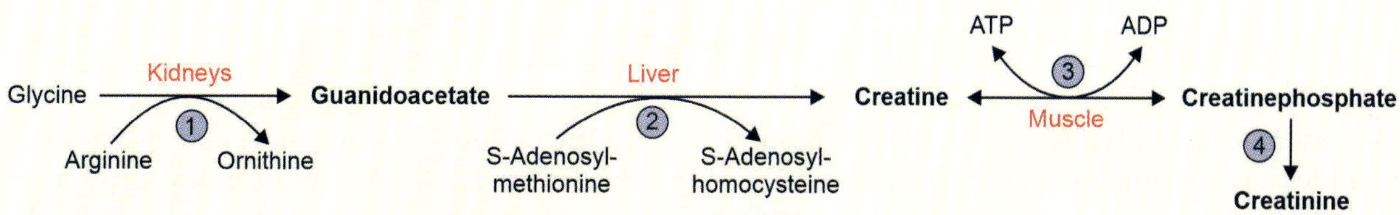

Fig. 14.8: Synthesis of creatine and creatinine: (1) Transaminidase; (2) Methyltransferase; (3) Creatine phosphokinase; (4) Nonenzymatic reaction

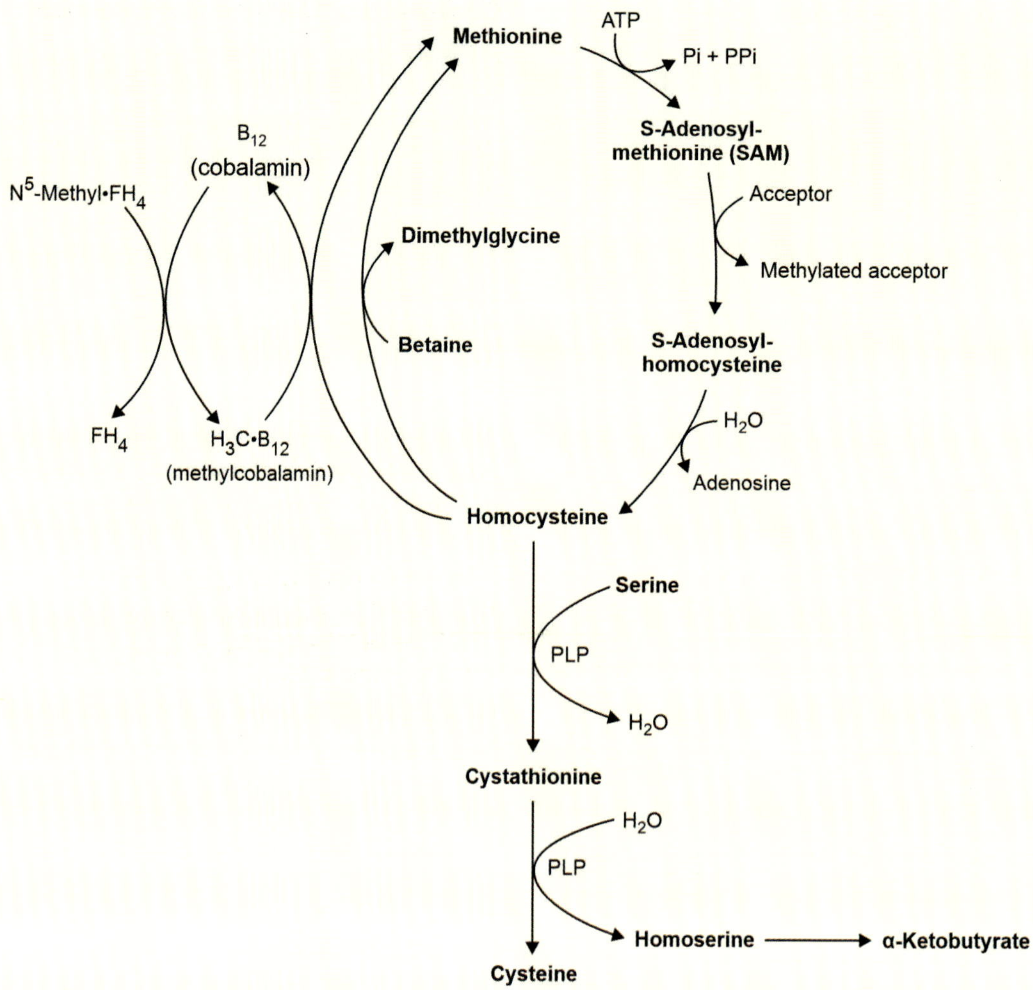

Fig. 14.9: Conversion of methionine to S-adenosylmethionine (active methionine), homocysteine and cysteine

Table 14.4: Use of S-adenosylmethionine (SAM) as a methyl donor

Methyl acceptor	*Product formed*	*Biological significance*
Ethanolamine	Choline	Synthesis of choline-containing phospholipids
Guanidoacetate	Creatine	Synthesis of creatine-phosphate, a high-energy reserve
N-acetylserotonin	Melatonin	Neurotransmitter
Norepinephrine	Epinephrine	Synthesis of catecholamines
Epinephrine	Metanephrine	Metabolite of epinephrine
Bases in DNA and RNA, and amino acids in proteins	Methylated bases in nucleic acids, and methylated amino acids in proteins	Regulation of gene expression

- S-Adenosylmethionine is also used in the synthesis of polyamines, i.e. spermidine and spermine.
- After the transfer of the methyl group, S-adenosylmethionine is converted to S-adenosylhomocysteine.
- In the next step, S-adenosylhomocysteine is converted to homocysteine.
- When cells need to resynthesize methionine, homocysteine-methyl-transferase transfers a methyl group from N^5-methyltetrahydrofolate (N^5-methyl•FH_4) and convert homocysteine to methionine.

Formation of Cysteine

- After removal of the active methyl group, by a methyl-transferase (as discussed above), S-adenosylmethionine is converted to S-adenosylhomocysteine.
- Thereafter, adenosyl-homocysteinase, cleaves the adenosyl moiety (a molecule of adenosine) and forms homocysteine, which has one carbon more than cysteine.
- In the next step, homocysteine is coupled with serine and forms cystathionine. The reaction is catalyzed by the enzyme cystathionine synthase, which also requires pyridoxal phosphate as a coenzyme.
- Thereafter, cystathionine is cleaved by a splitting enzyme, cystathione lyase, also called cystathionase, and forms cysteine and α-keto-butyrate.

FORMATION OF BIOGENIC AMINES

Amines **(biogenic amines or biologically active amines)** are a group of compounds of diverse origins and functions. These are **synthesized from amino acids,** such as serotonin from tryptophan, catecholamines from tyrosine, tyramine from tyrosine, etc.

Catabolism of Tyrosine and Synthesis of Catecholamines

Aromatic amines with a catechol ring (3,4-dihydroxyphenyl ring), i.e. **dopamine, norepinephrine and epinephrine,** are collectively called catecholamines. They have general modulatory effects on overall brain functions, such as mood and arousal.

Dopamine: Dopamine is an intermediate in the synthesis of norepinephrine. It is a **neurotransmitter in nerves** that interconnect nuclei of the basal ganglia in the brain, and **controls voluntary movement**. Damage to these nerves causes Parkinson's disease, which is characterized by tremor and difficulties in initiating and controlling movement.

Norepinephrine: Norepinephrine is a major **transmitter in sympathetic nervous system**. Stimulation of these nerves is responsible for the various features of **fight or flight response** such as stimulation of heart rate, sweating and vasoconstriction in skin, and bronchodilation.

Epinephrine: It is **produced by adrenal medulla** under the influence of acetylcholine-containing nerves analogous to the sympathetic pre-ganglionic nerves. It has **stimulatory effect on glycogen metabolism in the liver.**

Both, norepinephrine and epinephrine are released from the storage vesicles **in adrenal medulla, in response to stress, exercise, cold and low levels of blood glucose.**

Biosynthesis of Catecholamines

In the adrenal medulla, tyrosine is converted to norepinephrine (noradrenaline) and epinephrine (adrenaline), the two hyperglycemic hormones, secreted by the gland.

- First, **tyrosine** is converted **to** dihydroxyphenylalanine **(DOPA)** by the enzyme tyrosine hydroxylase.
- Thereafter, DOPA-decarboxylase converts **DOPA to dopamine**, which enters the storage granules as an active neurotransmitter.
- In the next step, **dopamine** is converted to norepinephrine by dopamine-β-hydroxylase.

  Norepinephrine is a hormone, present in sympathetic nerve endings. Its synthesis is regulated by plasma tyrosine in the brain.
- In the next step, methylation of **norepinephrine** by the enzyme phenyl-ethanolamine-N-methyl-transferase (PNMT), converts it **to epinephrine**. In this reaction active methionine (S-adenosylmethionine) is used as a methyl donor (Fig. 14.10).

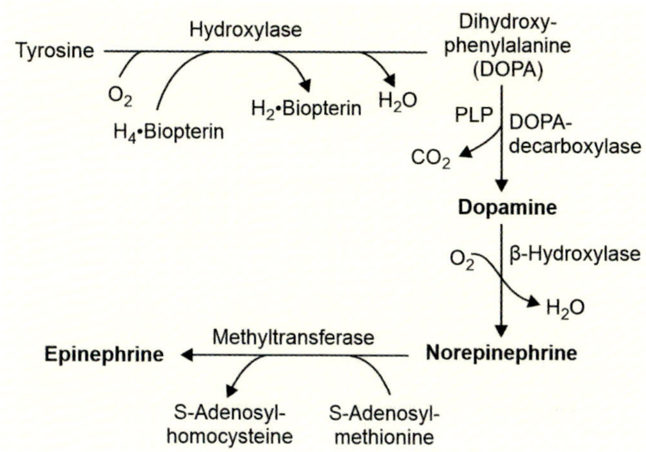

Fig. 14.10: Synthesis of catecholamines from tyrosine in the adrenal medulla

Metabolism of Tryptophan and Synthesis of Serotonin

Serotonin, also called **5-hydroxy-tryptamine** (5-HT), is derived **from tryptophan**. It is a neurotransmitter (in the brain), a **vasoconstrictor** and **bronchoconstrictor**. It has multiple physiological roles, including **pain perception and regulation of sleep, temperature and blood pressure**. It also **increases mobility of the gastrointestinal tract.**

Serotonin-producing tumor cells in the intestine result in a condition referred to as **malignant carcinoid syndrome**, also called **argentaffinoma,** because this tumor arises from the intestinal argentaffin cells, that normally secrete serotonin. There is an **increased production of serotonin** that causes **flushing, anxiety and gastrointestinal upset.** Since serotonin is normally catabolized to 5-hydroxyindoleacetic acid (5-HIAA), in this condition, urinary excretion of 5-HIAA is increased by more than 50-fold and its estimation is used to establish the diagnosis.

- **In the platelets, brain and intestinal epithelium, tryptophan** is hydroxylated by tryptophan hydroxylase, **to** form **5-hydroxytryptophan.**
- **5-Hydroxytryptophan** is subsequently decarboxylated **to 5-hydroxytryptamine,** also **called serotonin,** by a decarboxylase (Fig. 14.11).

Synthesis of Melatonin

Melatonin is a **sleep-inducing substance and maintains circadian rhythm of sleep wake cycle**. It also **inhibits synthesis and secretion of other neurotransmitters,** such as dopamine and GABA.

It is synthesized from serotonin in the pineal gland and retina, where acetyltransferase converts serotonin into **N-acetyl-5-methoxytryptamine,** also called melatonin (Fig. 14.12).

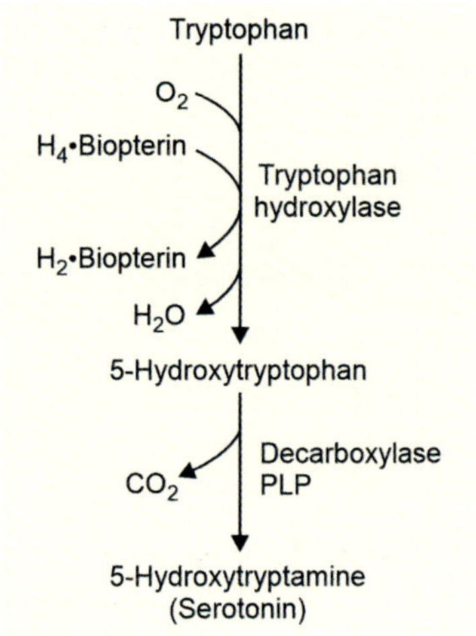

Fig. 14.11: Synthesis of serotonin from tryptophan

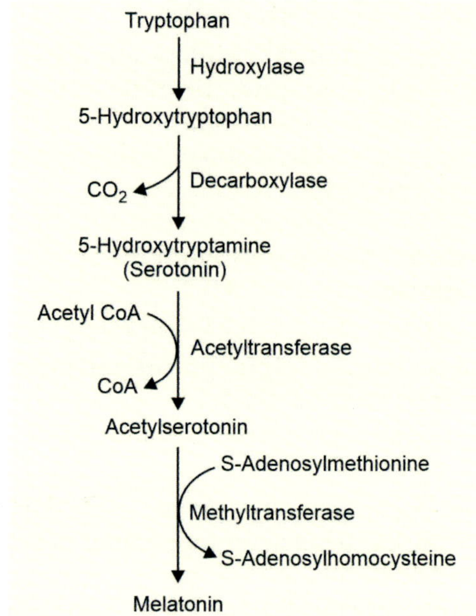

Fig. 14.12: Synthesis of melatonin from tryptophan

ONE-CARBON TRANSFER

Amino acids, such as histidine, serine and methionine, also **serve as a source of one-carbon moiety** whereas **tetrahydrofolate** (FH_4) **serves,** both, **as acceptor as well as donor of one-carbon** (1-C) unit, in a variety of reactions involved in amino acid and nucleotide metabolism. For example:

1. **Folic acid** is, firstly, converted to **N^5-formyl-tetrahydrofolic acid** (N^5-CHO–FH_4) or folinic acid in the liver and is, thus, used in the transfer of one carbon (one carbon moiety) from a donor to the acceptor molecule (Fig. 14.13).
2. Besides formyl (–CHO), 1-C may be transferred in the form of formate (–HCOO–), methenyl (= CH–),

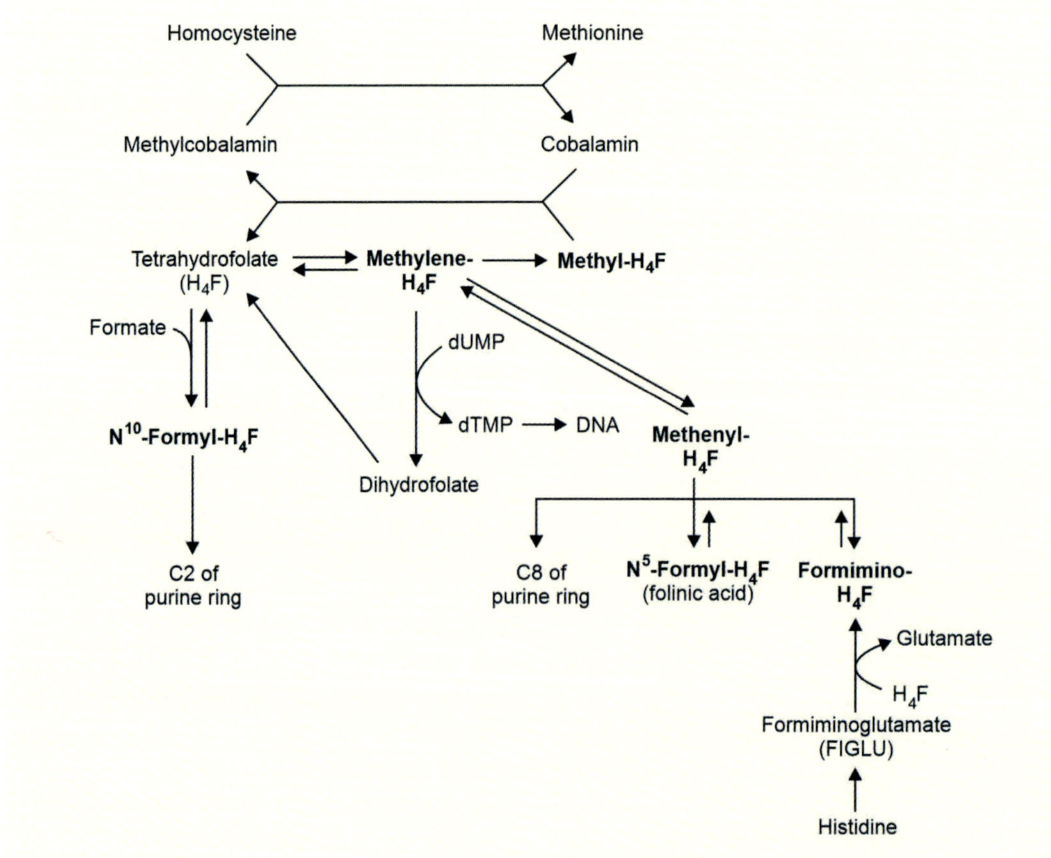

Fig. 14.13: Interrelationships between cobalamin, folate and 1–C metabolism

methylene ($-CH_2-$), methyl ($-CH_3$), hydroxymethyl ($-CH_2OH$) or formimino ($-CH = NH$) groups.

3. The various forms are interconvertible to one another by $NADP^+$ or NAD^+-dependent dehydrogenases.
4. The **one-carbon** moiety carried by FH_4 may be **utilized** in many reactions, such as it acts as **in the conversion of glycine to serine, homocysteine to methionine,** as **carbon atom 2 and 8 in** biosynthesis of a **purine** ring, in the conversion of **uracil to thymine**, and in the biosynthesis of choline.
5. In some of these reactions, vitamin B_{12} (cobalamin) is also used.

INBORN ERRORS OF AMINO ACID METABOLISM

Phenylketonuria

Phenylketonuria **(PKU)** is an **inborn error of phenylalanine metabolism**. It is an autosomal recessive disorder due to the **deficiency of hepatic phenylalanine hydroxylase**. As a result of it, phenylalanine cannot be converted to tyrosine, and thus, in PKU tyrosine becomes dietary essential.

In PKU, due to the deficiency of phenylalanine hydroxylase, phenylalanine is utilized an alternate pathway, where:

- **Phenylalanine** is first **converted to phenyl-pyruvic acid** by the enzyme phenylalanine transaminase.
- Subsequently, phenylpyruvate is also reduced to **phenyl-lactic acid** as well as decarboxylated to **phenylacetic acid** (Fig. 14.14).

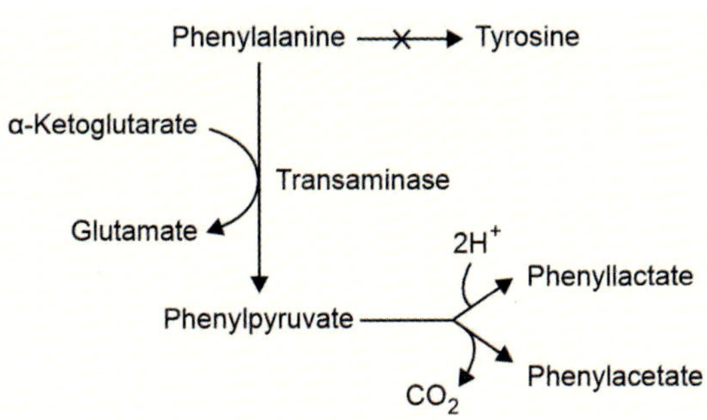

Fig. 14.14: Conversion of phenylalanine to phenylketoacids in phenylketonuria

Due to increased urinary excretion of phenyl-pyruvic acid (a phenyl-ketone), this disease is called phenylketonuria. Increased levels of phenyl-keto acids in blood cause **mental retardation and convulsions.** Such infants (patients with PKU) are given diets which are low in phenylalanine but contain tyrosine.

Tyrosinemias

Complete or partial deficiency of tyrosine amino-transferase results in tyrosinemia, which, in turn, leads to the accumulation and excretion of tyrosine and its metabolites.

There are two types of tyrosinemias:

- **Tyrosinemia type I:** It is also called **hepatorenal tyrosinemia**. It is caused by the **deficiency of fumarylacetoacetate hydrolase** and is characterized by **liver failure, renal tubular dysfunction, rickets and polyneuropathy**.
- **Tyrosinemia type II:** It is also called **oculocutaneous tyrosinemia**. It is due to the **deficiency of tyrosine transaminase**. It results in **eye and skin lesions**, and **mental retardation**.

Alkaptonuria

Alkaptonuria is due to hereditary **deficiency** of the enzyme **homogentisic acid oxidase.** These individuals excrete homogentisic acid in their urine. **Homogentisic acid**, in turn, gets **auto-oxidized** and is, subsequently, **polymerized** to form intensely dark substance, referred to as **alkapton**. Dark urine is the only consequence of this condition, in early life.

Homogentisate is slowly **oxidized** and **deposited in the bone, connective tissue and other organs**. This condition is called **ochronosis** because of ochre color of the pigment.

Albinism

Lack of tyrosinase in melanocytes affects the synthesis of melanin and leads to the **formation of white patches on the skin and iris** in the eyes. This condition is referred to as albinism.

Lack of the pigment in the skin makes the albinos more **sensitive to sunlight and increases the risk** of carcinoma of skin. Lack of the pigment in the eyes contributes to **photophobia**.

Some Important Questions

1. **Outline urea cycle. What is the site of urea synthesis? What is the need for urea synthesis in the body?**
2. **Describe various mechanisms of the removal of ammonia from amino acids.**
3. **How is ammonia removed from the body?**
4. **Explain how tyrosine is metabolized. Describe biologically important compounds derived from it?**
5. **Describe fate of phenylalanine in the body.**

6. Name enzymes and coenzymes of the following reactions:
   i. Synthesis of carbamoylphosphate
   ii. Conversion of serotonin to melatonin.

7. Name important biologically active compounds derived from:
   i. Tyrosine
   ii. Tryptophan

8. Discuss briefly:
   i. Biosynthesis of phosphocreatine
   ii. Utilization of proteins for energy
   iii. Reactions of urea cycle
   iv. Synthesis of urea and its inborn errors
   v. Transamination and its importance
   vi. Transmethylation
   vii. Processes of the removal of NH_3 from amino acids

9. Write notes on:
   i. Alkaptonuria
   ii. Catabolism of tyrosine
   iii. Phenylketonuria
   iv. Removal of ammonia from the body
   v. Deamination
   vi. Active methionine

Chapter 15

Metabolic Integration

Metabolism is the sum of all chemical changes in the body. It consists of the sum of anabolism (synthesis) and catabolism (degradation) with the release of energy, and achieving a fairly constant internal environment referred to as homeostasis, the state of steady internal, physical and chemical conditions maintained by the living systems. The central theme of metabolism is to extract energy from food, store excess of the energy for future needs, and to maintain tissue proteins for performing various vital functions.

METABOLIC PROCESSES THAT OCCUR IN SPECIFIC ORGANS DURING FED AND FASTING STATE

The homeostatic range of blood sugar is regulated within fairly narrow limits, despite changes in the environment, diet or level of physical activity. In humans, the primary sensors for this are the beta cells of the islets of pancreas, which secrete insulin.

- **In the fed state** there is an **increase in blood sugar** concentration, which in turn, **stimulates the beta cells to secrete insulin** into the blood and, simultaneously, **inhibits** the alpha cells from **secreting glucagon**.
- **In the fasting state** there is a **fall in blood glucose** concentration, which causes **insulin secretion to be stopped**, and **glucagon to be secreted** from the alpha cells into the blood. This, in turn, **inhibits the uptake of glucose** from the blood by the insulin sensitive cells.

This combination, i.e. **high blood insulin and low glucagon** levels, **act on** the effector tissues, chief of which are the **liver**, fat cells **(adipocytes)** and **muscle cells.**

THE LIVER

Liver occupies a central position and maintains circulating levels of all the fuels for their oxidation by the other tissues, mainly brain and muscle. One of the important functions of the liver is to maintain blood glucose homeostasis. After a carbohydrate rich meal, i.e. in the postabsorptive state, when blood glucose concentration is high, liver takes up glucose from circulation and converts it to glucose-6-phosphate, which is used through various routes, depending upon the need of the body.

Metabolic Integration in the Liver in the Fed State

In the fed state, when **blood glucose concentration is high**, the liver is **inhibited** from **producing glucose**. For this purpose:

- Liver **converts glucose into glycogen and triglycerides.**
- **Glycogen is stored in the liver**, whereas the **triglycerides are secreted into the blood as VLDL** particles (very low-density lipoprotein).
- VLDL particles are **taken up by the adipose tissue** and **stored** there **as** triacylglycerols **(fat)**
- **Amino acids,** which are absorbed from the gut, are **taken up by the muscle** and **stored** there **as proteins** (Fig. 15.1).

Metabolic Integration in the Liver During Fasting

In the fasting state, a **fall in blood glucose** concentration causes **insulin secretion** to be **stopped** and **glucagon** to be **secreted** from the alpha cells into the blood. This, in turn, **inhibits the uptake of glucose** from the blood **by the liver, fat cells and muscle**. For this purpose:

- Liver is stimulated to **release glucose from glycogen, through glycogenolysis.**
- **Glucose synthesis is** also stimulated from noncarbohydrate sources, such as glucogenic amino acids (received by the liver as a result of proteolysis of tissue proteins, mainly the muscle) and glycerol (obtained from adipose tissue, as a result of hydrolysis of triacylglycerols), **by** the process of **gluconeogenesis.**
- **Glucose,** thus produced, is **released into the blood,** thereby, **correcting hypoglycemia** and is also **transported to the brain for its use** there.
- A **fall in** the circulating concentration of **insulin** also **results in** the **release of free fatty acids** (from triacylglycerols) from the adipose tissue. These are **taken up by the liver and muscle.**

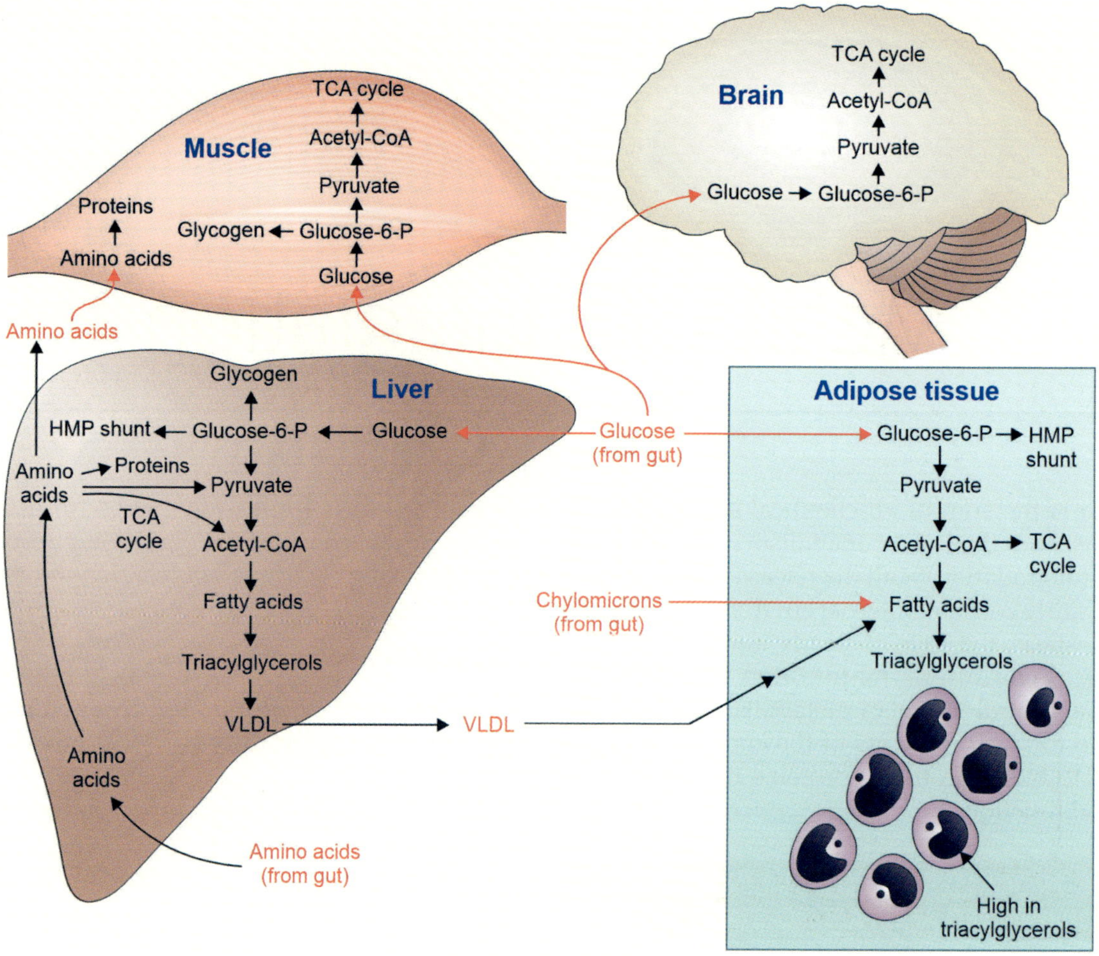

Fig. 15.1: Metabolic processes that take place in the specific organs in the fed state

- **Peripheral muscles and liver consume**, progressively, less glucose and switch-over to **fatty acids as the main source of energy.**
- This, in turn, **promotes β-oxidation of fatty acids,** increases the production of acetyl CoA and stimulates ketogenesis. As a result of it, plasma concentration of **ketone bodies is increased**.
- **Ketone bodies are** released into the blood are **used by many tissues, including muscle and brain** (Fig. 15.2).

THE ADIPOSE TISSUE

The adipose tissue, also known as fat cells, is a loose connective tissue composed, mostly, of adipocytes that are specialized in storing energy, as triacylglycerols (fat).

There are **two types of adipose tissue,** known as **white adipose tissue** (which **stores energy**) and **brown adipose tissue** (which **generates body heat**).

White adipose tissue is widely distributed throughout the body, but is most prominent **under the skin**, and in the **abdominal cavity and skeletal muscle**.

The **main role of the white adipose tissue is to store energy** (in the form of triacylglycerols) and release fatty acids, when needed.

Metabolic Integration in the Adipose Tissue in the Fed State

- **Adipocytes take up glucose** through GLUT4 (the special glucose transporters, whose number in the cell wall is increased as a direct effect of insulin acting on these cells).
- **Glucose that enters the fat cells**, in this manner, is **converted into triglycerides** (via the same metabolic pathways as used by the liver), which are stored there, together with the VLDL-derived triglycerides (from the liver) as well as in chylomicrons from the gut (Fig. 15.1).

Metabolic Integration in the Adipose Tissue During Fasting

- **A fall in** the circulating concentration of **insulin promotes lipolysis in the adipose tissue and releases free fatty acids and glycerol** (from triacylglycerols), which enter liver.
- **Fatty acids** also **enter muscle** and are **consumed** there **as the main source of energy** (Fig. 15.2).

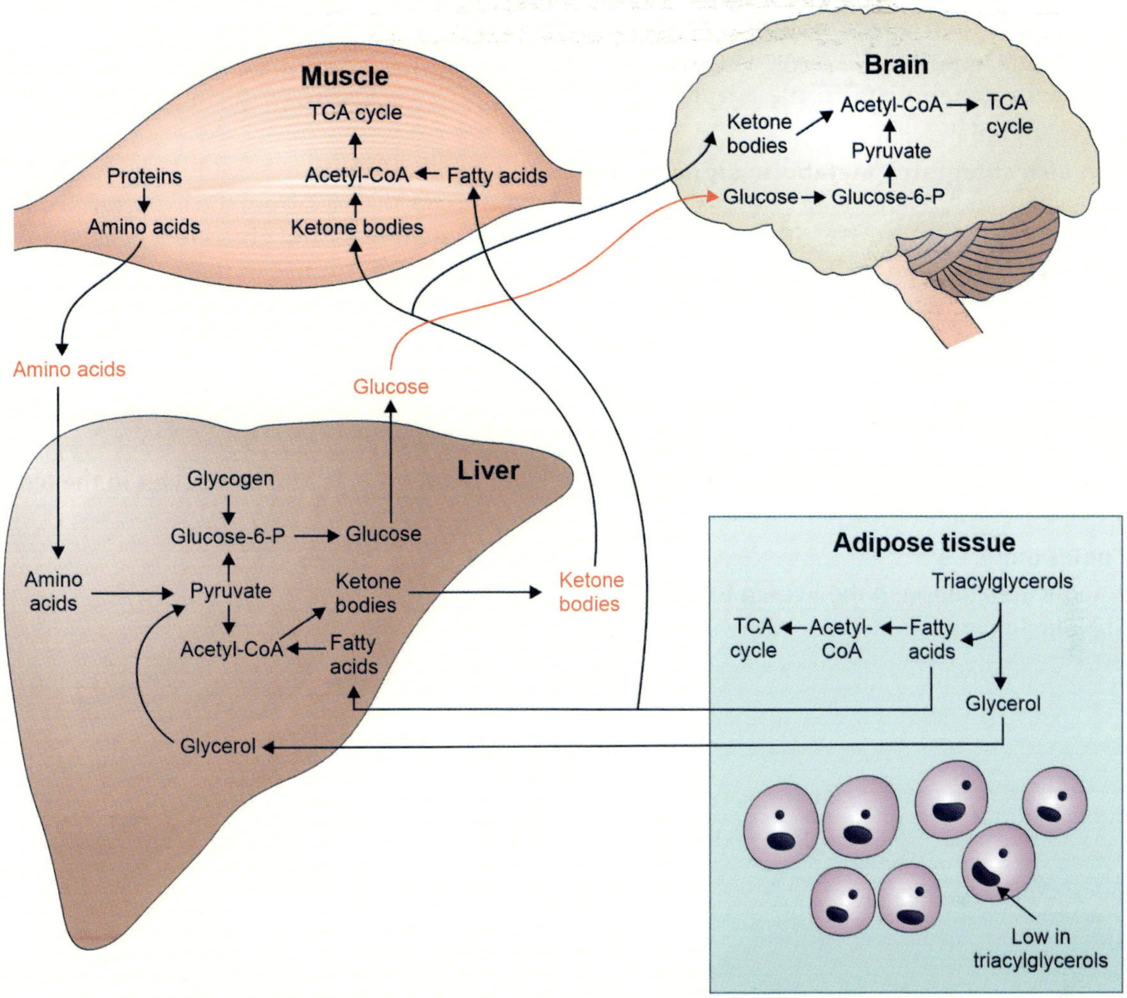

Fig. 15.2: Metabolic processes that take place in the specific organs in the fasting state

THE MUSCLE

The muscle cell, also known as **myocyte**, is the type of cell found in muscle tissue. Myocytes develop from myoblasts to form muscles in a process known as myogenesis. There are two specialized forms of myocytes with distinct properties, **cardiac and smooth muscle cells**. On the other hand, **skeletal muscles** are formed by morphological units referred to as muscle fibers.

- **Cardiomyocytes** are the cells that form the chambers of the heart, and have a single central nucleus.
- **Skeletal muscle fibers** help support and move the body.
- **Smooth muscle cells** control involuntary movements, such as the peristalsis contractions in the esophagus and stomach.

Metabolic Integration in Muscles in the Fed State

- **Skeletal muscle,** similar to live, **takes up glucose,** through insulin-sensitive GLUT4, and **converts it to glycogen,** which is **stored** there. The glycogen stored in the muscle remains in the muscle, and is only **broken-down during exercise,** to glucose-6-phosphate and thence, to pyruvate (to be used in the citric acid cycle) and lactate (which is returned to the blood, taken up by the liver and converted to glucose by gluconeogenesis).
- Via liver, **amino acids enter the muscle** and are **stored as proteins** (Fig. 15.1).

Metabolic Integration in Muscles During Fasting

- **Free fatty acids** (released from triacylglycerols) are **taken up by the muscle** and are **used as the source of energy**.
- **Ketone bodies,** released from liver into the blood, **are also used by muscle as a source of energy.**
- **Proteins are degraded** and the **amino acids are** transported to the liver, where they are **used for the synthesis of glucose, by** the process of **gluconeogenesis** (Fig. 15.2).

THE BRAIN

The brain, particularly, the **hypothalamus, plays a key role in** the homeostatic **regulation of energy and**

glucose metabolism. It **modulates** various aspects of metabolism, such as **food intake, energy expenditure, insulin secretion, hepatic glucose production and glucose/fatty acid metabolism in the adipose tissue and the skeletal muscle**.

The brain also **integrates metabolic signals from peripheral tissues** (such as the liver, pancreas, adipose tissue, gut and muscle) and **modulates various processes that consume energy** (such as locomotor activity, fatty acid oxidation in the skeletal muscle, and thermogenesis).

Metabolic Integration in the Brain in the Fed State

Glucose, as we know, is the **primary fuel of the brain** under normal conditions and that it requires a steady supply of glucose from the blood.

Metabolic Integration in the Brain During Fasting

- **Glucose,** released from the liver (formed **as a result of glycogenolysis and gluconeogenesis), is transported to the brain, for use** in there.
- **Ketone bodies, released from liver** into the blood, **are also used by the brain as a source of energy** (Fig. 15.2).

Some Important Questions

1. **Discuss the metabolic processes that take place in the liver, brain, muscle and adipocytes in the fed and fasting states.**
2. **Write notes on:**
   i. Metabolic integration in the liver in the fed state
   ii. Metabolic integration the liver in the fasting state

Unit V

Special Aspects of Metabolism

Chapter

16

Detoxication

Detoxification refers to the **ability of the body to abolish or reduce toxicity of a chemical substance to its excretory metabolite**. Though not always true, majority of the metabolites are comparatively, more acidic, less toxic and more water-soluble than the original compound. Since most of these chemical substances are foreign to our life, so generally, these chemical substances are also referred to as **xenobiotics**.

DETOXICATION REACTIONS

Most of the toxic **compounds** are highly lipophilic. They **accumulate within the cells** and **interfere with the normal cellular functions**, over a period of time.

Generally, these toxic substances are **metabolized in the liver** and the metabolites so produced are relatively more water-soluble and **pass** via blood **to the kidney for excretion**. Besides, some of the metabolites may also be excreted **via feces, bile or the expired air**.

A small portion of the metabolite may, however, also return to the intestine, by enterohepatic circulation. The xenobiotic or its metabolite may also bind to a cellular macromolecule, such as DNA, RNA or protein, and may be retained in the tissues. The binding of a xenobiotic or its metabolite, however, can cause serious consequences, such as mutations.

Typical Detoxification Reactions can be Divided into Phase I and Phase II

Phase I Reactions

Lipophilic xenobiotics are often first metabolized in phase I, by the enzymes which function to make xenobiotics more polar and provide sites for conjugation reactions. In the phase I of reactions, a xenobiotic may undergo **oxidation (hydroxylation), reduction or hydrolysis** and the metabolite so produced may either be excreted as such or undergoes phase II of metabolism.

- **Oxidation:** Compounds detoxified by the oxidative processes include alcohols, aldehydes, amines and their derivatives, aromatic hydrocarbons, and certain drugs.
  - **Alcohols:** Aliphatic as well as aromatic alcohols are oxidized to their corresponding acids. For example:
    Methanol → Formic acid
    Ethanol → Acetic acid
    Benzyl alcohol → Benzoic acid
  - **Aldehydes:** Aldehydes are also oxidized to their corresponding acids. For example:
    Benzaldehyde → Benzoic acid
    Trichloro-aldehyde → Trichloro-acetic acid
  - **Amines:** ***Primary aliphatic amines*** are oxidized to their acids and liberate ammonia. For example:
    $RCH_2–NH_2$ → R–COOH + Ammonia
    On the other hand, aromatic amines are oxidized to phenols.
  - **Anilides:** Anilides are oxidized to the corresponding phenols. For example:
    Acetanilide → p-Acetyl-aminophenol
  - **Aromatic hydrocarbons:** These are oxidized to phenols, e.g. oxidation of benzene produces several aromatic alcohols, such as phenols, quinols and catechols. The process, thus, involves the introduction of an –OH group (hydroxylation) onto the aromatic ring. This, in turn, provides a site for the attachment of a conjugating group in the phase II reaction.
    Some **epoxides** formed during the oxidation of xenobiotics are strong electrophiles and hence are very reactive. These may be converted to relatively inactive hydroxyl compounds by the enzyme epoxide hydrolase, which in turn, provides an –OH group for the conjugating molecule.
  - **Drugs:** Some drugs may be oxidized to their hydroxy derivatives. For example:
    Meprobamate → Hydroxy-meprobamate.
- **Reduction:** Some of the xenobiotics during the course of their detoxification undergo reduction. For example:
  Picric acid → Picramic acid
  Trichloroacetaldehyde → Trichloro-ethanol

Sometimes, a reduced metabolite may be more toxic than the original xenobiotic, e.g. prontosil (an azo red dye) is reduced to the more toxic sulfanilamide.

- **Hydrolysis:** Some of the xenobiotics, particularly certain therapeutic compounds, undergo hydrolysis during the course of their detoxification, e.g. aspirin, procaine, etc.
  Aspirin (acetylsalicylic acid) → Acetate + Salicylic acid
  Procaine → ρ-Aminobenzoic acid + Diethyl-aminoethanol
  Aspirin (acetylsalicylic acid) undergoes hydrolysis and produces acetate and salicylic acid. Acetate so formed may be either oxidized or used for the synthesis of various physiological compounds. On the other hand, salicylic acid is excreted by the kidneys after conjugation with glucuronic acid.

Though some xenobiotics may undergo conjugation directly and the conjugate, so produced, is excreted as such without undergoing a preliminary reaction in phase I but conjugation, more often, occurs as a phase II reaction (Fig. 16.1).

Phase II Reactions

Phase II reactions are the conjugation reactions which are catalyzed by the conjugating enzymes that directly interact with the xenobiotics, but more commonly with the metabolites produced in phase I reactions. The metabolite of the phase I reaction is subsequently conjugated with some other compound (such as glycine) or group (like a methyl group) in the phase II reaction.

By conjugation the molecule becomes more polar and highly water soluble, which can be easily excreted from the body. Most of the conjugation reactions are synthetic processes and thus require energy.

The conjugation of a xenobiotic (X) with the conjugating molecule (Y) can occur via two different pathways, i.e. either the X or the Y gets activated and subsequently conjugates with the other molecule:

$$X \rightarrow X{\sim}Y \rightarrow X{\sim}Y$$
$$Y \rightarrow Y{\sim}X \rightarrow X{\sim}Y$$

Compounds Used for Conjugation in Phase II

Compounds used for conjugation in phase II include readily available reactants, such as glutathione, amino acids like glycine or glutamine, glucuronate (as UDP glucuronic acid), a sulfate group, an acetyl group or a methyl group:

- **Glucuronic acid:** Glucuronic acid is an oxidation product of glucose. It participates in detoxification reactions as UDP-glucuronic acid, which gets conjugated with a xenobiotic (X-OH) and forms a highly soluble excretory glucuronide (X-O-glucuronide). This reaction is catalyzed by UDP-glucuronyl-transferase present, both, in the endoplasmic reticulum as well as cytosol of many tissues, but mainly in the liver (Fig. 16.2).

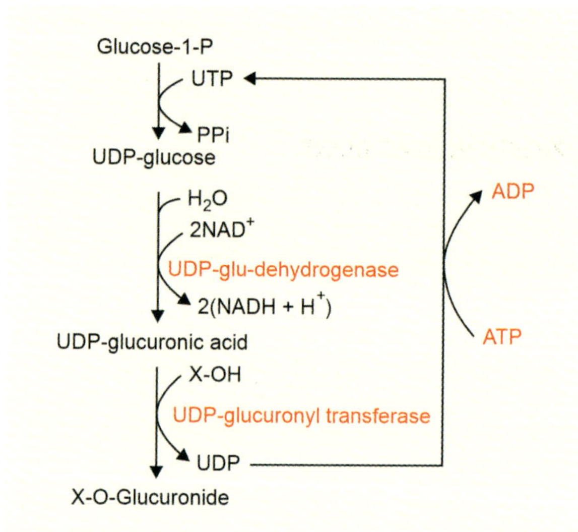

Fig. 16.2: Conjugation of xenobiotic (X-OH) with glucuronic acid

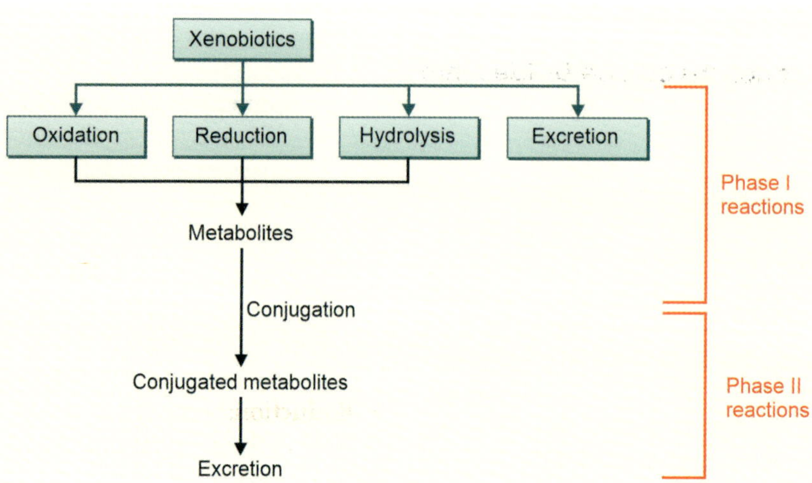

Fig. 16.1: Mechanisms of biotransformation of xenobiotics

Various compounds, such as benzoic acid, morphine, methanol and camphor are excreted in conjugation with glucuronic acid. Endogenously produced bilirubin is also conjugated in the liver with glucuronic acid.

Benzoic acid + UDP-glucuronic acid → Benzoyl-glucuronide + UDP

Bilirubin + UDP-glucuronic acid → Bilirubin monoglucuronide

Bilirubin monoglucuronide + UDP-glucuronic acid → Bilirubin diglucuronide + UDP

- **Glutathione:** A wide range of organic compounds, which are toxic electrophiles such as aromatic halogenated compounds, aliphatic halides, sulfates, nitro-compounds and carcinogenic epoxides (formed from polycyclic hydrocarbons), are excreted after conjugation with the cysteinyl moiety of glutathione (a tripeptide of glutamate, cysteine and glycine).

  A xenobiotic (H–X) after conjugation with glutathione forms mercapturic acid. This reaction is catalyzed by a group of enzymes referred to as glutathione-S-transferases. These are present in various tissues with high amounts in the liver cytosol.
  - In the initial reaction, reduced glutathione (GSH) reacts with an electrophilic center on the xenobiotic.
  - The glutamyl and glycinyl groups are sequentially removed.
  - Subsequently, an acetyl group is added (from acetyl-CoA) to the amino group of the remaining cysteinyl residue which is bound to the xenobiotic (X-cysteine).
  - The resulting compound, a mercapturic acid, i.e. a conjugate of acetylcysteine, is excreted in the urine (Fig. 16.3).

  Due to conjugation with glutathione, large doses of some of the drugs such as paracetamol, leads to depletion of glutathione in the liver.

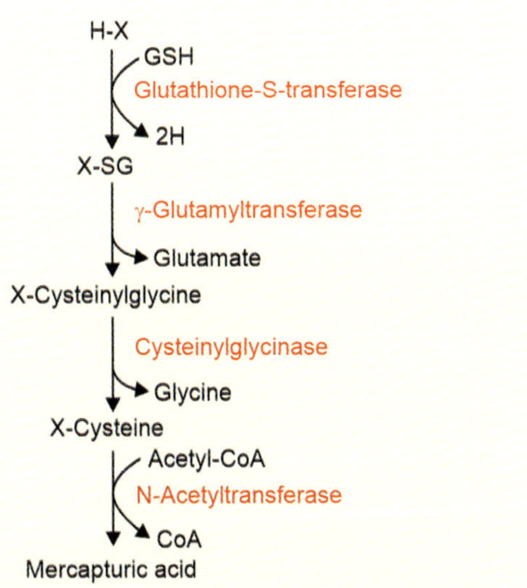

Fig. 16.3: Conjugation of xenobiotic (H-X) with glutathione (GSH)

- **Glycine:** Glycine conjugates with many aromatic carboxylic acids, e.g. benzoic acid, cholic acid, etc. Glycine conjugates are harmless compounds and are excreted in the urine.

  Benzoic acid + Glycine → Benzoyl glycine (hippuric acid)

  Cholic acid + Glycine → Glycocholic acid
- **Glutamine:** Phenylacetic acid is detoxified by conjugation with glutamine.

  Phenylacetic acid + Glutamine → Phenylacetyl-glutamine
- **Sulfate:** Biosynthesis of a sulfate ester requires some high energy sulfate donor, i.e. 3′-phosphoadenosine-5′-phosphor-sulfate (PAPS or active sulfate). Transfer of the sulfate group, from active sulfate, to various acceptors, such as phenol and indole, is catalyzed by specific sulf-transferases.
- **Acetate:** As for other acetylation reactions, active acetate (acetyl-CoA) is used as an acetyl donor. Acetylation of a xenobiotic is catalyzed by acetyltransferases present in the cytosol of various tissues, mainly in the liver. Many drugs such as sulfanilamide and isoniazid are metabolized by acetylation.
- **Methyl group:** The methyl group of S-adenosylmethionine (SAM or active methionine) is used by methyltransferases to methylate a xenobiotic, mainly various pyridine derivatives. Many of the methylated products though are less toxic than the parent xenobiotic, some of these however, are more toxic, e.g. excess dose of nicotinamide after methylation is converted to a more toxic product (methyl-nicotinamide).

EXAMPLES OF TOXIC COMPOUNDS

Toxic compounds (xenobiotics) include foreign substances or **exogenous chemicals** (excluding antigen) which our body does not recognize, such as **drugs, pollutants, some food additives and cosmetics**, etc. (Table 16.1).

Table 16.1: Sources of xenobiotics

Sources	*Examples*
Industrial chemicals	Solvents (benzene, carbon tetrachloride) Detergents Bleaching agents
Air pollutants Food additives and contaminants	Tobacco smoke Colors (butter yellow, azo dye) Sweeteners (saccharin) Insecticides
Bacterial metabolites Cosmetics Drugs	Bacterial toxins Lipstick, hair dyes, body sprays Aspirin, tranquilizers, oral contraceptives

A xenobiotic **may enter the body by various routes,** such as by:

- **Inhalation of the polluted air**, e.g. industrial chemicals and automobile exhaust
- **Ingestion of contaminated food**, such as those contaminated with pesticides, insecticides or herbicides
- **Food additives** including colors and sweeteners, like butter yellow, azo dye or saccharin
- **Cosmetics**, such as hair dyes, sprays or lipstick
- **Drugs, such as aspirin**, tranquilizers or oral contraceptives
- **Some of the toxic metabolites**, which are formed by the action of bacteria on food in the gastrointestinal tract, such as amines produced by the decarboxylation of the unabsorbed amino acids.
- **Certain endogenous substances**, which are produced in the body, e.g bilirubin (produced during normal metabolism of the red blood cells) or phenols (produced in large intestine by the action of bacteria on tryptophan).

Some Important Questions

1. **What is detoxification? Describe various types of xenobiotic detoxification reactions.**
2. **Write note on:**
   i. Detoxification of xenobiotics.
   ii. Reactions of xenobiotic detoxification.
   iii. Phase I reactions of xenobiotics detoxification.
   iv. Phase II reactions of xenobiotic detoxification.
   v. Role of glucuronic acid in xenobiotic detoxification.
   vi. Role of glutathione in xenobiotic detoxification.

Chapter

17

Oxygen Toxicity

Oxygen is **essential for our life** as **we know that we cannot survive without oxygen**. All the **living beings** on earth **use oxygen** and **produce carbon dioxide**. Carbon dioxide, in turn, is **utilized by plants to regenerate oxygen**.

- In our body **most of the oxygen** (more than 90%), we inhale, **is utilized in oxidative phosphorylation** for the **generation of** energy, in the form of **ATP**.
- A **small percentage** of oxygen (5–8%) in our body is also **utilized in several enzymatic reactions for** the **hydroxylation and oxygenation of various compounds** during their metabolism.
- A **very small quantity of oxygen**, however, **is** also **used in biological redox reactions**, where **oxygen is activated by the redox active metal ions**, such as iron and copper. These metal ions form **components of** the **various metal-containing enzymes** and proteins, e.g. cytochrome oxidase, hemoglobin, etc.

In some of the reactions, these metal ions **provide one electron**, at a time, **to oxygen** and **activate it to** various **strong oxidizing forms**. It is **the last fraction of oxygen** which **form oxygen toxicity products**, that are **potentially harmful. These damaging molecules** are called **reactive oxygen species** (ROS) and **reactive nitrogen species** (RNS), including **free radicals** and **nonradicals** (Table 17.1).

REACTIVE OXYGEN SPECIES

Partial reduction of the molecular oxygen leads to formation of a number of ROS, including free radicals and nonradicals (Fig. 17.1).

- **The first product** formed, **due to the reduction of molecular oxygen, is** called **superoxide anion** ($O_2^{\bullet-}$), which is **a free radical**.

Table 17.1: Oxygen toxicity products

Reactive oxygen species
Superoxide anion ($O2^{\bullet-}$)
Hydrogen peroxide (H_2O_2)
Hydroxyl radical ($OH^{\bullet-}$)
Reactive nitrogen species
Peroxy-nitrite ($ONOO^-$)
Nitric oxide (NO)

- **Reduction of the superoxide anion yields hydrogen peroxide** (H_2O_2), which is a **nonradical ROS.**
- **Reduction of H_2O_2** by a cleavage reaction result in the **formation of hydroxyl radical** ($OH^{\bullet-}$), which is **a free radical**.
- **Reduction of hydroxyl free radical** results in the **formation of water**, which is the end product of complete reduction of oxygen.

REACTIVE NITROGEN SPECIES

Reduction of various nitrogenous compounds such as sulfhydryl proteins and several nitrogenous compounds lead to the **formation of** a number of nitrogen-based reactive species called reactive nitrogen species **(RNS)**. These include:

- **Peroxy-nitrite** ($ONOO^-$), and
- **Nitric oxide** (NO).

FREE RADICALS

The reactive chemical species **(ROS and RNS)** which have a **very short life span** and **one or more unpaired electron**(s) are referred to as free radicals.

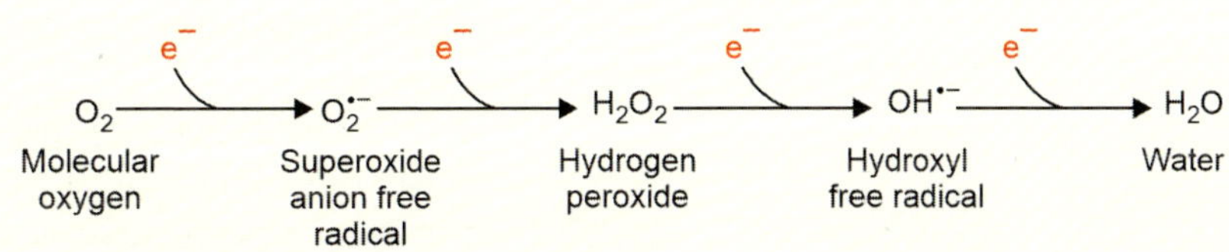

Fig. 17.1: Formation of reactive oxygen species from molecular oxygen (e^- = electron)

Sources of free Radicals

Both, **exogenous** as well as **endogenous substances** can produce free radicals with in the cells and their surroundings. These are continuously produced within the cells due to:

- **Nonenzymatic reactions of various organic compounds with oxygen.**
- **Ionizing radiation**.
- Result of **electron transfer processes in mitochondria** (mitochondrial electron transport chain).
- **Activities of various oxidizing enzymes** such as NADPH oxidase, nitric oxide synthase, xanthine oxidase, myeloperoxidase, lipoxygenase and cyclooxygenase, which are linked to the inflammatory processes, e.g. synthesis of prostaglandins and respiratory burst in phagocytosis.

Free radicals **lead to a chain of reactions** which, in turn, by passing the unpaired electron, result in the oxidation of various cellular macromolecules such as lipids, proteins and DNA, and induce damage to the cells and tissues.

In order to detoxify the harmful effects of the various oxygen toxic species (free radicals), also designated as pro-oxidants, our body generates several enzymes and nonenzymatic compounds referred to as antioxidants.

ANTIOXIDANTS

Antioxidants are the compounds, both enzymes and non-enzymes which counter the toxic effects of free radicals and/or inhibit their generation (Table 17.2).

Table 17.2: Antioxidants
• **Enzymes** Superoxide dismutase (SOD) Glutathione peroxidase (GPx) Catalase (CAT) Glutathione reductase (GR) Thioredoxin reductase (TrxR)
• **Nonenzymatic antioxidants** – **Reduced substances** Reduced glutathione (GSH) Reduced thioredoxin (TrxR) – **Vitamins** β-Carotene Vitamin A Vitamin C Vitamin E – **Trace elements** Zinc (Zn) Selenium (Se) – **Other Compounds** Uric acid Bilirubin Lycopene Flavonoids Albumin

Antioxidant Enzymes

Several enzymes are known to detoxify various ROS and RNS species, and help our body to prevent us from the harmful effects of free radicals, referred to as oxidative stress. These include:

- **Superoxide dismutase (SOD):** Superoxide dismutase is an enzyme that detoxifies superoxide anion ($O_2^{\bullet -}$) which is formed as a result of the reduction of molecular oxygen. SOD **converts superoxide anion to hydrogen peroxide** (H_2O_2).

  SOD is a metal-containing enzyme and **has three isoenzymes**, which are designated as:
  - **SOD_1** – SOD_1 **contains Cu and Zn**, and is **found in cytosol** of the cell.
  - **SOD_2** – SOD_2 is a **Mn-containing enzyme**. It is **found in mitochondria**.
  - **SOD_3** – SOD_3 **contains Cu and Zn**, and is **found** in the **extracellular matrix**.
- **Catalase (CAT):** Catalase is an enzyme which **removes hydrogen peroxide** (H_2O_2) and converts it to water and oxygen. It is **iron-containing** enzyme **found in peroxisomes** of all the cells of the living organisms which utilize oxygen.
- **Glutathione peroxidase (GPx):** GPx is an enzyme that **detoxifies lipid peroxides** as well as **H_2O_2 with the help of reduced glutathione** (GSH). It is a **Se-containing enzyme and has various isoenzymes**.
- **Glutathione reductase (GR):** In the GPx catalyzed reaction, **GSH is converted** to its **oxidized form** (GSSG). GR reduces GSSG back to GSH with the help of NADPH (Fig. 17.2).

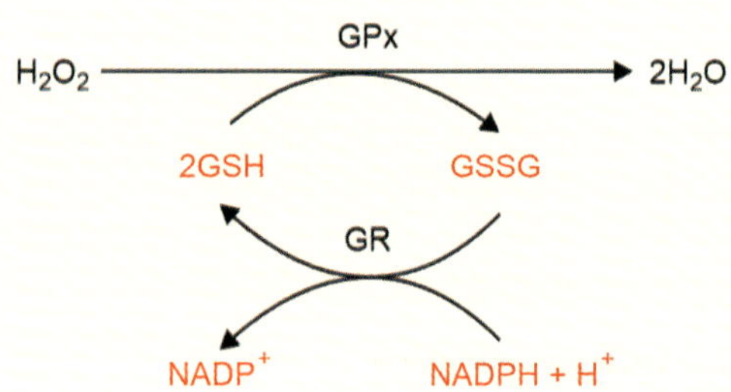

Fig. 17.2: Detoxification of H_2O_2 by glutathione peroxidase (GPx) catalyzed reaction with reduced glutathione (GSH). Oxidized glutathione (GSSG) is reduced by glutathione reductase (GR) to regenerate GSH

- **Thioredoxin reductase:** Similar to glutathione reductase, thioredoxin reductase (TrxR) **reduces oxidized thioredoxin** and converts it back to reduced thioredoxin.

  Thioredoxin protects disulfide bonds in proteins and catalyzes the reduction of protein mixed disulfides. Thioredoxin, specifically is important in the repair of DNA and proteins by reducing ribonucleotide reductase and methionine sulfoxide reductases.

Nonenzymatic Antioxidants

Nonenzymatic antioxidants include several endogenous substances such as reduced glutathione **(GSH), uric acid, bilirubin and ceruloplasmin**, besides some dietary micronutrients like vitamins **(β-carotene and vitamin A, vitamins C and vitamin E), flavonoids and polyphenols,** and trace elements **(zinc and selenium)**. These substances are referred to as the fundamental antioxidants, since these detoxify various ROS and RNS, and repair the oxidized compounds, directly.

- **Reduced glutathione:** Glutathione (GSH or reduced glutathione) is a **tripeptide** consisting of glutamate, cysteine and glycine. Due to the presence of cysteine, it has a thiol group which reacts with various oxidizing species (ROS and RNS) such as **hydroxyl-, perchlorate-** and **peroxy-nitrite radical**.
- **Reduced thioredoxin (TrxR):** TrxR provides reducing equivalents for thioredoxin reductase, which is also involved in the removal of peroxides.
- **Antioxidant vitamins:**
  - **β-Carotene (provitamin A):** It is a powerful antioxidant which **reduces singlet oxygen**. It is highly reactive to **peroxyl-radicals** and **prevents DNA damage**.
  - **Vitamin A**—Being fat-soluble, vitamin A is a **lipophilic antioxidant**. It is a potent **scavenger of singlet oxygen** and **protects retina and skin against damage from UV light (sunlight)**.
  - **Vitamin C**—Vitamin C or ascorbic acid **reduces** potentially damaging **hydroxyl-, alkoxyl-, peroxyl-** and **α-tocopheroxyl-radicals**. Physiological concentration of ascorbic acid also **inhibits oxidation of LDL, lipids** and **proteins.** Ascorbic acid **acts synergistically with vitamin E** and protects vitamin E from oxidative damage.
  - **Vitamin E**—It is a lipid-soluble antioxidant found in LDL and biological membranes. Vitamin E acts as a radical-scavenging antioxidant against lipid peroxidation.

    Vitamin A, vitamin C and vitamin E, collectively are referred to as **antioxidant vitamins**.
- **Trace elements:** Zinc (Zn) and selenium (Se) are essential components of superoxide dismutase (SOD) and glutathione peroxidase (GPx), respectively.
- **Uric acid:** Uric acid is an endogenous compound synthesized as the **end product of purine metabolism**. It is a **strong ROS and RNS scavenger**.
- **Bilirubin: Unconjugated bilirubin** is a powerful antioxidant. It protects proteins from ROS- and RNS-mediated oxidative damage.
- **Other antioxidants: Lycopene, flavonoids** and serum **albumin** (containing –SH groups) also act as scavengers of ROS and RNS.

OXIDATIVE STRESS

An **imbalance between the levels of prooxidants and antioxidants**, either **due to increased generation of free radicals** (which cannot be detoxified by the antioxidants) **or reduced concentration of antioxidants**, result in oxygen toxicity. This, in turn, **put stress on normal physiological functions of cells** leading to its damage, is referred to as oxidative stress.

As discussed above, when concentration of free radicals is increased, it leads to **oxidative stress and causes cell damage.**

Mechanism of Oxidative Damage

- One of the most sensitive sites of free radical damage is the **cell membrane**, since cell membrane is **rich in polyunsaturated fatty acids** (PUFA). ROS accepts a hydrogen atom from PUFA thereby causing a **chain of lipid peroxidation reactions** and cell damage.
- These **lipid peroxides are** further **metabolized and produce** aldehyde products such as **malondialdehyde** (MDA), which, in turn, **reacts with proteins**, and **form** adduct and cross-links that are designated as **advanced lipoxidation end products** (ALE).
- ROS also react **with carbohydrates** and produce dicarbonyl compounds, which, in turn, also react with proteins, and **form** adduct and cross-links that are designated as glycoxidation products, also called **advanced glycation end products** (AGE).
- ROS also damage the genome and cause mutations in DNA.

Role of Oxidative Damage in Pathogenesis of Diseases

Increased concentrations of ALE and AGE lead to several pathological conditions including metabolic, degenerative and inflammatory diseases such as ischemia-reperfusion injury, cancer, atherosclerosis, Alzheimer's disease, alcoholic liver disease and diabetes mellitus.

Some Important Question

1. Write notes on:

i. Reactive oxygen species
ii. Oxidative stress
iii. Free radicals
iv. Superoxide dismutase
v. Antioxidant vitamins
vi. Antioxidant enzymes
vii. Antioxidants

Unit VI

Biochemical Genetics, Protein Synthesis and Carcinogenesis

Unit V

Special Aspects of Metabolism

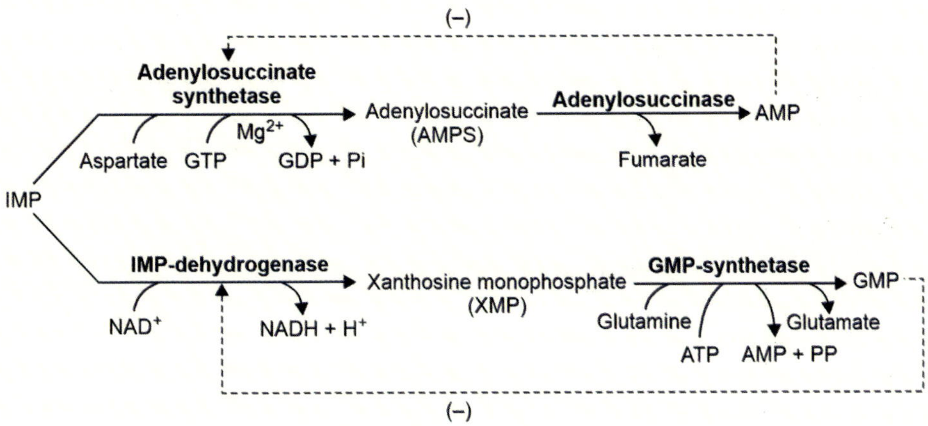

Fig. 18.3: Synthesis of AMP and GMP

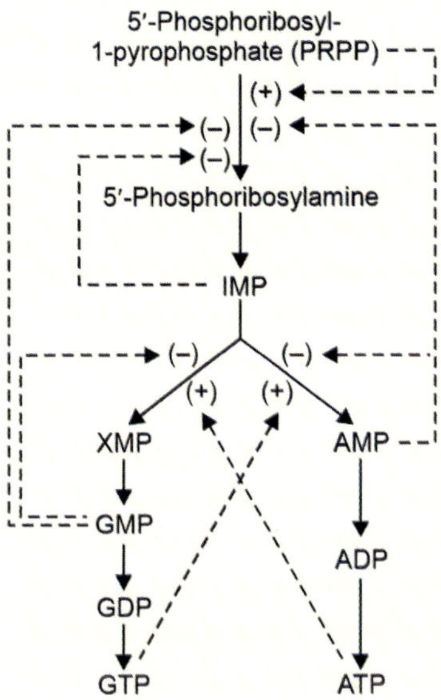

Fig. 18.4: Regulation of the synthesis of purine nucleotides

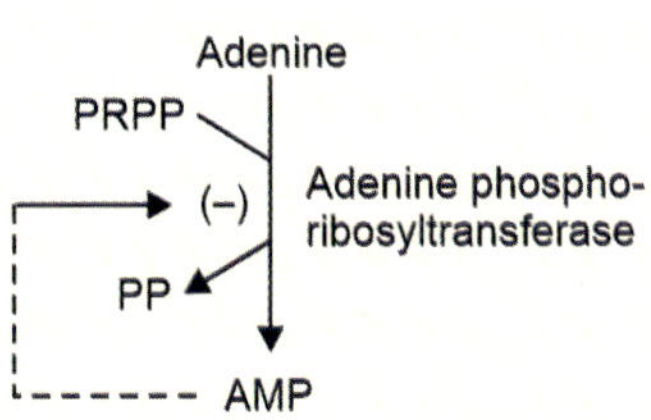

Fig. 18.5: Synthesis of AMP from adenine by APRTase

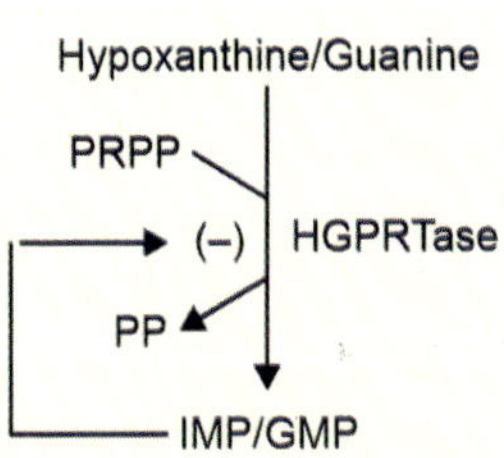

Fig. 18.6: Synthesis of IMP/GMP from hypoxanthine/guanine by HGPRTase

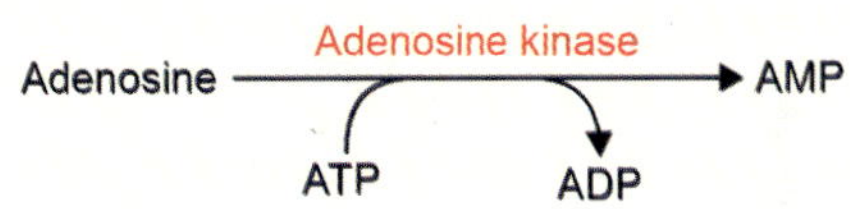

Fig. 18.7: A nucleoside kinase reaction

- For their interconversion, GMP or AMP is first degraded to IMP, which, then, depending upon the need of the cell, can form any of the two nucleotides:
- By reductive deamination, GMP is converted to IMP. The reaction is catalyzed by GMP reductase. GTP activates this step, whereas XMP competitively inhibits the reaction.
- Conversion of AMP to IMP is catalyzed by AMP deaminase (5′-AMP amino-hydrolase). This reaction is activated by K^+ and ATP, but inhibited by Pi, GDP and GTP (Fig. 18.8).

DEGRADATION OF PURINE NUCLEOTIDES

Degradation of purine nucleotides, i.e. AMP and GMP, leads to the formation of **uric acid**, in humans (Fig. 18.9).

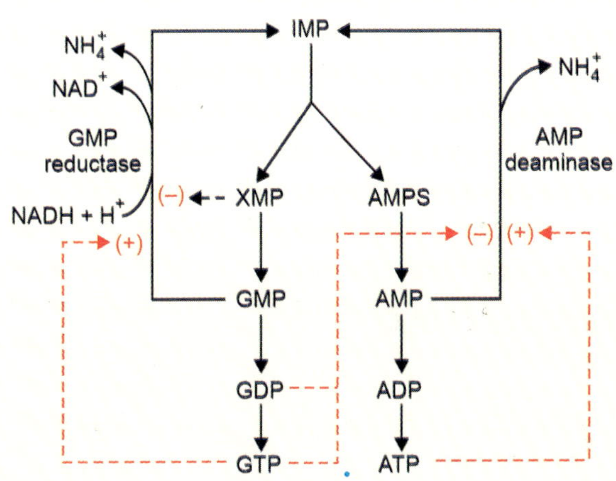

Fig. 18.8: Interconversion of purine nucleotides. (+) = Stimulation; (–) = Inhibition

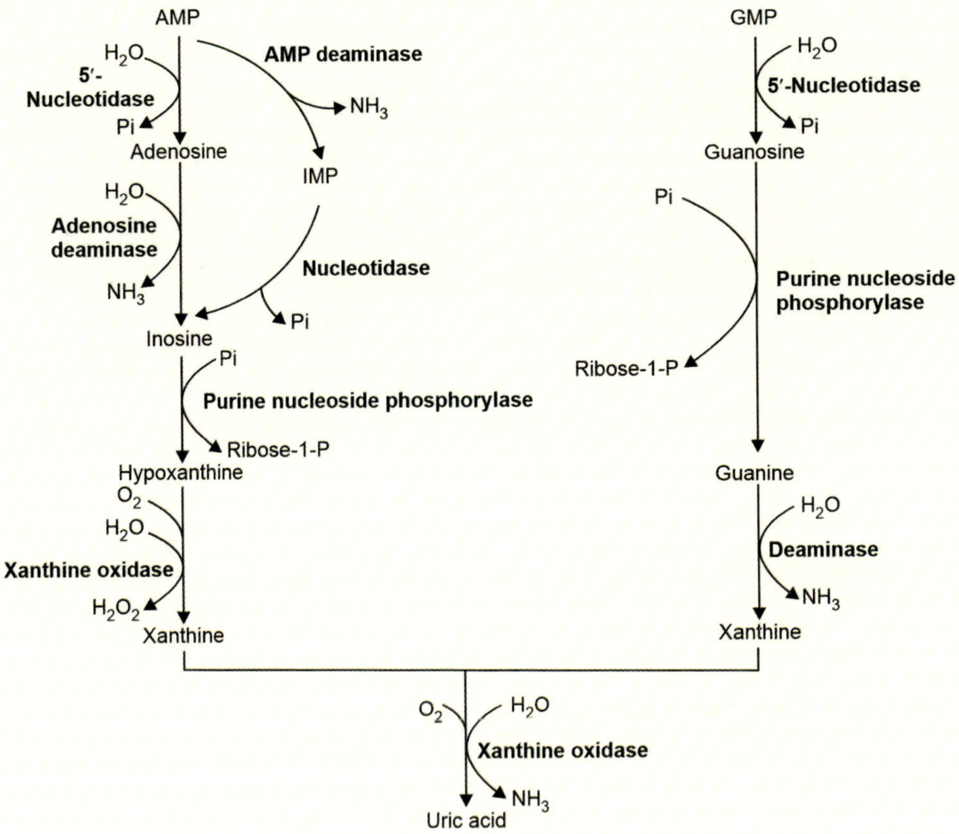

Fig. 18.9: Degradation of purine nucleotides

Degradation of AMP

- **AMP** is converted **to adenosine, by 5'-AMP-nucleotidase** which has high specificity for its substrate.
- Thereafter, **adenosine deaminase (ADA) converts** adenosine as well as deoxyadenosine **to inosine.**
- Alternatively, AMP deaminase, which is specific for AMP, removes ammonia and converts AMP to IMP. Subsequently, nucleotidase removes phosphoric acid and converts IMP to inosine.
- Activities of the above three enzymes, i.e. AMP-nucleotidase, ADA and AMP deaminase are several folds higher in muscle than in other tissues.
- **Purine nucleoside phosphorylase** (PNP) then removes the ribose moiety from **inosine** and converts it **to hypoxanthine**.

Degradation of GMP

- In the first step, phosphoric acid is removed by **5'-nucleotidase** and **GMP** is converted **to guanosine**.
- With the removal of the ribose moiety by PNP, guanosine is converted to guanine.
- **Guanase** (an amino-hydrolase), removes amino group from guanine and **converts it to xanthine**.

Immunodeficiency Diseases Associated with Degradation of Purine Nucleosides

Severe Combined Immunodeficiency

A **deficiency in ADA** is associated with severe combined immunodeficiency (SCID) **involving both T-cell and B-cell functions**. Thus, proliferation and differentiation of immune cells are compromised. Treatment of such children includes blood transfusion, bone marrow transplantation, enzyme replacement therapy with ADA-polyethylene glycol and gene therapy.

Purine Nucleoside Phosphorylase Deficiency

It is associated with **immunodeficiency involving T-cell functions**, i.e. a defective T-cell immunity but **with normal B-cell functions**.

In both the conditions, i.e. SCID and PNP deficiency, there is a **decrease in uric acid formation** which is accompanied with **increased levels of purine nucleosides and nucleotides**. Overwhelming infection in such children results in death within 2 years of age.

Formation of Uric Acid

In human beings and other primates, the end product of purine degradation is uric acid which is excreted in the urine. Hypoxanthine and xanthine, produced as above, are catabolized by the enzyme **xanthine oxidase** and are converted to uric acid.

Serum uric acid: Uric acid is **sparingly soluble in an aqueous medium**. Normal serum uric acid is maintained between **3 and 7 mg/dL. Males** have physiologically **higher values** because of higher rate of tubular urate reabsorption, and the uricosuric effect of estrogen in females.

HYPERURICEMIA

Elevated level of uric acid in the serum (>7 mg/dL) is referred to as **hyperuricemia**. Hyperuricemia is often asymptomatic. It may be primary or secondary.

Primary Hyperuricemia

This is due to some metabolic defect that results in increased synthesis of purine nucleotides via *de novo* pathway, such as:

- **Increased PRPP synthetase activity:** This results in increased intracellular concentration of PRPP which acts as a positive effector of the enzyme amidotransferase. This, in turn, increases *de novo* synthesis of purine nucleotides as well as their subsequent degradation to uric acid.
- **HGPRTase deficiency:** Deficiency of HGPRTase, as in Lesch-Nyhan syndrome, causes a decrease in the salvage pathway of hypoxanthine and guanine to reform nucleotides. This, in turn, spares PRPP and results in overproduction of purine nucleotides and their degradation to uric acid.
- **Glucose-6-phosphatase deficiency (glycogen storage disease I or von Gierke's disease):** It results in increased levels of glucose-6-phosphate which is diverted to HMP shunt. This, in turn, increases availability of ribose-5-phosphate and enhances the generation of PRPP. Raised levels of PRPP increase *de novo* synthesis of purine nucleotides and the overproduction of uric acid. In addition, associated lactic acidosis elevates renal threshold for urate which further leads to hyperuricemia.

Secondary hyperuricemia: It is secondary to some disease other than a metabolic disorder, such as a kidney disease or a disease associated with excessive cell turnover and increased breakdown of nucleic acids, e.g. radiation therapy/cancer chemotherapy, or psoriasis.

Hyperuricemia may result in deposition of uric acid as sodium urate crystals primarily, in joints, in a clinical condition called gout.

GOUT

It is a disease characterized by elevated levels of uric acid in the blood **(hyperuricemia)** and its increased excretion in the urine **(uric aciduria)** due to a variety of metabolic abnormalities. Most of the clinical conditions with hyperuricemia arise due to the poor aqueous solubility of uric acid. As a result, sodium urate crystals are deposited in joints of the extremities **(gouty arthritis)** and/or in the renal interstitial tissue **(gouty nephropathy)**. The crystals activate the complement pathway resulting in the recruitment of neutrophils, macrophages, release of inflammatory mediators and free radicals. In the affected joint, hyaluronic acid is reduced both due to decreased production and increased degradation. Hyperuricemia is, thus, associated with recurrent attacks of painful arthritic joints and inflammation, most often of big toe, caused by the deposition of insoluble sodium urate crystals, called **tophi** (Fig. 18.10).

DE NOVO SYNTHESIS OF PYRIMIDINE NUCLEOTIDES

Unlike purine nucleotides, a pyrimidine nucleotide is synthesized differently. During the synthesis of the pyrimidine nucleotides, firstly, a pyrimidine ring is synthesized as orotate (orotic acid).

1. During this process, the first step is the synthesis of carbamoyl phosphate from glutamine and HCO_3^-. This reaction consumes two molecules of ATP. This

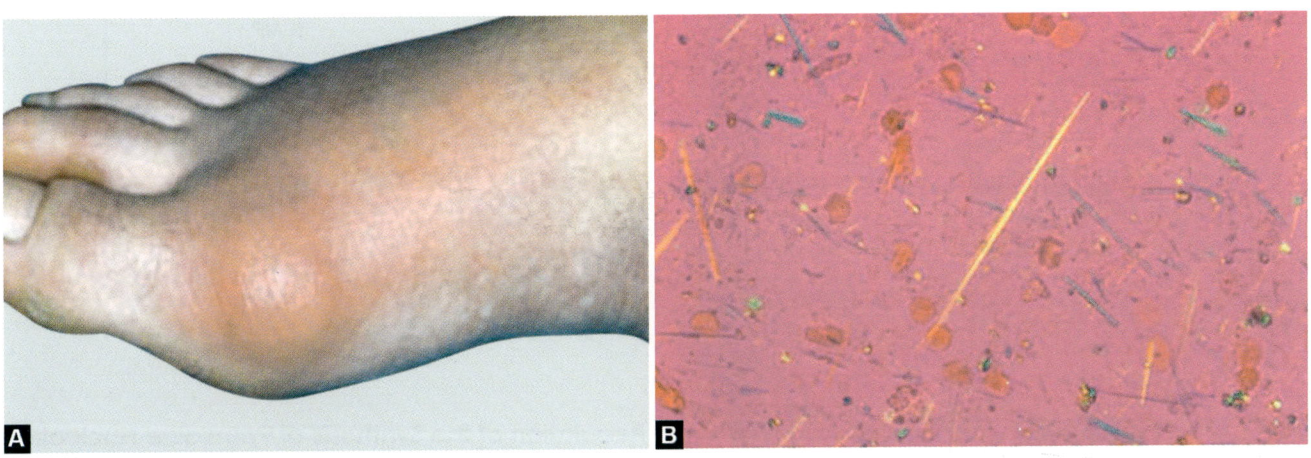

Fig. 18.10: Gout. (A) The condition most commonly affects the great toe (first metatarsophalangeal joint) when it is also called podagra; (B) Under polarized microscope, negatively birefringent needle-shaped monosodium urate crystals of various sizes and colors are seen in the joint aspirate

is a regulated step in the pathway and is catalyzed by carbamoyl phosphate synthetase II (CPS II), in the cytosol.

2. In the next step, carbamoyl phosphate condenses with aspartate and forms carbamoyl aspartate.

   This reaction is catalyzed by aspartate transcarbamoylase (aspartate carbamoyl-transferase). This is the committed step in the synthesis of pyrimidine nucleotides.
3. Dihydro-orotase results in ring closure and forms dihydro-orotate.
4. Dihydro-orotate dehydrogenase, a mitochondrial enzyme, oxidizes dihydro-orotate to orotate (Fig. 18.11).

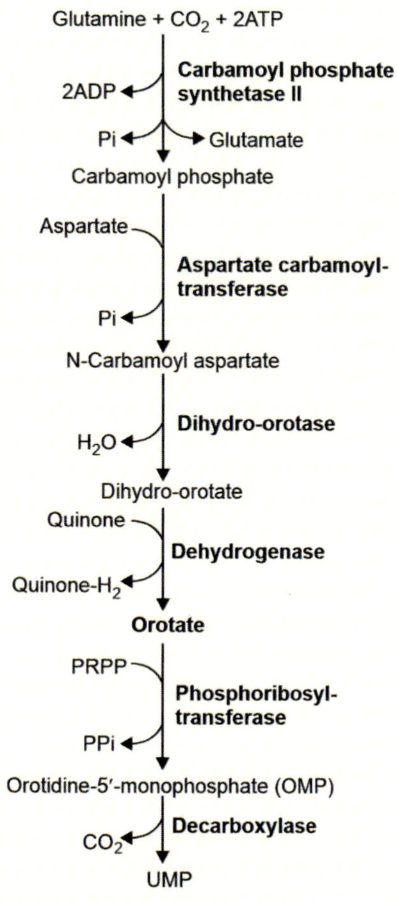

Fig. 18.11: Synthesis of UMP

Thus, a pyrimidine ring is synthesized as orotate (orotic acid), using aspartate (C4, C5 and C6, and N1), glutamine (N3) and carbon dioxide (C6; Fig. 18.12).

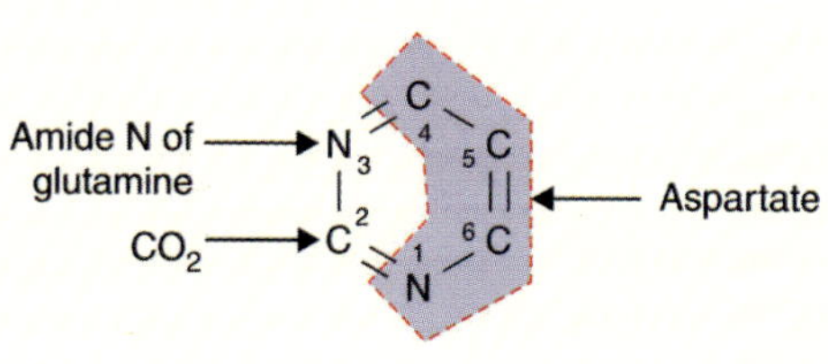

Fig. 18.12: Sources of carbons and nitrogens in a pyrimidine ring

Synthesis of UMP

Thereafter, orotate phosphoribosyl-transferase transfers ribose-5-phosphate from PRPP and converts the pyrimidine base orotate to its nucleotide, orotidine monophosphate (OMP).

OMP is converted to UMP, by OMP decarboxylase (orotidylate decarboxylase; Fig. 18.11).

Orotate phosporibosyl-transferase and **OMP decarboxylase** activities are present on a single **bifunctional protein**, termed **UMP synthase.**

Orotic Aciduria

It is due to a **defect in *de novo* synthesis of pyrimidine nucleotides**. There is a genetic deficiency of both the activities of the bifunctional protein **UMP synthase.** High levels of **orotic acid excretion in the urine** and deficiency of enzymes in erythrocytes confirm the diagnosis.

Synthesis of CMP

CMP is synthesized from UTP via CTP. Firstly, UTP is converted to CTP by the enzyme CTP-synthetase, which uses glutamine as a donor of the amino group. ATP is used as a source of energy. CTP is a negative effector of the reaction. Thereafter, CTP is converted to CMP.

Synthesis of TMP

TMP is synthesized from CDP and UDP, which are first converted to dUMP (as discussed below). Thereafter, by transmethylation of dUMP, TMP (thymidylate or deoxy-thymidylate) is synthesized. The reaction is catalyzed by thymidylate synthase. In this reaction, N^5, N^{10}-methylene-tetrahydrofolate (N^5, N^{10}-methylene-FH_4) is used as a source of the methyl group (one carbon moiety) and also as a reducing agent (Fig 18.13).

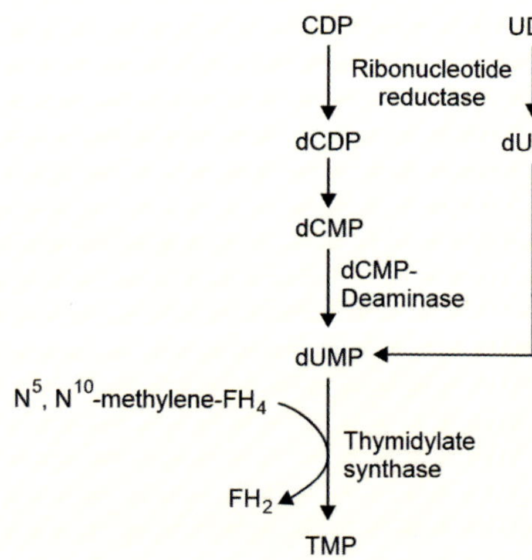

Fig. 18.13: Synthesis of TMP

Regulation of the Synthesis of Pyrimidine Nucleotides

- Pyrimidine synthesis is regulated by CPS II. The enzyme is inhibited by CTP and is activated by ATP and PRPP.

- OMP decarboxylase is competitively inhibited by UMP.
- CTP synthetase is inhibited by CTP. This is an example of feedback inhibition. This, in turn, regulates the conversion of UTP to CTP.

Thus, cells maintain a balance between uridine and cytidine nucleotides.

SALVAGE PATHWAY FOR THE SYNTHESIS OF PYRIMIDINE NUCLEOTIDES

Pyrimidine bases, i.e. orotate, uracil and thymine but not cytosine, can be salvaged and converted to the corresponding nucleotides by pyrimidine phosphoribosyl-transferase. The enzyme utilizes PRPP as a source of ribose-5-phosphate (Fig. 18.14).

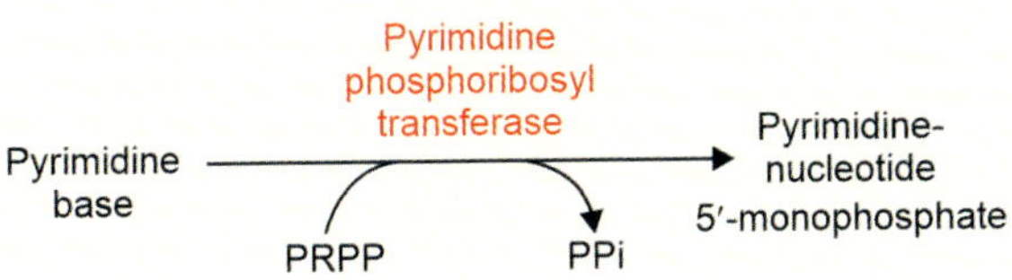

Fig. 18.14: Salvage pathway for pyrimidine nucleotides synthesis

DEGRADATION OF PYRIMIDINE NUCLEOTIDES

Pyrimidine nucleotides are, firstly, converted to free bases, which are subsequently, degraded to form the end products.

- Pyrimidine **nucleotides** (CMP, UMP, dCMP and dTMP), released as a result of the degradation of nucleic acids, **are converted to** the corresponding **nucleosides, by** the nonspecific **phosphatases**.
- **Cytidine and deoxycytidine** are, thereafter, deaminated **by** pyrimidine nucleoside **deaminase to uridine and deoxyuridine**, respectively.
- **Uridine, deoxyuridine and deoxythymidine** are degraded **by uridine phosphorylase** and converted **to uracil** (from uridine and deoxyuridine) **and thymine** (from deoxythymidine).
- **Uracil and thymine** produced as above **are further degraded to β-alanine and β-amino-isobutyric acid**, respectively.

SYNTHESIS OF NUCLEOSIDE DI- AND TRIPHOSPHATES

- Various nucleoside monophosphates, i.e. AMP, GMP, CMP, UMP as well as dAMP, dGMP, dCMP and dTMP are sequentially converted to their nucleoside triphosphates.
- Firstly, a nucleoside monophosphate **(NMP) is converted** to the corresponding nucleoside diphosphate **(NDP)**. The reaction is catalysed by the base specific nucleoside monophosphate **kinase**.
- Thereafter, nucleoside diphosphate **kinase converts** a nucleoside diphosphate **(NDP) to** the corresponding nucleoside triphosphate **(NTP)**.

SYNTHESIS OF DEOXYRIBONUCLEOTIDES

Purine and pyrimidine ribonucleotides, formed by the respective *de novo* pathways, **are converted to** their **deoxyribonucleotides during DNA replication**.

- Ribonucleoside diphosphates **(NDP)**, i.e. ADP, GDP, CDP and UDP are reduced at C2′ position **to** their deoxy forms, i.e. dADP, dGDP, dCDP and dUDP **by ribonucleotide reductase** (ribonucleoside diphosphate reductase.
- Phosphorylation of **dNDP** convets them to **dNTP** which, in turn, is used in the biosynthesis of DNA. The reaction is catalyzed **by nucleoside diphosphate kinase**. Any of the NTP or dNTP, such as ATP, can function as the phosphoryl donor for this reaction.

Some Important Questions

1. **Explain the process of *de novo* synthesis of purine nucleotides.**
2. **Describe the process of degradation of purine nucleotides.**
3. **Describe the process of *de novo* synthesis of pyrimidine nucleotides.**
4. **Describe briefly:**
   i. Synthesis of IMP
   ii. Regulation of purines biosynthesis
   iii. Inter-conversion of purine nucleotides
   iv. Immunodeficiency diseases associated with purine degradation
   v. Formation of uric acid
   vi. Primary hyperuricemia
   vii. Secondary hyperuricemia
5. **Write notes on:**
   i. Salvage pathway for purines
   ii. Lesch-Nyhan syndrome
   iii. Severe combined immunodeficiency disease
   iv. Gout
   v. Hereditary orotic aciduria

Chapter 19

DNA Replication

As discussed in Chapter 4, **DNA is a genetic material**. The process of DNA synthesis is referred to as **replication**.

Replication is **a semiconservative process**, since during replication, each strand of the double-stranded DNA serves as a template for the synthesis of a new strand, in a very accurate manner. In this process, both the strands of the parental DNA double helix serve as template and produce two daughter DNA molecules. Therefore, after each round of replication, out of the two newly formed double-stranded DNA, one strand is a parental strand while the other one is a newly synthesized complementary strand. This process of DNA replication where after each round of replication, one strand in a double helix is maintained intact (parental strand) and combines with the other one which is a newly synthesized daughter strand, is called semiconservative replication (Fig. 19.1).

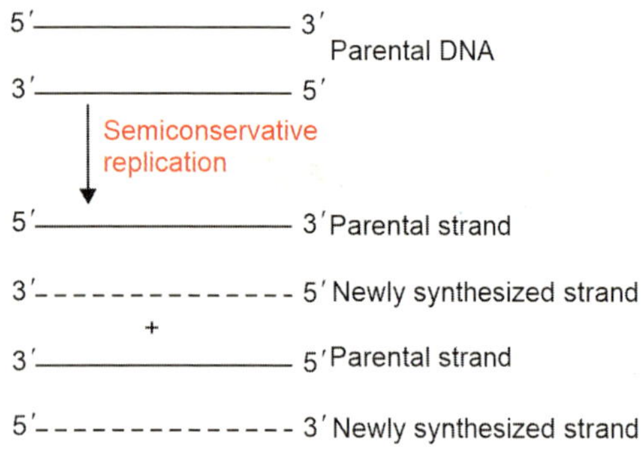

Fig. 19.1: Semiconservative replication

REQUIREMENTS FOR DNA REPLICATION

The following proteins/enzymes are required by the cell for the process of replication:

DnaA protein: DnaA is a protein that binds at the origin of replication. It is also called the origin-binding protein. Nearly, 20–50 monomers of DnaA bind at the specific nucleotide consensus sequence that is present at the origin of replication. This binding in turn requires ATP and results in separation (melting) of two strands of the DNA.

Single strand DNA-binding protein: Single strand DNA-binding (SSB) protein binds to the singlestranded DNA and prevents the two strands from rejoining. They are stripped-off the SSB-protein, before the replication begins. In eukaryotes, the two strands of DNA, after their separation, are covered with another protein, which is referred to as replication protein A, also called replication factor A. It is functionally similar to the SSB-protein, which occurs in prokaryotes.

Helicases: Helicase is the enzyme that separates two strands of the DNA. This enzyme initiates the unwinding of the double helix, at the single-stranded region, adjacent to the duplex and functions in a particular polarity only. In eukaryotes, helicase activity is associated with the enzyme DNA polymerase δ.

Topoisomerases: As we know, chromosomes of many bacteria and viruses are the circular molecules of the double helix DNA and have a peculiar twisted appearance. This is referred as supercoiling or super-helicity. If the topological problems are not corrected, it may stop unwinding of the parent DNA and hence, DNA replication.

The group of enzymes, called **topoisomerases overcome supercoiling**. They are endonucleases, which alter topological coiling of the circular DNA. They introduce nicks in one or both the strands, remove supercoils, and reseal the ends.

There are several types of topoisomerases (Table 19.1).

Topoisomerase II inhibitors

Topoisomerase II inhibitors are in common clinical use as drugs. For example, antimicrobials of the quinolone category such as norfloxacin, ciprofloxacin, ofloxacin, etc. and some anticancer agents such as doxorubicin and etoposide, block topoisomerase II activity. These compounds, thus, **arrest DNA replication as well as RNA transcription**, which explains the high clinical potency of these drugs.

Type	Target DNA	Activity		ATP required	Effects in	
		Endonuclease	Ligase		Prokaryotes	Eukaryotes
I	One strand	Yes	Yes	No	Relax negative supercoils	Relax both negative and positive supercoils
II	Both strands	Yes	Yes	Yes	Relax both negative and positive supercoils. Introduce negative supercoils into relaxed DNA	–
III	One strand	Yes	Yes	No	Remove circular DNA products called catenates which are generated just prior to the completion of DNA replication	–
Reverse gyrase	Both strands	Yes	Yes	Yes	Found in archaebacteria: Introduce positive supercoils into DNA and prevent denaturation from high temperature and acidity	–

Table 19.1: Topoisomerases: Salient features

Other drugs, like camptothecin, anthracycline, etc. interfere with the enzyme-catalysed resealing of the DNA strands. They do not affect the overall activity of the enzyme but convert these topoisomerases into the DNA-breaking agents. Since DNA degradation leads to cell death, these drugs **are used in the treatment of certain hematological neoplasms**, e.g. leukemias and lymphomas.

DNA polymerases: DNA polymerases (DNA-dependent DNA polymerases) are the enzymes that catalyse the synthesis of the complementary strand, on the single-stranded DNA template. They add nucleotides at the free 3′-OH group and extend the chain in 5′ → 3′ direction (Fig. 19.2).

Different types of the DNA polymerases are found in prokaryotes and eukaryotes.

- **DNA polymerases in eukaryotes:** Five different types of DNA polymerases are found in eukaryotes. These are designated as DNA polymerase α, β, γ, δ and ε. All have 5′ → 3′ synthetic activities. With the exception of the polymerase γ, which occurs in mitochondria, they are involved in the chromosomal DNA synthesis as well as its repair.
- **DNA polymerases in prokaryotes:** Three distinct forms of the enzyme are found in prokaryotes. These are designated as DNA polymerase I, II, and III.
- **Reverse transcriptase:** RNA-dependent DNA polymerase, designated as reverse transcriptase, **is also a** member of the **polymerase** family of enzymes. It is found in retroviruses (RNA-containing eukaryotic viruses), such as human immunodeficiency virus (HIV), which is the causative agent of the acquired immunodeficiency syndrome (AIDS). Reverse transcriptase catalyses synthesis of the double-stranded DNA, from the single-stranded RNA template.

PROCESS OF DNA REPLICATION

DNA replication is a complex process, which involves initiation, elongation and termination Initiation of DNA

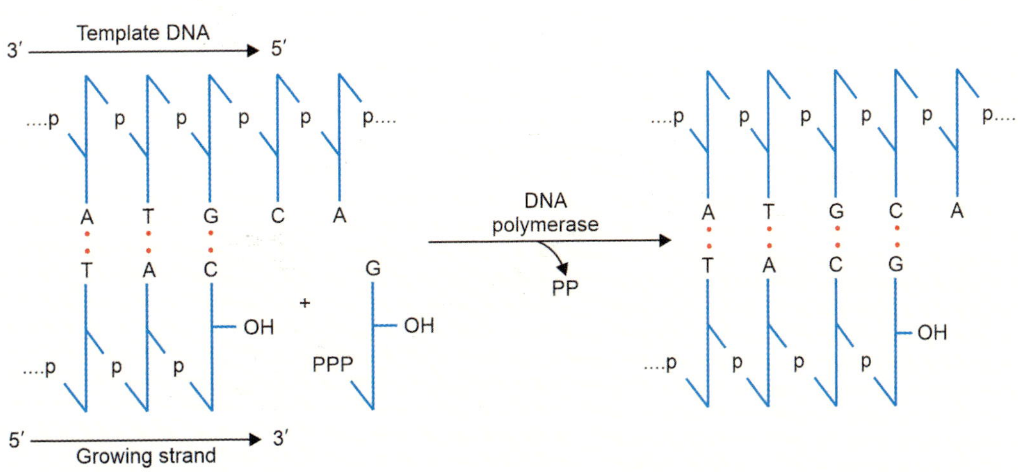

Fig. 19.2: Action of DNA polymerase

Replication initiation of DNA replication involves formation of the replication fork and synthesis of the RNA primer.

Formation of Replication Fork

- **Replication starts at the** site referred to as **origin of replication**. It is designated as ori C, in *E. coli*. The sequence of nucleotides at the origin is **rich in AT**.
- The **DnaA protein binds** at the origin.
- Binding of DnaA at the AT-rich region **promotes unwinding of the two strands** of the parent DNA. After the two strands get separated, the circular chromosome exhibits a bubble-like structure, called replication bubble **(replication eye).** The branch point in the replication bubble, at which DNA synthesis begins, is called **replication fork.**
- Formation of the replication fork **initiates stepwise assembly of various proteins and enzymes** that are **required for DNA replication** (Fig. 19.3).

With the movement of the enzyme **helicase two single-stranded regions of the parent DNA are generated.** Subsequently, the **SSB-protein covers the two strands and keeps them apart** from each other. Thereafter, synthesis of RNA primer starts.

Synthesis of RNA Primer

- Synthesis of RNA primer begins with the formation of **pre-priming complex** (also called **pre-priming assembly**), which **consists of DnaB, DnaC** and four other proteins referred to as **n, n′, n″ and i proteins.**
- After the **pre-priming complex associates with** the enzyme **primase** (called RNA polymerase), it **forms primosome** (the priming complex).
- The primosome **interacts with the template** (at the replication fork) and begins the synthesis of the RNA primer.

Whereas, **only one priming complex** is required to **initiate the synthesis of the leading strand, multiple copies** of the complex are **required for the synthesis of the lagging strand.**

After the site of the primer, initiation has been recognized, SSB-proteins are displaced and the primase lays down the primer.

During the process of replication, two antiparallel DNA strands are simultaneously replicated at the two advancing replication forks, in the 5′ → 3′ direction, but differently.

One of its strands is synthesized continuously (in the direction of the movement of the replication fork). This is **called the leading strand.** On the other hand, the **second strand is synthesized discontinuously** (i.e. in small fragments, though in the 5′ → 3′ direction only). This strand is **called** the **lagging strand.**

Okazaki fragments: The **small fragments synthesized discontinuously, on the lagging strand** are called as Okazaki fragments. They vary in size from about 100–200 deoxyribonucleotides (in eukaryotes) to nearly 1000–2000 deoxyribonucleotides (in prokaryotes).

Chain Elongation

Chain elongation is **carried out by** an assembly referred to as **replisome** (replicase system).

Various components of the replisome are shown in Table 19.2.

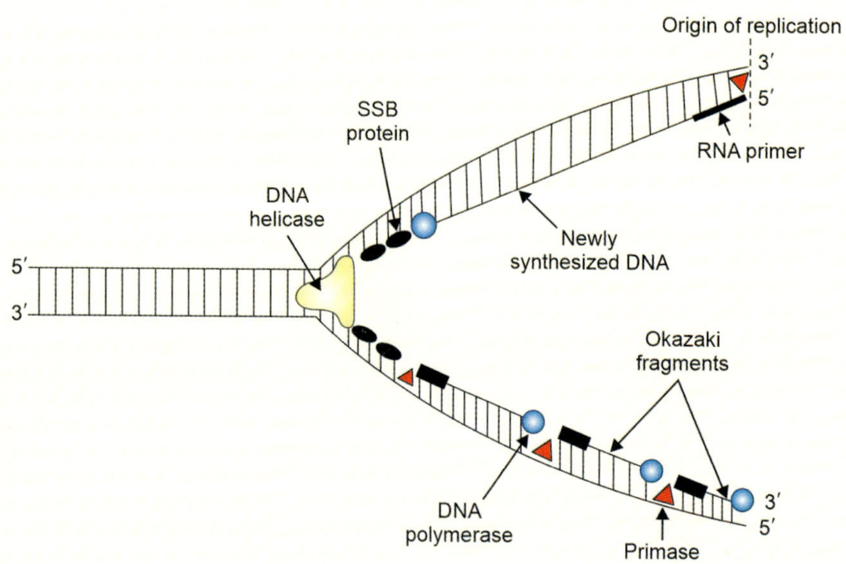

Fig. 19.3: A replication fork

Table 19.2: Components of a replisome

Component protein/ enzyme	*Functions*
DnaA	Unwinding of two strands of DNA at the origin of replication
DnaB	Helicase activity, unwinds DNA for creation of the initiation bubble
Topoisomerase II	Removal of supercoils
SSB-protein	Binds to single strands of the DNA, to keep two strands apart from each other.
DnaC	Binding with the SSB-protein at the origin of replication
Primase	Synthesis of the RNA primer
n, n′, n″ and i proteins	Primosome assembly
DNA polymerase III	Chain elongation on the 3′-OH group of the primer
DNA polymerase I	Excision of the primer and gap-filling
DNA ligase	Ligation of the polynucleotide fragments

A **replisome exists** only **as a protein complex**, which is associated with the particular structure that DNA takes at the replication fork.

- The replisome, which contains two polymerase III holoenzymes, **synthesizes the leading strand as well as the lagging strand**.
- It moves, as a single unit, in the 5′ → 3′ direction along the leading strand, whereas the lagging strand template loops around to permit the holoenzyme to extend the primed lagging strand.
- After completing the synthesis of an Okazaki fragment, holoenzyme (on the lagging strand) is relocated to the new primer, near the replication fork, and extends the RNA primer to form a new Okazaki fragment. At each location, DNA polymerase uses RNA primer, for the synthesis of DNA.
- After the polymerase reaches the end of the single-stranded template, it takes over the next primer that is annealed to the template, as DNA–RNA hybrid.
- **In eukaryotes, the primers may be formed at several locations**, which are determined by nucleosome spacing. This, in turn, results in continuous synthesis of the leading strand and several RNA primed Okazaki fragments (which are separated from each other by the single-stranded nicks) on the lagging strand. In this process, synthesis of the leading strand is always ahead of the synthesis of the lagging strand.
- Thereafter, DNA polymerase I replaces ribonucleotides (from RNA primer) with the deoxyribonucleotides and finally, the nicks are sealed by DNA ligase.

Termination of DNA Replication

DNA replication is terminated by a protein designated as the **Tus protein** (terminator utilization substance), which arrests movement of the replication fork and terminates DNA replication.

- The Tus protein acts **as a contra-helicase** and **binds to** a region called **ter site**, which has GT-rich termination sequence. This, in turn, prevents advancement of the replication fork, by arresting the action of DnaB.
- Finally, delinking of the parent strands, from the daughter strands, is catalysed by the enzyme topoisomerase.

DIFFERENCES IN DNA REPLICATION BETWEEN PROKARYOTES AND EUKARYOTES

DNA replication in eukaryotes differs from the process in prokaryotes in several ways (Table 19.3).

Table 19.3: Differences in DNA replication between prokaryotes and eukaryotes

Prokaryotes	*Eukaryotes*
Replication begins at the origin	Replication begins at multiple sites, simultaneously
SSB-protein keeps two strands separate	Replication protein A keeps two strands separate
Only negative supercoils are relaxed	Both negative and positive supercoils are relaxed
There are three types of DNA polymerases, called polymerase I, II and III	There are five types of DNA polymerases, called polymerase α, β, γ, δ and ε
Helicase is a specific enzyme	Helicase activity is associated with DNA polymerase α
Primase is a specific RNA polymerase	Primase activity is present in DNA polymerase α
Both the DNA strands are synthesized by DNA polymerase III	Leading strand is synthesized by DNA polymerase δ while lagging strand is synthesized by DNA polymerase α
Very long Okazaki fragments are synthesized	Small sized Okazaki fragments are synthesized
The process is simple, rapid and error-prone	The process is complex, slow but accurate

TELOMERES

Telomeres are 1000 or more nucleotides long tandem repeats (copies of short G- and T-rich oligonucleotide sequences) present at the 3′-end of the strand (at the end of each chromosome). A telomere also has a 12–16 nucleotides long single strand overhang, which serves as a template for the primer that initiates the synthesis of the final Okazaki fragment on the lagging strand (Fig. 19.4).

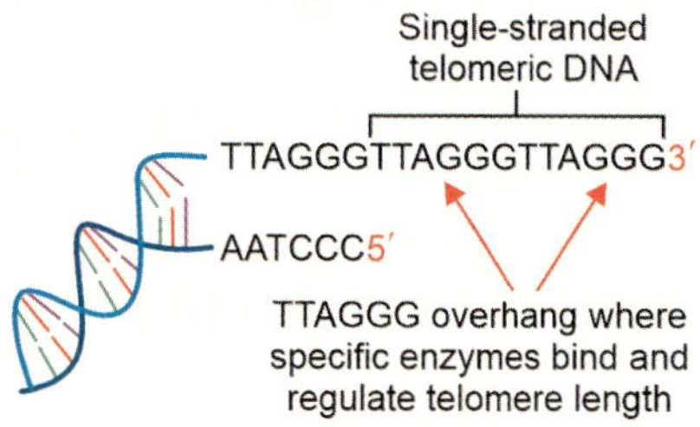

Fig. 19.4: Telomere

In most of the eukaryotes, telomere replication is carried out by a specialized reverse transcriptase, designated as telomerase.

Telomerases: These are ribonucleoproteins whose RNA components have enzyme activity. Such a component contains a segment that is complementary to the repeating telomeric sequence and acts as an internal template. Its function, therefore, is similar to that of reverse transcriptase. Absence of the telomerase shortens the chromosome with each round of replication and contributes to normal senescence of the cell. Maintenance of the chromosomal length thus depends on the action of telomerase.

DNA REPLICATION IN MITOCHONDRIA

Mitochondrial chromosome of the mammals is a 15 kb segment. It is circular and contains 500–600 nucleotides long D-loop that undergoes frequent cycles of degradation and resynthesis.

NUCLEOSOMES

Nucleosomes are the lowest level of chromosome organization.

- **Eukaryotic DNA** being large **is packed in chromatin** in association **with the** basic proteins called **histones**, which are rich in lysine and arginine.
- **Histones** are positively charged molecules and **form ionic bonds with the DNA** which is negatively charged.
- There are **five classes** of histones, designated as **H1, H2A, H2B, H3 and H4**.
- Two molecules each of H2A, H2B, H3 and H4 form an octamer-structured core of the individual nucleosome around which a segment of the DNA double helix is wound twice, forming a negatively super-twisted helix. These DNA segments are small (approximately, 50 nucleotides), and are called **linker DNA** (Fig. 19.5).
- Histones-octamer joined by the linker DNA, forms a **nucleosome** (nucleofilament).
- Synthesis of the new histones occurs mainly during the S phase, simultaneously with the replication of DNA.
- Newly synthesized DNA inherits some parental histones which combine with an equal amount of the new histones, to complete the structure of the nascent nucleosomes that are formed behind the moving replication fork.

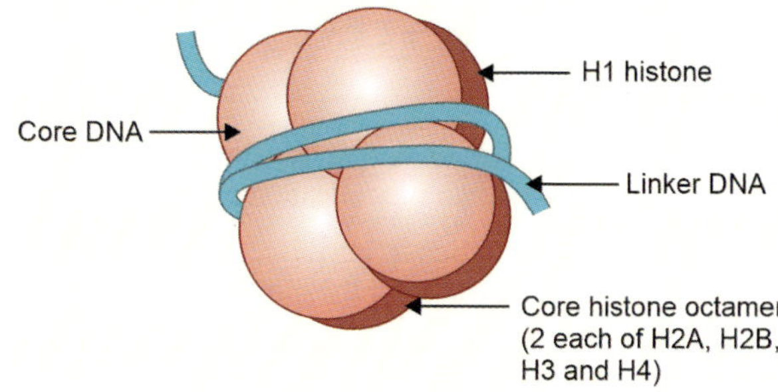

Fig. 19.5: A nucleosome

GENE MUTATIONS

Mutations are **inheritable, irreparable and permanent alterations in DNA sequence** which **may be phenotypically silent** (hidden) **or expressed** (visible). They can be detected only by gene sequence determination.

CAUSES OF GENE MUTATIONS

Mutations **may arise by** a number of means, such as due to **an error in replication during proofreading**, by **UV or ionizing radiation** (X-rays and γ-rays), or **by a chemical mutagen** (an alkylating agent). Besides, DNA may also undergo **certain spontaneous changes**, such as deamination of cytosine (to form uracil), depurination, etc.

CLASSIFICATION OF GENE MUTATIONS

Mutations are classified into two categories, i.e. a **point mutation** and **frameshift mutation**.

Point Mutation

A point mutation involves a **change in a single base-pair in the DNA**, resulting in a single base change in the corresponding mRNA. This type of mutation may **also** be **referred to as base substitution mutation**. This may result in **transition** or **transversion** types of mutation (Fig. 19.6).

- **Transition mutation:** The substitution where a purine-pyrimidine pair is replaced by another such pair is called transition. It may occur spontaneously, induced chemically by a base analog (e.g. 5-bromouracil) or by a mutagen (such as nitrous acid). For example, if 5-bromouracil gets incorporated into DNA (in place of a thymine), it may induce **AT → GC transition**. On the other hand, treatment of DNA with nitrous acid may result in, both, AT → GC as well as **GC → AT transitions**.
- **Transversion mutation:** The substitution where a **purine-pyrimidine pair is replaced by a pyrimidine-purine pair** is called transversion. This may **occur spontaneously** and is common in human beings.

Frameshift Mutation

Frameshift mutations are the **result of insertion or deletion of a base-pair**.

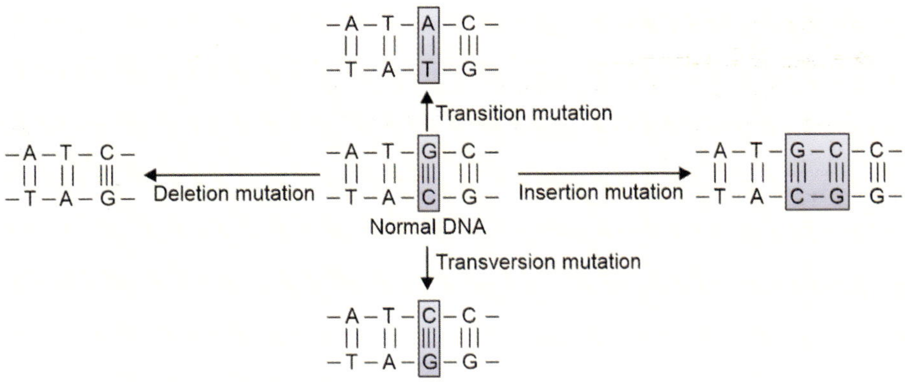

Fig. 19.6: Gene mutations

- **Deletion: Deletion of a base-pair** from the DNA base sequence of the gene **may change its reading frame** and **result in** a **nonfunctional gene product.** For example, a frameshift mutation as a result of base deletion **may lead to the production of abnormal hemoglobin** such as **hemoglobin Wayne**. Deletion **may be caused by deaminating agents.**
- **Insertion:** Insertion of a base-pair into the gene sequence **can lead to the synthesis of abnormal chain length of a protein**. Some insertions can be **caused by mutagens**, such as acridines, ethidium bromide, etc.

EFFECTS OF GENE MUTATION

Mutations **may be expressed** phenotypically (visible) or **remain silent.**

Visible Mutation

A visible or expressed **mutation** may be a missense mutation or a **nonsense** mutation.

- **Missense mutation:** It is the result of a base change that **causes the incorporation of a different amino acid in the encoded protein.** An example of missense mutation is a change in second base of the codon GAA (or GAG) which codes for glutamate in the sixth position of the α-chain of hemoglobin. The change from A to U results in GUA (or GUG) which codes for valine. This, in turn, results in sickle cell anemia, one of the most common forms of hemoglobinopathies.
- **Nonsense mutation:** It may be a result of a **change in the base of the codon,** which **may destroy a termination codon,** or result in the **formation of a new termination codon.**
  - **The formation of a new termination codon** may result in premature termination and, thus, **reduce chain length of the protein.** For example, the codon UAU or UAC normally encodes for tyrosine, as the 145th amino acid in the β-chain of hemoglobin. A single base mutation from UAU to UAA or UAC to UAG results in a termination codon, which in turn, reduces the chain length from 146 to 144 amino acids. This results in the synthesis of hemoglobin McKees Rocks which has a higher oxygen affinity and decreases oxygen delivery to the tissues.
  - On the other hand, **mutation of a base in the termination codon to a codon which encodes for an amino acid result in a protein that has larger chain length than the normal**. For example, a normal α-globin chain has 141 amino acid residues. When the stop codon UAA mutates, it results in the incorporation of an amino acid at 142nd position and increases the chain length to nearly 172 amino acids, i.e. until another stop codon is reached. Abnormally long α-globin chain has been shown to result in many instances of α-thalassemias.
- **Silent mutation:** This is a result of a **base change that occurs in the third position of a codon**, e.g. UUA to UUG. Since both the codons code for leucine and there is no change in the specified amino acid, such mutations are called silent mutations.

Certain mutations, which may otherwise be silent, require the presence of another mutation in a neighbouring gene to become clinically manifested, as observed in polycystic kidney disease (PKD), a disorder in which numerous cysts (fluid-filled epithelial sacs) develop in both the kidneys (Fig. 19.7).

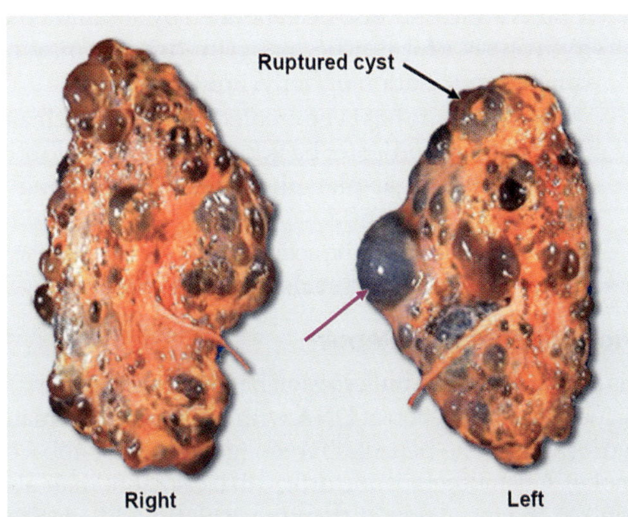

Fig. 19.7: Bilateral polycystic kidneys. Purple arrow indicates the largest cyst

DNA REPAIR

As mentioned above, DNA is a genetic material. It is essential that the newly synthesized DNA should be error free. Even with less than 1 out of 1000 accidental changes may result in a mutation. Hence, any error that may occur during replication is immediately repaired. DNA repair is a high-priority process for the maintenance of integrity of the genetic information and other cellular functions.

There are several processes for DNA repair, each one of which can repair a certain type of the damage.

REPLACEMENT OF THE DAMAGED SEGMENT

A segment of the damaged DNA is repaired by the process called **excision repair**. The process includes **incision at the site of damage, excision of the damaged segment, resynthesis of the new strand at the site of damage** and **ligation of the two ends**. Such systems exist both in eukaryotes and prokaryotes.

Excision Repair

Excision repair is carried out by the replacement of the damaged DNA, depending upon the extent of the damage in the two strands. It includes **base excision repair** and **nucleotide excision repair**.

- **Base excision repair:** It eliminates the modified bases, like those that have been deaminated, methylated or modified chemically.
  - The **modified bases are hydrolytically removed by** the enzymes termed **DNA glycosylases**, e.g. deaminated cytosine (uracil) is removed by uracil DNA glycosylase.
  - This, in turn, **produces a deoxyribose-phosphate residue** (i.e. having only the sugar moiety which is linked with a phosphate but is without a base). Such a site is designated as an apurinic-apyrimidinic site **(AP site)**.

    Such a site may also be generated by spontaneous hydrolysis of a purine or pyrimidine. It may be called depurination or depyrimidination.
  - After an AP site has been created, **AP endonuclease nicks phosphodiester backbone** at the AP site and **excises the sugar-phosphate residue**, creating a gap of one nucleotide.
  - This **gap is filled by** the action of **DNA polymerase I.**
  - Finally, **DNA ligase seals the ends** (Fig. 19.8).

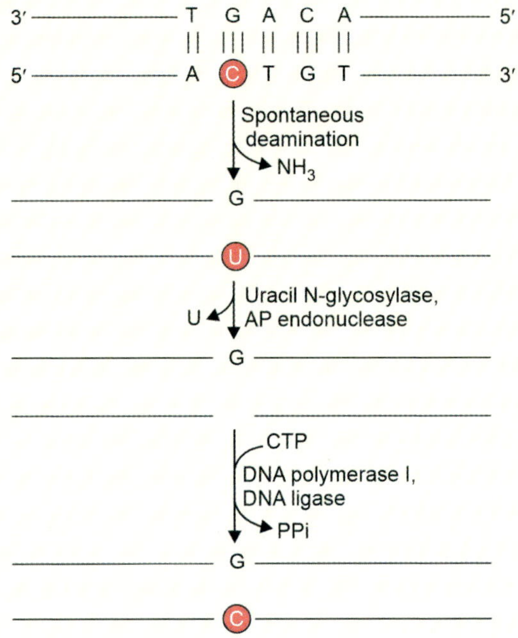

Fig. 19.8: Base excision repair in prokaryotes

Nucleotide Excision Repair

It is activated when a bulky lesion has been produced, such as due to the interaction of **DNA with a polycyclic aromatic hydrocarbon**, like benzo(a)pyrene (generated by tobacco smoke). Chemotherapeutic drugs, like cisplatin, may also result in the formation of **thyminecisplatin adducts**. The **dimerization of the adjacent pyrimidines**, induced by UV light, may also result in generation of a bulky lesion.

In *E. coli*, such a repair is initiated by recognition of the distortion of DNA by an endonuclease system which is a product of three genes, i.e. UvrA, UvrB and UvrC. This endonuclease system is designated as excision nuclease or exci-nuclease. In this process:

- A tetramer, consisting of **two UvrA and two UvrB proteins**, is formed. This, in turn, causes local melting of DNA (at the expense of ATP) and **locates the bulky lesion.**
- **UvrB makes 3′ incision**, followed by a **5′ incision by** UvrC.
- It leads to the **release of an oligonucleotide including the bulky lesion,** e.g. the pyrimidine dimer.
- Thereafter, **UvrD** (a helicase) **unwinds DNA** and releases the above excised oligonucleotide.
- **DNA polymerase** then **displaces UvrB** and **fills the gap.**
- The repair is **completed by DNA ligase** (Fig. 19.9).

Excision Repair in Eukaryotes

In eukaryotes, the endonuclease activity of human cells consists of 16–17 different polypeptides.

- Nucleotide excision repair of human DNA begins with the **binding of** a protein designated as xeroderma pigmentosum A **(XP-A) to a dimer** which consists of two other proteins, i.e. **XP-F and ERCC-1** (excision repair component).
- **XP-A binds** to the dimer between **XP-F and ERCC-1** and **forms a complex (XP-F: XP-A: ERCC-1).** Its **XP-A** component recognizes the damaged site and binds to the complex.
- **Thereafter**, a replication protein **(HSSB)** also binds to **XP-A** and gets associated to the damaged site.

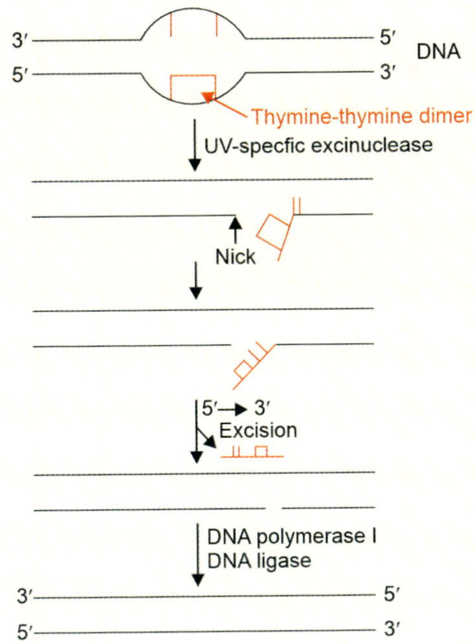

Fig. 19.9: Nucleotide excision repair in prokaryotes

- The additional enzyme complex, known as general transcription factor TFIIH interacts with XP-C and the whole complex gets associated to the damaged site through XP-A.
- Subsequently, **XP-G also gets associated with this complex** to complete the exci-nuclease system.
- The **3′ nick is introduced by XP-G** while **XP-F in association with ERCC-1 makes the 5′ nick**. This, in turn, results in excision of an oligonucleotide.
- The **gap is filled by polymerases γ and ε.**
- Finally, **DNA ligase seals the nick.**

Defects in nucleotide excision repair have been shown to result in various hereditary disorders, such as xeroderma pigmentosum.

Xeroderma pigmentosum: This is a condition characterized by varying levels of UV sensitivity and corresponding **deficiencies in DNA repair system,** such as a **mutation in XP-V gene**. These patients exhibit sunlight-induced photo-dermatosis characterized by severe skin reactions that range from skin ulceration to the development of skin cancer. Some of its forms are also accompanied by neurological abnormalities due to abnormal gene expression and DNA deterioration caused by the accumulation of the damaged DNA (Fig. 19.10).

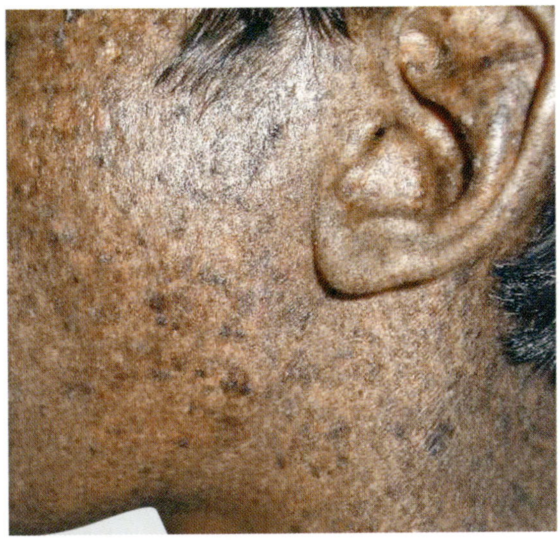

Fig. 19.10: Xeroderma pigmentosum: An inherited disease characterized by photosensitivity, epithelial atrophy and hyperpigmentation

Some Important Questions

1. **What is replication? Describe the process of DNA replication in prokaryotes. How it differs from eukaryotes?**
2. **What is mutation? Describe various types of mutations.**
3. **Discuss differences between DNA polymerases found in prokaryotes and eukaryotes.**

2. **Describe briefly:**
   - i. Origin of replication
   - ii. Semi-conservative replication
   - iii. Topoisomerase inhibitors
   - iv. Role of RNA primer in replication

3. **Write notes on:**
   - i. DnaA protein
   - ii. Topoisomerases
   - iii. DNA polymerases
   - iv. Reverse transcriptase
   - v. Replication fork
   - vi. Okazaki fragments
   - vii. Point mutation
   - viii. Frame-shift mutation
   - ix. Nonsense mutation
   - x. Silent mutation
   - xi. Primosome
   - xii. Telomeres
   - xiii. Histones
   - xiv. DNA repair
   - xv. Xeroderma pigmentosum
   - xvi. Single-stranded DNA-binding proteins
   - xvii. DNA helicases
   - xviii. Telomerases

Chapter 20

RNA Transcription

Transcription refers to the **process of RNA synthesis**, by which a DNA sequence is transcribed into the RNA transcript. The process of RNA synthesis **requires an appropriate sequence of DNA as a template**, and the enzymes called **RNA polymerases**.

As discussed in Chapter 4, **there are three different forms of RNA.** These are referred to as **tRNA, mRNA and rRNA. Each form has a specific function** and is essentially required **in protein synthesis**.

Each cycle of transcription begins as well as ends with the recognition of some specific sites in the DNA template.

PROMOTER REGION

The **site, where RNA polymerase binds** is called promoter.

The **nucleotide** in the promoter region **is assigned a negative number, if it is present** towards the 5′-site (i.e. **prior to the transcription start site**). **This position is also referred to as upstream**. On the other hand, a nucleotide is assigned a **positive number**, if it is **present towards the 3′-site** (i.e. after the transcription start site). This position is called **downstream**. Accordingly, the **first nucleotide at the transcription start site is referred to as +1**.

Certain conserved sequences have been shown to occur in the promoter region, both in prokaryotes and eukaryotes.

In Prokaryotes: The promoter region, where **RNA polymerase binds**, is the site which is **extending**, nearly, **45 base pair (bp) upstream and 10 bp downstream**, of the transcription start site. It has two highly conserved short (oligonucleotide) sequences, called **pribnow box** (–10 sequence) and **–35 sequence** (Fig. 20.1).

In Eukaryotes: The promoter region in eukaryotes, **has three different** highly conserved **sequences**, which are referred to as the **TATA box**, the **GC box** and the **CAAT box**.

In addition, **transcription in eukaryotes is also affected by** certain other promoter elements, called enhancers.

RNA POLYMERASES

RNA polymerases are the enzymes, which are required to **synthesize RNA** in the 5′→3′ direction, **using a DNA template**. They initiate polymerization of the ribonucleotides at the consequence sequence on a promoter site and do not need a primer.

Different types of RNA polymerases are found in prokaryotes and eukaryotes.

- **In prokaryotes:** A **single type of RNA polymerase** synthesizes all forms of RNAs (tRNA, mRNA and rRNA) in bacteria. It is a **multienzyme complex**. The core enzyme **consists of four peptides** (two a, one b, and one b′) subunits. It also requires another protein,

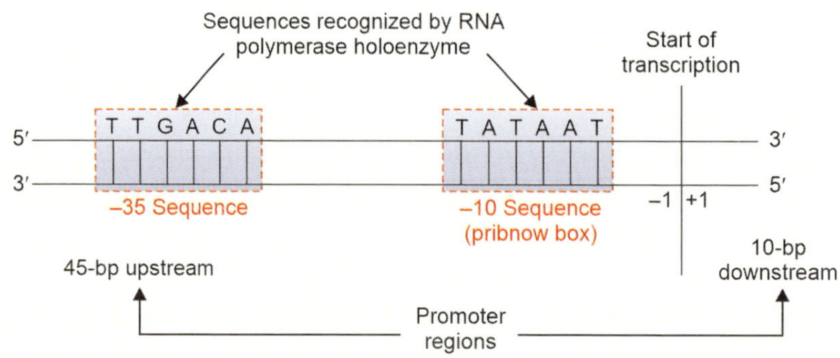

Fig. 20.1: Promoter regions in prokaryotes

i.e. the fifth subunit, which is designated as the **sigma (σ) factor**. This RNA polymerase cannot recognize the promoter region on the DNA template without the addition of the σ factor.

Binding of the σ factor with the core enzyme results in the **formation of holoenzyme**, which, in turn, **initiates RNA synthesis** in prokaryotes.

- **In eukaryotes: Three** different **types of RNA polymerases** have been identified in eukaryotes. These are referred to as **RNA polymerase I, II and III**.
  - **RNA polymerase I transcribes** ribosomal RNA **(rRNA)**, genes for which are located within the nucleolus.
  - **RNA polymerase II transcribes mRNA**. It synthesizes large RNA particle, which is the precursor of the mRNA and the small nuclear RNAs (snRNAs).
  - **RNA polymerase III produces** small RNA molecules, which are processed to give various types of tRNA and some snRNAs.

In addition, to the above three types of RNA polymerases, eukaryotes also have another type of RNA polymerase, called **mitochondrial RNA polymerase** (mtRNA polymerase), which is responsible for the synthesis of all forms of RNAs (mRNA, tRNA and rRNA) within the mitochondria.

PROCESS OF TRANSCRIPTION

The process of RNA synthesis occurs in 3 steps, which are referred to as **initiation, elongation and termination**.

Initiation of Transcription

- **RNA polymerase holoenzyme** (RNA polymerase with the sigma factor) **locates the promoter** on the DNA template.
- After the holoenzyme has recognized the promoter, it **binds** there **and forms a complex**.
- This, in turn, results in **unwinding of nearly 10 nucleotide base pairs of the DNA double helix**.
- The **unwound DNA then binds to the initiating** ribonucleotide triphosphate, usually a **purine ribonucleotide** (GTP or ATP) and, thus, forms the first phosphodiester bond.

Elongation of the RNA Transcript

- After the holoenzyme enzyme has begun to synthesize RNA transcript, its σ **subunit is released** and the core enzyme (RNA polymerase) translocates to the next position and continues the process.
- The **template strand gets attached to the growing RNA chain**, by base pairing. The enzyme topoisomerase, which is a component of the transcription complex, helps in the process of unwinding and restoring the DNA double helix (Fig. 20.2).

Termination of Transcription

- After the desired RNA transcript has been synthesized, RNA polymerase complex recognizes the termination sequence, which is present at the end of the gene, and terminates the process.
- Termination of the transcription process can occur in either of the two modes, i.e.:
  - The enzyme, RNA polymerase, itself recognizes the termination region on the DNA template. This process is referred to as **rho (ρ) independent termination**.
  - Alternatively, **termination of the process may require** an additional protein which is designated

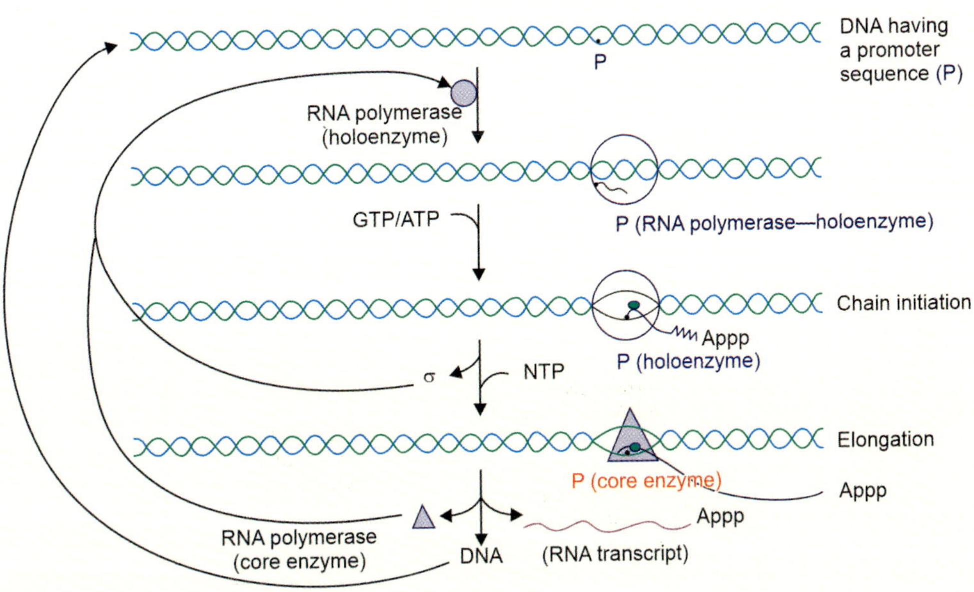

Fig. 20.2: Process of RNA transcription

as ρ **factor, for the release of the RNA transcript.** This is termed as the **ρ-dependent termination**.

DIFFERENCES IN TRANSCRIPTION PROCESS IN PROKARYOTES AND EUKARYOTES

Transcription in eukaryotes is more complex than prokaryotes.

- Transcription in prokaryotes requires only an appropriate sequence of the DNA as a template, the enzyme RNA polymerase (holoenzyme) and ribonucleoside triphosphates as the substrates,
- Initiation of the process in eukaryotes requires several additional molecular events:
  1. **Chromatin**, though is organized in the nucleosomes, however, some of its part which is containing the promoter sequences, is not well organized and is not accessible to the transcription machinery. Such a nucleosomal organization **requires DNase activity** for proper access by the transcription machinery.
  2. Certain gene-specific sequences, referred to as **enhancers, are also needed**. These sequences stimulate transcription as well as binding of various transcription factors.
  3. Besides RNA polymerases certain additional proteins called **transcription factors are required**. They bind to some sequences in the promoter region, for the initiation of the process. These transcription factors also facilitate binding of the RNA polymerase.

Differences in the process of transcription between prokaryotes and eukaryotes are shown in Table 20.1.

POST-TRANSCRIPTIONAL MODIFICATIONS OF RNA TRANSCRIPTS

In prokaryotes, the **mRNA is**, generally, identical to its primary transcript and does **not** require any modification while primary transcripts of **tRNA and rRNA are processed, post-transcriptionally**.

In eukaryotes, all the three types of RNA transcripts undergo extensive modifications, post-transcriptionally.

- **Post-transcriptional modifications of the mRNA** transcript in eukaryotes-Post-transcriptional modifications of the mRNA transcript in eukaryotes include:
  - **Addition of poly(A) tail:** The poly(A) tail of 40–200 adenine nucleotides is added to the free 3′-end of the mRNA primary transcript by a polymerase. This polyadenylation (poly A tail) does not require a template and helps in stabilization of the mRNA and facilitates its exit from the nucleus (Fig. 20.3).

Table 20.1: Differences in the process of transcription between prokaryotes and eukaryotes

Prokaryotes	*Eukaryotes*
No nucleosomal organization is required as chromatin is easily accessible to the transcription machinery	Nucleosomal organization is required, which is done by the enzyme DNase. This is essential for proper access by the transcription machinery
Promoter region, for the binding of the RNA polymerase, is simple	Promoter region is complex, and binds RNA polymerase with other transcription factors
There is only one type of RNA polymerase	There are three distinct forms of the enzyme RNA polymerase, one for each class of the RNA. These are referred to as RNA polymerase I, II and III
Introns are rarely found in the primary transcript	Introns very commonly occur in the primary transcript
Post-transcriptional modifications are restricted to tRNA and rRNA only	Post-transcriptional modifications take place in all the three types of RNAs

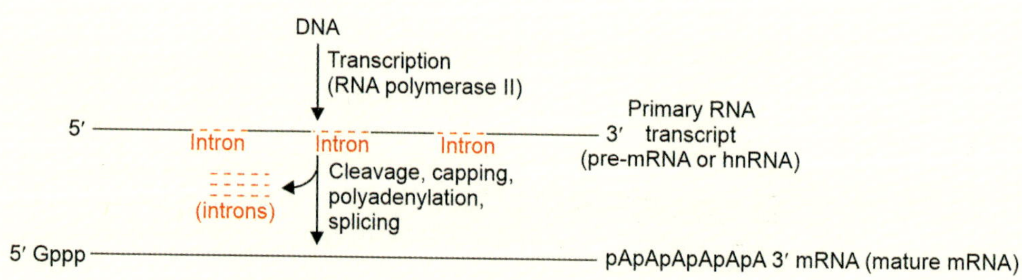

Fig. 20.3: Post-transcriptional processing of mRNA

- **Splicing:** The primary mRNAs transcript, called **pre-mRNA** or heterogenous nuclear RNA **(hnRNA)**, contains two types of sequences called **introns** and **exons**.
  - **Introns**, also called **intervening sequences**, are the **noncoding sequences** that are present in pre-mRNA but **not in mature mRNA**.
  - The other sequences, which are **expressed** or **retained**, are called **exons**.
  - As pre-mRNA is extruded from the RNA polymerase complex, it is rapidly bound by small nuclear ribonucleoproteins (snRNPs or **snrnps**). Different snrnps **bind to the RNA precursor** and **form** a large complex, termed **spliceosome**. This, in turn, carries out dual steps of the **RNA splicing**, i.e. **breakage of the intron** at the 5′-site, and **joining of the exon** sequences together. After removal of the introns, fully functional mature mRNA leaves the nucleus and passes into the cytosol.
  - **Mutations in the β-globin gene interfere** with the removal of introns. This, in turn, **leads to** a condition called **β-thalassemia**.

- **Post-transcriptional modifications of the rRNA transcript in eukaryotes:** Ribosomal RNAs are synthesized from the long precursor molecules, called **pre-rRNAs** or **45S RNA**, which contains sequences for **28S, 5.8S and 18S rRNAs. During post-transcriptional modifications**, each **pre-rRNA is cleaved to** yield the required rRNA species (Fig. 20.4).

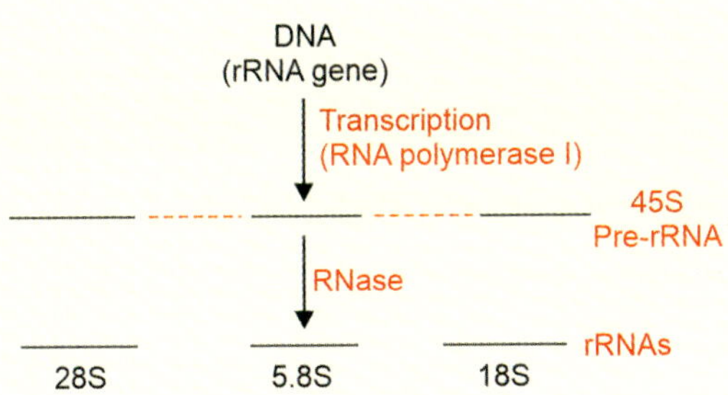

Fig. 20.4: Post-transcriptional processing of rRNA

Some of the proteins, which are destined to become components of ribosomes, also get associated with the pre-rRNAs, prior to and during post-transcriptional modifications in the nucleolus.

- **Post-transcriptional modifications of the tRNA** transcript in eukaryotes: tRNA undergoes following modifications:
  - **Trimming:** The primary transcript of tRNA has large number of nucleotide sequences on both the ends which are removed, and the tRNA molecule is trimmed, non-specifically. From the 5′-end, the primary tRNA transcript undergoes endo-nucleolytic cleavage **by ribonuclease P** (a ribozyme), while the 3′ extension is removed by the exonucleolytic cleavage.

    Sometimes, the primary transcript may also contain introns, which are removed by the two-component enzyme system, whereas one of the enzymes removes introns, the other rejoins the remaining exon chains.
  - **Addition of the terminal CCA sequence:** Each functional tRNA, both in the cytosol and the mitochondria, has a sequence of three nucleotides, CCA at the 3′ terminus. These nucleotides are **added, sequentially, by** the enzyme **tRNA-nucleotidyl-transferase**.
  - **Modifications of some of the bases:** As we know, the tRNA molecules have several modified nitrogenous bases. These modifications are done by various enzymes, which are either site specific or nucleotide sequence specific.

ANTIBIOTICS THAT INHIBIT TRANSCRIPTION

Some of the antibiotics are known to inhibit the process of transcription, e.g. rifampicin. It is used in the treatment of tuberculosis and inhibits RNA polymerase activity in several bacteria.

RNA INTERFERENCE

Specific cellular mRNAs can be degraded by introducing mammalian cells to a double-stranded RNA (dsRNA), derived from a virus or a transposon, or artificially prepared in the laboratory, in which one of the strands is complementary to the mRNA being targeted. This phenomenon is called RNA interference (RNAi).

Several potential clinical applications of RNAi are currently being evaluated, e.g. in the treatment of cancer, AIDS and other infections. Further, RNAi is currently the method of choice for eukaryotic gene inactivation. The consequences of loss of gene function reveal the role played by the gene product (RNA or protein) in the cell.

RNA interference is employed in post-transcriptional gene silencing or gene knockdown, as follows:

- A dsRNA is introduced into a target cell. One strand of the dsRNA is designed to be an antisense RNA because its sequence is complementary to the RNA transcript of the gene selected for silencing.
- Inside the cell, an ATP-dependent RNase III called **dicer** (ribo-endonuclease), catalyses cleavage of both the strands to produce a double-stranded small interfering RNA (ds-siRNA), 21–23 nucleotides long and having 2-nucleotides long 3′-overhangs on each strand.
- The ds-siRNA is passed onto another protein complex called **RNA-induced silencing complex (RISC)**.

- In an ATP-dependent manner, RISC unwinds the ds-siRNA and selects the antisense strand, now called the **guide strand**. The other strand called the passenger strand is discarded.
- RISC pairs the single guide strand with a complementary region on the target gene transcript (mRNA).
- The RNase H activity of RISC performs its slicer function by cleaving the RNA transcript so that it can no longer be translated by ribosomes.
- The guide strand remains associated with RISC hence, it can be used for multiple cycles of mRNA cleavage, i.e. post-transcriptional gene silencing (Fig. 20.5).

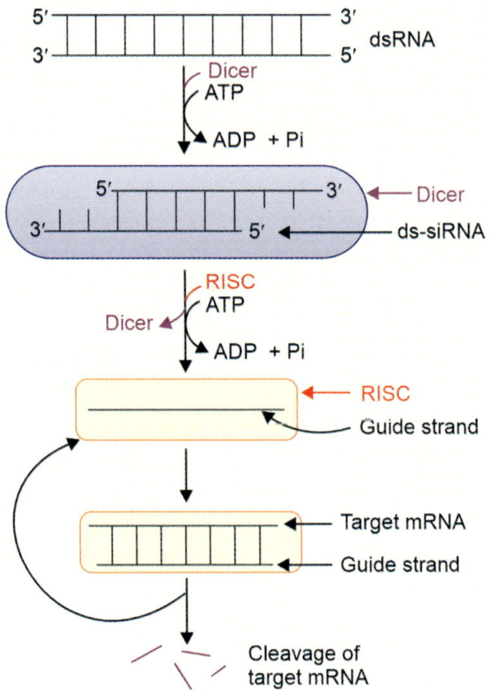

Fig. 20.5: RNA interference

Some Important Questions

1. Describe the process of transcription in prokaryotes. How it differs from eukaryotes?

2. Write notes on:

i. Promoter region
ii. RNA polymerases
iii. Post-transcriptional modifications
iv. DNA template
v. Upstream nucleotide sequence
vi. Pribnow box
vii. TATA box
viii. Enhancers
ix. Rho-dependent termination of transcription
x. Rho-independent termination of transcription
xi. RNA interference

Chapter 21

Genetic Code and Protein Synthesis

The **process of protein biosynthesis** is called translation. It is the **biochemical translation of the genetic information, from the four-letter language of nucleotides to the twenty-letter language of amino acids**, as **defined by the genetic code**.

GENETIC CODE

Genetic code is **a dictionary that gives a correspondence between the sequences of four nucleotide bases** that are **found in mRNA to the sequence of twenty amino acids,** which occur **in peptides.**

- Each word of the genetic code is **composed of three letters** (nucleotide bases) and is referred to as **codon.**
- This is due to the reason, that **if one nucleotide codes for an amino acid, four nucleotides will code for** $(4)^1$, i.e. **four amino acids only. If** there are **two** nucleotides in a code, **it will translate** $(4)^2$, i.e. **16 amino acids only**. Hence, a **3:1 correspondence of nucleotides to amino acids** with $(4)^3$, i.e. 64 combinations, is there **to code 20 amino acids.**
- Codons are present on the mRNA language as the nucleotides (U, C, A and G) and are written in a sequence from the 5′-end to the 3′-end.
- Thus, **codons are the permutations of four bases,** which are **taken in the sets of three.**
- These 64 combinations of three bases each define genetic code (Table 21.1).

Stop Codons

As shown in Table 21.1, out of the 64 codons, **only 61** are known to **code for 20** amino acids while the remaining **3 are used as stop codons**. Since these 3 codons **stop the process of translation**, these are also referred to as **termination codons**.

Table 21.1: Genetic code

5′-Base	*Middle-base*								*3′-Base*
	U		*C*		*A*		*G*		
U	UUU	Phe	UCU		UAU	Tyr	UGU	Cys	**U**
	UUC		UCC	Ser	UAC		UGC		
	UUA		UCA		UAA	Stop	UGA	Stop	
	UUG		UCG		UAG		UGG	Trp	
C	CUU	Leu	CCU		CAU	His	CGU		**C**
	CUC		CCC	Pro	CAC		CGC	Arg	
	CUA		CCA		CAA	Gln	CGA		
	CUG		CCG		CAG		CGG		
A	AUU		ACU		AAU	Asn	AGU	Ser	**A**
	AUC	Ile	ACC	Thr	AAC		AGC		
	AUA		ACA		AAA	Lys	AGA	Arg	
	AUG	Met	ACG		AAG		AGG		
G	GUU		GCU		GAU	Asp	GGU		**G**
	GUC	Val	GCC	Ala	GAC		GGC	Gly	
	GUA		GCA		GAA	Glu	GGA		
	GUG		GCG		GAG		GGG		

Salient Features of the Genetic Code

Genetic code has some salient features which have been described in Table 21.2.

Table 21.2: Salient features of the genetic code

Degeneracy	Multiple codons code for the same amino acid
Unambiguous	A specific codon codes for only a single amino acid
Nonoverlapping	Reading of the genetic code occurs without overlapping
Punctuation	Message is read continuously without any break between the sequence of codons until a nonsense codon is reached
Universality	The same codon is used in all the living organisms with only few exceptions in the mitochondria

Variations in Codon-Anticodon Interaction

As discussed in Chapter 4, there are 3 types of RNA present in cells which are referred to as mRNA, tRNA and rRNA.

- The mRNA is a group of RNAs which is synthesized within the nucleus as a result of transcription. Each **mRNA** transcript has 5′→3′ polarity, which **is complementary to the coding strand of gene** (DNA molecule), and **conveys the message** (information) **from the gene to the protein-synthesizing machinery**.
- **The information** from mRNA, i.e. the sequence of nucleotides (U, C, A and G) **is read from 5′-end to 3′-end**, in combination of three nucleotides (at a time) **in the form of codons**.
- There are about **50 different types of tRNAs** and that each tRNA fulfils its role as an adapter molecule.
- Each **tRNA** (in the anticodon arm) **has** a sequence of three nucleotides called **anticodon**.
- The **tRNA binds an amino acid** and **locates itself at the correct codon**, for the translation of the information present in the sequence of nucleotides on mRNA into the sequence of amino acids.
- So, there are **50 anticodons** (tRNAs) to recognize **61 codons** which define **20 amino acids** each one of which is specifically carried by a tRNA.
- **This**, in turn, **suggests** that a **single tRNA may recognize more than one codon**.
- As shown in Table 21.1, there are more than one codon for one amino acid.
- This is referred to as degeneracy of genetic code (Table 21.2).
- To explain the possible cause of degeneracy of codons, Crick proposed a hypothesis and designated it as **Wobble hypothesis**.

WOBBLE HYPOTHESIS

Crick explained that there occur certain variations in the standard base pairing rule in codon-anticodon interaction and that all the codons may not be used equally. Accordingly, he suggested that **only the first two bases of the codon have a precise pairing with the last two bases of the anticodon** of the tRNA while **the pairing between the third base of the codon to the first base of the anticodon may wobble (tremble or move unsteadily)**. Thus, the first two positions of the codon predominate in tRNA selection while the third position wobbles, i.e. the base at the 5′-end of the anticodon (i.e. the first base of the anticodon or the third base of the codon) is not as well defined.

PROCESS OF PROTEIN SYNTHESIS

Th process of protein synthesis involves **activation of amino acids** and **initiation, elongation and termination of translation** along with the **release of the polypeptide chain**.

Activation of Amino Acids

For their incorporation into the polypeptide chain, firstly, **amino acids are activated** and **attached to the appropriate tRNA** carrier molecules. Attachment of the amino acid to its tRNA requires ATP and the reaction is catalyzed **by** the enzyme **aminoacyl-tRNA synthetase**. Aminoacyl-tRNA synthetase is a group of enzymes, each one of which is specific for an amino acid and its appropriate tRNA (Fig. 21.1).

The enzyme also edits protein synthesis, as the wrong or inappropriate acylated-tRNA is recognized and removed. Furthermore, amino acids are incorporated in the polypeptide chain from the amino terminal end to the carboxy terminal end.

Initiation of Protein Synthesis

Initiation of protein synthesis, in eukaryotes, **involves** assembly of various components of the translation system, which include **two ribosomal subunits, mRNA, aminoacyl-tRNA** (specified by the codon), **GTP and** various **initiation factors**, which facilitate assembly of the initiation complex.

- Firstly, the **initiation codon** (AUG) **is recognized by the initiation tRNA** (that carries methionine). This is

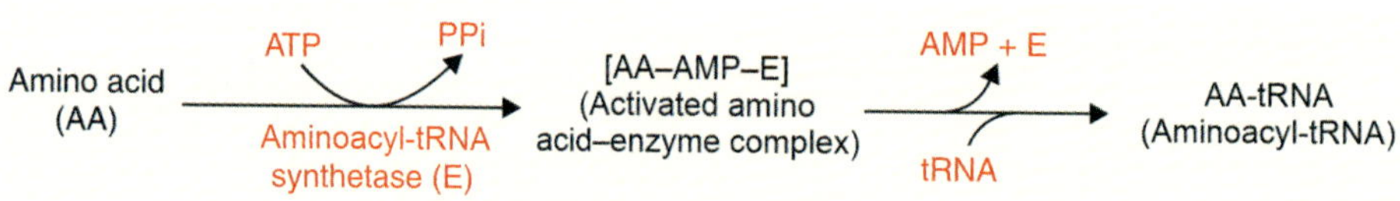

Fig. 21.1: Amino acid activation

facilitated by eIF-2a (eukaryotic initiation factor-2a), which binds to **GTP and methioninyl-tRNA** (Met-tRNAi^{Met}), and **forms a ternary complex**.

- Subsequently, the **ternary complex gets associated with mRNA** and **40S ribosomal subunit** and **eIF-3**.
- Thereafter, Binding of the various components **(eIF-2a.Met-tRNAi^{Met}.GTP, eIF-3.40S rRNA, eIF-4c** and some more protein factors) with **mRNA forms preinitiation complex**.
- The **40S.Met-tRNAi^{Met}.mRNA complex interacts with the 60S subunit** and eIF-4d to **form 80S ribosome**.
- The **initiating methioninyl-tRNA is** correctly **placed on the mRNA at** such a position that it occupies the donor site, also called the peptidyl site or **P-site**, on the ribosome, so that its methioninyl-residue may be transferred (donated) to the free α-amino group of the incoming aminoacyl-tRNA.
- With the **hydrolysis of GTP, eIF2a.GDP, eIF-3 and other factors are released** (Fig. 21.2).

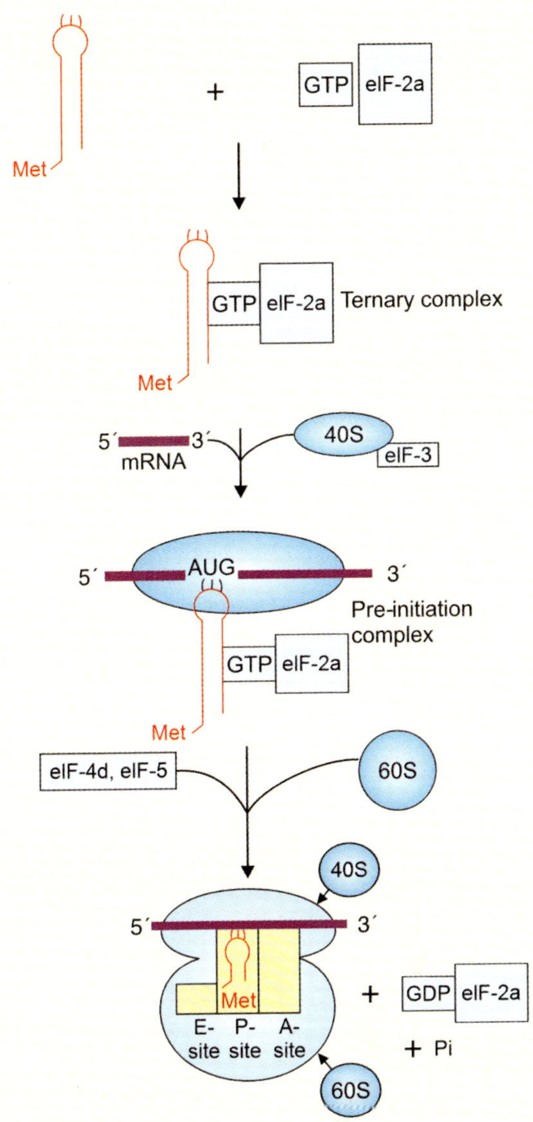

Fig. 21.2: Initiation of protein synthesis

In *E. coli*, binding and positioning of mRNA on the 30S ribosomal subunit is facilitated by complementary base pairing between the pyrimidine-rich sequence of 8 nucleotides in the 16S RNA and a purine-rich sequence of 10 nucleotides designated as Shine-Dalgarno Sequence, present on mRNA.

Elongation of the Polypeptide Chain

- Elongation of the polypeptide chain starts with the **incoming aminoacyl tRNA (specified by the next codon on the mRNA)** with the help of the elongation factor-1 (EF-1).
- **EF-1α** component of the EF-1 **forms a ternary complex (EF1α.aminoacyl-tRNA.GTP) with the incoming aminoacyl-tRNA and GTP.**
- **The aminoacyl-tRNA binds on the ribosome** and, if codon anticodon interaction is correct, the aminoacyl-tRNA is **placed at the A-site, GTP is hydrolyzed** and **EF-1α.GDP** complex **is dissociated.**
- The **initiating methioninyl-tRNA** (as discussed above) **and the incoming aminoacyl-tRNA** are now positioned on the ribosome on the **P-site and the A-site**, respectively.
- **Peptidyltransferase** catalyzes formation of the peptide bond and **transfers methionine on to the amino acid present on the aminoacyl-tRNA.**
- At this stage, **the aminoacyl-tRNA (attached with the polypeptide) occupies a hybrid position** (i.e. its **anticodon arm remains on the A-site** in the 40S subunit) while the **acceptor-arm along with the attached polypeptide is shifted towards the 60S subunit (P-site).** On the other hand, **anticodon of the deacylated tRNA remains on the P-site** (in the 40S subunit) while its **acceptor arm is shifted** in the 60S **towards the** exit site **(E-site).**
- **With** the help of elongation factor-2 (**EF-2,** also **called translocase), mRNA** and **the aminoacyl-tRNA (attached with the polypeptide) are now repositioned** (in the codon-anticodon register) **from A-site to P-site.**
- **GTP is hydrolyzed** and the **A-site becomes vacant.** Simultaneously, the **deacylated methioninyl-tRNA moves to the E-site** (which exists only in the 60S subunit; Fig. 21.3).

In each round, peptidyl-transferase transfers the growing polypeptide chain from the carrier tRNA to the α-amino group of the amino acid residue on the aminoacyl tRNA (specified by the next codon). The process of **chain elongation is stopped after the incoming aminoacyl tRNA finds a termination codon (stop codon) on the A-site.**

Termination of Protein Synthesis

- Termination of protein synthesis occurs with the presence of a stop codon (UAG, UAA or UGA) on the A-site on mRNA.

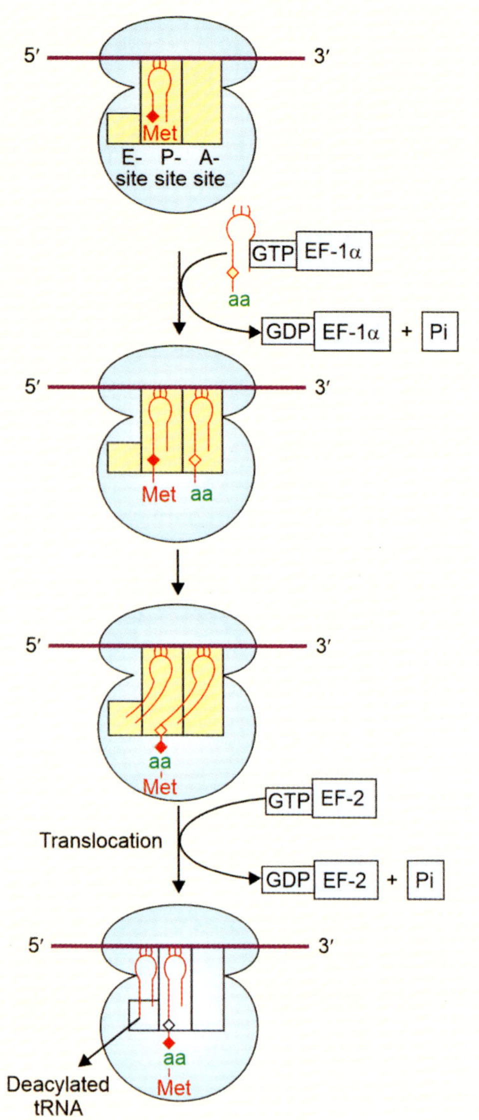

Fig. 21.3: Chain elongation

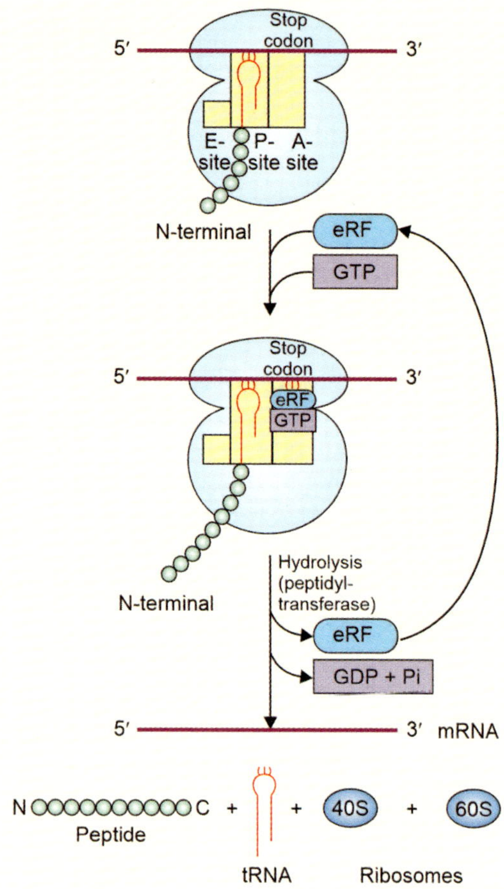

Fig. 21.4: Termination of protein synthesis

- At this point, a non-ribosomal protein called **releasing factor (eRF)** and **GTP** are attached.
- The **peptide-tRNA ester linkage is hydrolyzed by peptidyl-transferase and the polypeptide is released.**
- **Subsequently, hydrolysis of GTP** causes release of **eRF and dissociation** of the 80S **ribosome into two (60S and 40S) subunits**.
- The eRF and the ribosomes re-enter the new cycle at the initiation stage (Fig. 21.4).

Differences in the process of protein synthesis between prokaryotes and eukaryotes are shown in Table 21.3.

Table 21.3: Differences in the process of protein biosynthesis between prokaryotes and eukaryotes

Prokaryotes	*Eukaryotes*
The mRNA is usually polycistronic	The mRNA is monocistronic. It also contains a poly(A) tail
Ribosomes are present in the free form. These are 70S in size comprising of 50S and 30S subunits	Ribosomes are present in the free form as well as bound to endoplasmic reticulum. These are 80S in size consisting of 60S and 40S subunits
Three initiation factors are required in the process	One initiation factor is known to participate in the process
N-Formylmethioninyl-tRNA binds to the start codon	Met-tRNA is not formylated
Three elongation factors are required. These are referred to as EF-Tu, EF-Ts, and EF-G	Two elongation factors are required. These are referred to as eEF-1 and eEF-2
Termination of the process requires three releasing factors, which are referred to as RF-1, RF-2 and RF-3	Termination of the process requires one releasing factor, which is designated as eRF

INHIBITORS OF PROTEIN SYNTHESIS

As shown in Table 21.4, many antibiotics and toxins inhibit protein biosynthesis and are used in clinical practice, as therapeutic agents. For example:

- **Antibiotics:**
  - **Streptomycin:** Streptomycin binds to the smaller subunit of the prokaryotic ribosome and **interferes with the initiation of protein synthesis**. It also **causes misreading of the mRNA**.

Table 21.4: Inhibitors of the process of protein biosynthesis

Antibiotic/Inhibitor	*Inhibitory effect in*		*Inhibits the process of*
	Prokaryotes	*Eukaryotes*	
Streptomycin	30S subunit	—	Initiation and misreading of the mRNA
Tetracyclin	30S subunit	40S subunit	Binding of aminoacyl-tRNA
Puromycin/Chloramphenicol	70S ribosome	80S ribosome	Peptide transfer
Erythromycin	50S subunit	—	Translocation
Fusidic acid	EF-G	—	Translocation
Cycloheximide	—	80S ribosome	Elongation
Diphtheria toxin	—	60S subunit	Translocation
Ricin	—	60S subunit	Multiple processes in protein synthesis
α-Sarcin	—	60S subunit	Multiple processes in protein synthesis
Colicin E3	30S subunit	—	Initiation

- **Neomycin and Gentamycin:** Both of them interact with the small ribosomal subunit and **cause mistranslation.**
- **Tetracycline:** Tetracycline binds directly to the ribosome and **interferes in aminoacyl-tRNA binding.**
- **Puromycin:** It structurally, resembles an amino-acyl-tRNA. It thus, binds at the ribosomal A-site and acts as acceptor in peptidyltransferase reaction. Puromycin thus, **prematurely terminates translation,** leading to release of peptidylpuromycin complex.
- **Chloramphenicol:** It directly **inhibits peptidyltransferase,** by binding the transferase.
- **Erythromycin:** It **interferes with the translocation process**, on prokaryotic ribosomes.
- **Fusidic acid:** It interferes in the process of translocation, by **inhibiting EF-G** (GTP-dependent translocase), in prokaryotes.
- **Cycloheximide:** It **inhibits elongation process**, in eukaryotes.
- **Diphtheria toxin:** It is a protein, which is produced by *Corynebacterium diphtheriae* that **inhibits** the process of **translocation, in eukaryotes**.

• **Toxins:**
  - **Ricin:** It is obtained from the castor bean. It cleaves adenine from rRNA in the large subunit and, thus, **inactivates the ribosome in eukaryotes.**
  - **α-Sarcin:** It is a fungal toxin. It cleaves rRNA at the single site within the large subunit of the ribosome. Thus, it also **inactivates the ribosome in eukaryotes**.
  - **Colicin E3:** It is a toxin, which is obtained from *E. coli*. It has ribonuclease activity and cleaves 16S rRNA of the 30S ribosomal subunit near the mRNA-binding sequence and the decoding region. It, thus, inactivates small subunit of the ribosome and **stops initiation of protein synthesis**.

POST-TRANSLATION MODIFICATIONS

After synthesis of the polypeptide chain, several proteins undergo various modifications. Since these changes occur after translation, these are referred to as post-translation modifications. Post-translation modifications include **partial proteolysis of the protein chain** or **covalent modifications** with the addition of one or more groups on amino acids, in the protein chain.

• **Partial Proteolysis of the Protein Chain: Some proteins**, particularly, those destined for secretion from the cell, are synthesized as the large precursors that are not functionally active, e.g. insulin, zymogens, etc.

  A small portion of such a protein is removed by specialized endo-proteases, which, in turn, results in the release of a biologically active protein. Some of them are cleaved in endoplasmic reticulum or Golgi apparatus while others are cleaved in the developing secretory vesicles or after secretion. For example:
  - **Pre-pro-insulin to Insulin:** Insulin is **synthesized as pre-pro-insulin**, which enters endoplasmic reticulum where signal **peptidase** cleaves the signal peptide and **converts it to proinsulin**. Proinsulin is then transported to the Golgi apparatus where it is packed into the **secretory granules**. The **C-peptide** (connecting-peptide) **is removed** by proteolysis and mature **insulin is secreted**.
  - **Activation of Zymogen:** Inactive zymogen precursors are packed in the storage granules and activated by proteolysis, e.g. **trypsinogen** is cleaved **to trypsin**, or **chymotrypsinogen** is converted to **chymotrypsin**.

• **Covalent Modifications:** Post-translational modification of the amino acid may occur in several ways, such as:
  - **Phosphorylation:** Phosphorylation may occur **on the hydroxyl group of serine or threonine** in a

protein, e.g. reversible phosphorylation of glycogen phosphorylase and glycogen synthase by protein kinase and protein phosphatase, respectively

- **Glycosylation:** Plasma membrane proteins or some other proteins, which are to be secreted from the cell, have **carbohydrate chains attached to the hydroxyl group of serine or threonine by O-linkage or to the NH_2 group of asparagine by N-linkage**.

  Stepwise addition of sugar molecules (glucose, galactose, mannose, fucose, etc.) occurs in the endoplasmic reticulum and Golgi apparatus. Glycosylation of the protein forms a glycoprotein, such as membrane bound glycoproteins.
- **Methylation: Methylation of the α-amino group of lysine** occurs in histones. This, in turn, modulates their interaction with the DNA.
- **Hydroxylation: Proline and lysine** residues **in collagen are** extensively hydroxylated in the endoplasmic reticulum.

Some Important Questions

1. **Describe the process of translation in prokaryotes. How it differs from eukaryotes?**
2. **Describe briefly:**
   i. Salient features of the genetic code
   ii. Protein synthesis and its inhibitors
3. **Write notes on:**
   i. Promoter region
   ii. Post-translation modifications
   iii. Genetic code
   iv. Wobble hypothesis
   v. Inhibitors of protein synthesis

Chapter 22

Carcinogenesis

Carcinogenesis, also called **oncogenesis** or **tumorigenesis**, is the **formation of a cancer**, whereby normal cells are transformed into cancer cells. The process is characterized by **changes at the cellular, genetic and epigenetic levels,** and **abnormal cell division**.

An **agent that causes cancer** is termed as **carcinogen**, which may act directly or indirectly to change the genotype of the cell.

Carcinogenesis is a **multistep process**, where three types of changes occur:

1. **Immortalization:** It is the property of **indefinite growth without other changes** in the phenotype.
2. **Transformation:** It means **failure to observe normal constraints of growth**, e.g. transformed cells become independent of growth factors, which are, usually, needed for cell growth.
3. **Metastasis:** It is the stage at which **cancer cells gain ability to invade normal tissues**. They move away from the tissue of origin and establish new colony/colonies elsewhere in other parts of the body, where cancer grows as a secondary tumor by progressive infiltration, invasion, destruction and penetration. It is referred to as metastasis and marks the development of secondary implants (called **secondaries**), discontinuous with the primary tumor, in remote tissues. It is a complex phenomenon, due to a failure in cell–cell interaction and is a major problem presented by the disease.

EPIDEMIOLOGY

Epidemiological studies have correlated several environmental, racial and cultural influences to the occurrence of specific neoplasms, such as:

- **Smoking:** Though all smokers may not get cancer, a **close link between smoking and lung cancer has been well established.** Moreover, the risk increases with the increasing number of cigarettes/bidis smoked per day as well as the duration of smoking.
- **Diet:** A **high-fat low-fiber diet** has been shown to be a causative factor in **colon cancer**.
- **Age:** The frequency of occurrence of **many types of cancer increases with age**, may be **due to accumulation of somatic mutations, a decline in immune competence and age-related hormonal changes** (e.g. prostate cancer).
- **Inherited susceptibility:** It plays a role in the genesis of several types of cancer, such as **retinoblastoma**.
- **Preneoplastic disorders:** These are the conditions which predispose to the development of malignant neoplasia, e.g. **leukoplakia of the oral cavity** has been shown to increase the risk of squamous cell carcinoma.

INITIATION AND PROMOTION

Carcinogens, sometimes, are divided into those that initiate and promote tumor formation, implying the existence of difference stages in cancer development.

Initiation of Cancer

It **involves mutation**, a small but significant **change in DNA of the cell**. Initiation is an **irreversible process**. Such **cells may remain dormant for years within the body without undergoing proliferation**. This period is a gap between the exposure to a carcinogen (initiator) and the appearance of a full-blown tumor, and is referred to as the **latent period**, which may vary from 5 to 6 years for the induction of leukemia by radiation to as long as 35–40 years for the asbestos-induced lung cancer. Reasons for this long lag period are not known.

Promotion of Cancer

Carcinogenicity of an initiator (I) may be augmented by the subsequent administration of some other agent(s) called promoter (P), e.g. croton oil. Croton oil contains phorbol ester (a promoter of carcinogenesis). If it is applied after benzopyrene (mutagen) application, it results in a tumor.

An application of initiator (I) → No tumor

An application of promoter (P) → No tumor

An application of I followed by several applications of P → Tumor

An application of P followed by several applications of I → No tumor.

It is due to the reason that **application of the initiator**, as mentioned above, **causes mutational activation of some cells** and converts them to potential tumor cells. **Subsequent applications of the promoter lead to clonal expansion** of the initiated (mutated) cells to **produce a tumor** (Fig. 22.1).

CHEMICAL CARCINOGENS

Nearly 80% of the human cancers are caused by environmental factors, mainly chemicals. Exposure to such chemicals can be due to a person's occupation, diet, lifestyle or use of therapeutic drugs. While some of the carcinogens are **direct reacting substances**, majority of them are **indirect reacting substances** (Table 22.1).

Table 22.1: Some chemical carcinogens

Direct reacting substances
• Cyclophosphamide, nitrosourea
• Alkylating agents
• Acylating agents
Indirect reacting procarcinogens
• Polycyclic/heterocyclic aromatic hydrocarbons
– Benzo(a)pyrene
• Aromatic amines, amides, azo dyes
– 2-Naphthylamine
– 2-Acetylaminofluorene
– Dimethylaminoazobenzene
• Plant and microbial products
– Aflatoxin B1
– Griseofulvin
– Betel nuts
• Others
– Nitrosoamines and amides
– Vinyl chloride, nickel, chromium
– Insecticides, fungicides
– Polychlorinated biphenyls
– Arsenic
– Asbestos

- **Direct reacting substances:** These are referred to as direct carcinogens, since they **do not undergo any metabolic transformation** to become a carcinogen. As these substances enter the body in the mutagenic form, they are also referred to as **mutagens**, e.g. cyclophosphamide, nitrosourea, etc. The carcinogenic potential of a mutagen can be tested by a test referred to as Ame's test.
- **Indirect reacting substances:** Indirect reacting substances are also called **indirect carcinogens** or **procarcinogens**. These are not mutagenic in the form in which they enter the body, but are **converted in the liver to a more reactive form by** a family of enzymes referred to as **mixed function oxidases, through** an intermediate called proximate carcinogen. The final product of the conversion of procarcinogen, via **proximate carcinogen**, is called ultimate carcinogen. The **ultimate carcinogen** adducts with DNA and, subsequently, mutates it.

PRO-CARCINOGENS

Several compounds may act as pro-carcinogens, e.g.:

- **Polycyclic hydrocarbons:** Polycyclic hydrocarbons, such as benzo(a)pyrene, are **produced during high temperature combustion of tobacco**. These substances have been **implicated in the causation of lung cancer** in the smokers as well as in the nonsmokers, who are exposed to environmental tobacco smoke (i.e. passive smokers).

  Such compounds **can also be produced from animal fats** (e.g. in smoked cheese, meat or fish) and may be the **risk factors for colon cancer**.
- **Aromatic amines, amides and azo dyes:** Aromatic amines, amides and azo dyes are **present in the dyes and detergents**. They **increase the incidence of urinary bladder cancer** in workers in the aniline, dye and rubber industries (an occupational hazard).
- **Food additives and toxins:** Food additives and toxins, such as colors (butter yellow), sweeteners (saccharin) or certain plant and microbial toxins (such as aflatoxin B1), **may produce hepatocellular carcinoma**.
- **Nitrosamines and amides:** Nitrosamines and amides are endogenously **formed in the acidic environment of the stomach** and may **lead to gastric carcinoma**.

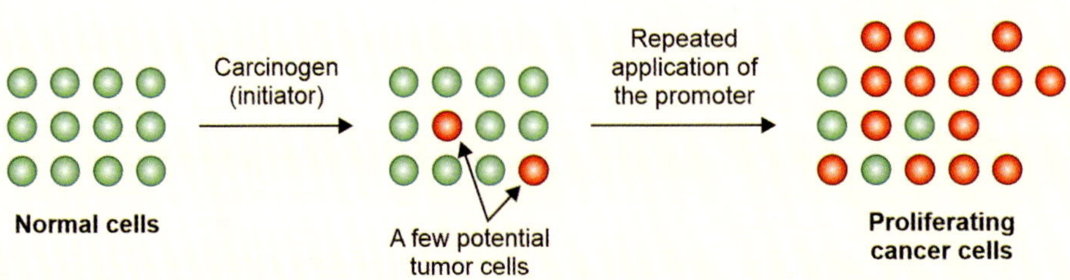

Fig. 22.1: Role of initiator and promoter in tumor development

Indirect carcinogens can also be tested by the Ames test, provided the medium is supplemented with the liver extract which serves as a source of mixed function oxidases.

RADIATION

Radiation, from whatever the source it may be (UV rays of sunlight, X-rays, nuclear fission or radionuclides), is strongly carcinogenic.

- Radiation **causes various mutagenic effects**, e.g. chromosomal break, translocation or point mutation, etc.
- It **may lead to leukemia, cancer of the skin, lungs, thyroid gland, breast or colon**.
- **UV rays** can also exhibit other biological effects, such as that it can **cause DNA damage by forming pyrimidine dimers.**
- Radiation also leads to the **formation of free radicals**, which, in turn, can interact with DNA and other macromolecules, thereby leading to their damage that further **contributes to the process of carcinogenesis**.

VIRUSES

Viruses which cause cancer are called oncogenic viruses or tumor viruses. These may be **DNA or RNA viruses** (Table 22.2).

Table 22.2: Oncogenic viruses

Type of virus	*Associated tumors*
DNA virus	
Epstein-Barr virus (EBV)	Nasopharyngeal carcinoma, Burkitt's lymphoma, B cell lymphomas
Hepatitis B virus	Hepatocellular carcinoma
Human papillomavirus	Anogenital cancer
RNA virus	
Human T cell leukemia-lymphoma virus type 1 (HTIV-1)	Adult T cell leukemia

These **viruses infect the host** either by inserting oncogenes in host chromosome, interfering protooncogene transcription factors/regulators or by inserting homologous sequences corresponding to normal proto-oncogene of host.

ONCOGENES

Oncogenes are the **tumor-causing genes** and have important role in development of many cancers. These genes are called oncogenes due to their ability to convert the normal cells to the oncogenic (tumorigenic) state. Oncogenes are **carried by viruses** that cause transformation of their target (host) cells.

Proto-oncogenes: The viral oncogenes have their cellular counterparts (in the host cells), which are involved in normal cell functions and are called proto-oncogenes (Table 22.3).

Table 22.3: Examples of proto-oncogenes associated with tumors

Proto-oncogene	*Tumor*
ras	Carcinoma of colon, lung, pancreas, genitourinary tract, acute lymphoblastic leukemia
erb	Squamous cell carcinoma
myc	Carcinoma of lung, breast
bcl-2	B cell lymphoma

Nomenclature of Oncogenes

Genomes of the acute transforming retroviruses (which cause rapid induction of tumor in animals) contain unique transforming sequences (genes) referred to as **viral oncogenes (v-onc)**. The v-onc sequences are not found in the genome of the non-transforming retroviruses.

Each v-onc is **designated by three letters** that **relates the v-onc to the virus** from which it was isolated. For example, **v-onc** contained **in** the **simian sarcoma virus** is referred to as **v-sis**, whereas the v-onc in **feline sarcoma virus** is designated as **v-fes**, etc.

The **cellular counterparts of these genes** (**protooncogenes** isolated from the host cells) are named by using the **prefix 'c'**, instead of the prefix 'v'. For example, the oncogene carried by **Rous sarcoma virus is called v-src**, whereas the **proto-oncogene** related to it, **in the cellular genome is referred to as c-src**.

ONCOGENESIS

Oncogenesis refers to the **expression of oncogenes**.

Oncogenes are activated through two mechanisms, i.e. either **by** the **infection of the cells by the tumor viruses** or by **mutation of the cellular proto-oncogenes** (which are usually normal).

- **During infection**, the transducing **virus carries with it the cellular gene(s)** that have been obtained by the recombination event. Thus, they mimic the behavior of **gain-of-function in proto-oncogenes**.
- On the other hand, when they specify proteins that inactivate tumor suppressor genes, their action, in part, mimics **loss-of-function of the tumor suppressor genes**.

Activation of Proto-oncogenes to Oncogenes

As discussed above, oncogenes are the deregulated form of the proto-oncogenes. As a result of some **mutation in** the otherwise **normal proto-oncogenes**, their

deregulation occurs and uncontrolled proliferation of cells starts, and **leads to cancer**. Besides, **chromosomal translocation, gene amplification, or insertion/deletion of promotor or enhancer** in the DNA sequence of certain **proto-oncogenes can alter their function** and **convert** them **into oncogenes**. Any of the following processes can result in the activation of a proto-oncogene to oncogene.

- **Point mutation: Substitution in the coding sequence can convert a cellular proto-oncogene into an oncogene. Any mutation at either position 12 or 61** has been shown to **convert a c-ras proto-oncogene into an active oncogene**. A large number of human tumors are known to carry ras mutations, e.g. urinary bladder cancer, carcinoma of the pancreas, colon, lungs and thyroid.
- **Chromosomal translocation: When a piece of one chromosome is split-off and joins the other chromosome**, it is called chromosomal translocation. It is a reciprocal event that exchanges parts of the two chromosomes. Chromosomal translocation has been shown to results in **overexpression of the proto-oncogene**, such as in certain cases of Burkitt's lymphoma.
- **Gene amplification:** Amplification of the DNA sequence may also result in the **activation of a protooncogene**. For example, **c-myc gene in neuroblastoma** and **c-erb B2 gene in breast cancer** are the examples of the activation of their proto-oncogenes, as a result of amplification of their DNA sequences.
- **Insertion of promoter/enhancer: Certain retroviruses**, e.g. avian leukemia virus, **when infect a cell**, the **DNA copy of their RNA genome** (called cDNA) **is synthesized by reverse transcriptase** and gets **integrated into the genome of the host**. The integrated double-stranded DNA is called provirus. These cDNA copies of the retroviruses are **flanked at both the ends** by the sequences termed as **long terminal repeats (LTR)**, which are important in the integration of a provirus. The provirus becomes **integrated near the myc gene and acts as a promoter**. This, in turn, **promotes transcription of the corresponding myc RNA** and subsequent **translation of the gene product in such cells**.

  In some cases, the **provirus may be inserted downstream as an enhancer**, instead of the upstream (Fig. 22.2).

BIOCHEMICAL CHANGES DURING TUMOR DEVELOPMENT

Once a cell becomes malignant, its composition and behavior does not remain static and that the **biochemical profile of a malignant cell is different from that of the normal cell** as it has a distinct type of metabolism (Table 22.4).

Table 22.4: Biochemical comparison of a normal cell with a tumor cell

Parameter	*Normal cell*	*Tumor cell*
Ribonucleotide reductase activity	Normal	Enhanced
RNA and DNA synthesis	Normal	Enhanced
Pyrimidine catabolism	Normal	Suppressed
Rate of glycolysis	Normal	Enhanced
Isoenzyme profile	Normal	Altered
Synthesis of fetal proteins	No	Yes
Synthesis of specialized proteins	Yes	No
Inappropriate synthesis of growth factors/hormones	No	Yes

TUMOR MARKERS

A tumor marker is defined as **a substance present in or produced by a tumor**, or **by the host cell in response to a tumor**. Such a substance can be used to differentiate

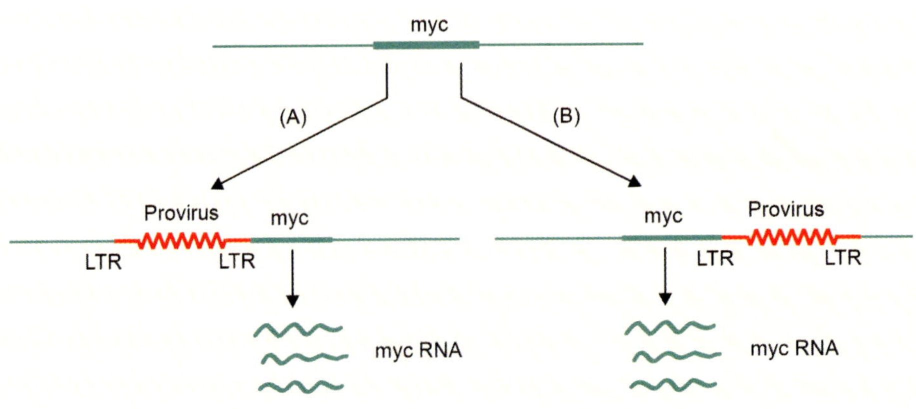

Fig. 22.2: Insertion of a promoter (A) or an enhancer (B)

Table 22.5: Selected tumor markers with the type of cancer in which these are increased in serum

Tumor marker	*Type of cancer*
Enzymes	
Alkaline phosphatase	Bone, liver
Heat stable alkaline phosphatase	Uterus, ovary
Acid phosphatase	Prostate
Amylase	Pancreas
Hormones	
ADH	Adrenal cortex, pancreas, small cell lung cancer
Calcitonin	Medullary thyroid carcinoma
Growth hormone	Pituitary adenoma, renal and lung cancers
β-hCG	Testes, trophoblasts
Oncofetal antigens	
α-Fetoprotein (AFP)	Hepatocellular carcinoma
CEA	Colorectal, GIT, lungs, breast
Squamous cell antigen	Head and neck, cervix, lungs, skin
PSA	Prostate
Carbohydrate markers	
CA 125	Ovary, endometrium
CA 15–3	Breast, ovary
CA 19–9	Pancreas, GIT, liver
Proteins	
β_2-microglobulin	Multiple myeloma, B cell lymphoma
C-peptide	Insulinoma
Ferritin	Liver, lungs, breast, leukemias
Immunoglobulins	Multiple myeloma, lymphomas
Oncogenes	
K-ras mutation	Leukemias, lymphomas
c-myc translocation	B and T cell lymphomas, small cell lung cancer
bcl-2	Leukemias, lymphomas
c-erb B2 amplification	Breast, ovary, GIT
Mutations in tumor suppressor genes	
BRCA-1	Breast, melanoma
p53	Breast, colorectal, lungs, liver
Rb1	Retinoblastoma, osteosarcoma
DCC	Colorectal
Others	
Estrogen and progesterone receptors	Breast
Hydroxyproline (in urine)	Bone metastasis, multiple myeloma
Polyamines (in CSF)	Brain

a tumor from the normal tissue or to determine the presence of a tumor based upon its measurement in the tissue, cells or body fluids. An ideal tumor marker is one which is both specific for a given type of cancer as well as sensitive enough to help in its early diagnosis.

Biochemical tumor markers can be classified into several groups such as **enzymes and isoenzymes, hormones, oncofetal antigens, carbohydrate-epitopes or oncogene products** (Table 22.5).

CHEMOPREVENTION

Chemoprevention is defined as the **introduction of some of the natural and/or synthetic substances in the diet, for preventing cancer.**

Chemo-preventive Agents

Bioactive phytochemicals, also called **nutraceuticals** (nutriceuticals), **present in edible plants** have been shown to **reduce the risk of various types of cancer,** particularly, those of the lungs, stomach, colon, breast, prostate, etc. Recent trend is to encourage enhanced consumption of fruits and vegetables, which are the natural sources of chemo-preventive agents (Table 22.6).

Table 22.6: Chemopreventive nutraceuticals

- Vitamins A, C and E ('big three' antioxidants)
- Flavonoids
- Curcumin (major colored component of turmeric)
- Lunasin (a soy peptide)
- Poppy seeds
- Diallyl sulfide (in garlic and onion)
- Aqueous extracts of decaffeinated green or black tea

Antioxidant Vitamins

Antioxidant vitamins include vitamin A and carotenoids, vitamin E and vitamin C, which have been shown to be the natural dietary inhibitors of carcinogenesis. They work by various mechanisms:

- Inhibit the formation of free radicals as well as increase their detoxification
- Stimulate immune system
- Inhibit nitrosamine formation
- Enhance cell-to-cell communication
- Metabolic detoxification of the carcinogen.

Some Important Questions

1. **What is carcinogenesis? Describe chemical carcinogenesis.**
2. **What are oncogenes? How proto-oncogenes are converted to oncogenes?**
3. **Differentiate between:**
   i. Direct reacting and indirect reacting carcinogens
   ii. Initiator and promoter
4. **Write notes on:**
   i. Metastasis
   ii. Carcinogenesis
   iii. Oncogenic viruses
   iv. Oncogenes
   v. Tumor markers
   vi. Chemoprevention
   vii. Antioxidant vitamins

Unit VII

Metabolic Regulation

Chapter 23

Hormones

Hormones are chemical messengers, which are produced and secreted by the ductless glands, also called endocrine glands. From the endocrine gland, they are released into the circulation and reach target tissues to exert their action. Accordingly, an endocrine hormone refers to the class of substances that arise in one tissue or gland and travel a long distance through circulation to reach the target cell, which expresses its receptors.

CLASSIFICATION OF HORMONES

According to their chemical nature, hormones are classified into three groups. These include:

1. Peptides and protein hormones
2. Steroids, derived from cholesterol
3. Amino acid derivatives, such as catecholamines and thyroid hormones, which are synthesized from tyrosine (Table 23.1).

MECHANISM OF ACTION OF HORMONES

Hormones act after **binding with** their **specific receptors,** which are located either **intracellularly** or within the cell membrane **(extracellularly)**.

A **hormone-receptor complex**, usually, **undergoes conformational changes**, due to interaction of the receptor with the hormone.

HORMONE RECEPTORS

Hormone receptors **are proteins** that differ by their specificity for the ligand as well as location within the cell. They are **present either intracellularly**, or **within the cell membrane (extracellularly)**. Depending upon the type of hormone, there are **two types of receptor systems,** which vary in their mechanism of action (Table 23.2).

Table 23.1: Various hormones, their sites of action and major physiological functions

Hormone	*Chemical nature*	*Site of action*	*Major physiological functions*
Hypothalamus			
Growth hormone-release hormone (GHRH)	Polypeptide	Anterior pituitary	Release of growth hormone
Growth hormone-release inhibitory hormone (GHRIH)	Peptide	Anterior pituitary	Suppression of GH and TSH
Luteinizing hormone-release hormone (LHRH)	Peptide	Anterior pituitary	Release of LH and FSH
Thyrotropin release hormone (TRH)	Tripeptide	Anterior pituitary	Release of TSH and prolactin
Corticotropin release hormone (CRH)	Polypeptide	Anterior pituitary	Release of ACTH and β-Lipotropin
Prolactin release factor (PRF)	Peptide	Anterior pituitary	Release of prolactin
Prolactin inhibitory factor (PIF)	Dopamine	Anterior pituitary	Suppression of prolactin secretion
Anterior pituitary			
Growth hormone (GH)	Protein	Several tissues	Overall growth
Follicle stimulating hormone (FSH)	Glycoprotein	Ovary	Growth of follicles
Luteinizing hormone (LH)	Glycoprotein	Ovary	Ovulation and secretion of progesterone
Thyroid stimulating hormone (TSH)	Glycoprotein	Thyroid gland	Stimulation of secretion of thyroid hormones

Contd...

Table 23.1: Various hormones, their sites of action and major physiological functions (*Contd...*)

Hormone	*Chemical nature*	*Site of action*	*Major physiological functions*
Adrenocorticotropic hormone (ACTH)	Polypeptide	Adrenal cortex	Stimulation of secretion of hormones of adrenal cortex
Prolactin	Protein	Mammary gland	Proliferation of mammary gland and milk secretion
β-Lipotropin	Polypeptide	—	Precursor of β-MSH and endorphins
α-Melanocyte stimulating hormone (α-MSH)	Peptide	Skin	Darkening of skin
Posterior pituitary			
Antidiuretic hormone (ADH)	Peptide	Arterioles and renal tubules	Elevation of blood pressure and reabsorption of water
Oxytocin	Peptide	Smooth muscle of the uterus and mammary glands	Contraction, sperm transport, parturition, and ejection of milk
Adrenal cortex			
Cortisol	Steroid	Several tissues	Metabolism of carbohydrates, proteins and lipids, and provide resistance to infections
Aldosterone	Steroid	Kidney	Electrolytes and water balance
Adrenal medulla			
Epinephrine and norepinephrine	Amino acid derivatives	Sympathetic receptors, and liver, muscle and adipose tissue	Stimulation of sympathetic nervous system, glycogenolysis and lipolysis
Thyroid gland			
Thyroxine (T_4)	Amino acid derivative	Most of the body tissues	Stimulation of O_2 consumption and regulation of metabolic rate
Calcitonin	Polypeptide	Skeleton	Lowering of plasma Ca^{2+} and P
Parathyroid gland			
Parathyroid hormone (PTH)	Polypeptide	Skeleton, kidney and GIT	Regulation of plasma Ca^{2+} and P
Pancreas			
Insulin	Polypeptide	Most of the cells	Regulation of blood glucose
Glucagon	Peptide	Liver	Glycogenolysis
Somatostatin	Peptide	Pancreas	Inhibition of insulin release
GIT			
Gastrin	Peptide	Stomach	Secretion of gastric acid
Secretin	Polypeptide	Pancreas	Secretion of bicarbonate from pancreas
Cholecystokinin-pancreozymin (CCK-PZ)	Polypeptide	Gallbladder and pancreas	Contraction of gallbladder
Motilin	Polypeptide	GIT	Stimulation of GIT motility
Vasoactive intestinal peptide (VIP)	Polypeptide	GIT	Neurotransmitter
Gastric inhibitory polypeptide (GIP)	Polypeptide	GIT	Inhibition of gastric secretion and gastric motility
Bombesin	Peptide	GIT	Stimulation of the release of various pancreatic hormones and enzymes
Neurotensin	Peptide	GIT and hypothalamus	Uncertain
Substance P	Peptide	GIT and brain	Sensory neurotransmitter and analgesic
Kidney			
1,25 $(OH_2).D_3$ (Calcitriol)	Sterol	Intestine, bone and kidney	Regulation of serum Ca^{2+}
Erythropoietin	Glycoprotein	Bone marrow	Stimulation of red cell formation

Table 23.2: Hormone receptors

Types of receptor	*Hormones*
Intracellular receptors	
• Cytosolic receptors	Steroids
• Nuclear receptors	Calcitriol, T_3
Cell surface (extracellular) receptors	
Tyrosine kinase-linked receptors	
• Intrinsic tyrosine kinase	Insulin, Insulin-like growth factor (IGF-1)
• Recruit tyrosine kinase	Growth hormone, prolactin
G-protein-linked receptors	
• Increase adenylate cyclase activity	ADH, catecholamines, epinephrine through adrenergic β-receptor and glucagon
• Increase phospholipase C activity	Oxytocin, PTH, Ca^{2+}, calcitonin, epinephrine through α-1 receptors

Intracellular Receptors

Lipid soluble hormones, such as **steroid hormones** and **thyroid hormones, can diffuse through the cell membrane** and **bind to their receptors (proteins)** which are **located either in the cytosol** or **in the nucleus**. These receptors are referred to as **intracellular receptors**.

Steroid hormones, such as glucocorticoids and mineralocorticoids, **are diffused into the cytosol and bind to their specific receptors (glucocorticoid/ mineralocorticoid receptors) with in the cytoplasm.**

Similarly, progesterone, estradiol, vitamin D_3 or androgens diffuse into the nucleus and bind to their receptors within the nucleus **(the nuclear receptors)**.

- These **receptors have two regions**, i.e. **hydrophobic hormone-binding region** and DNA-binding region that consist of two zinc fingers which are rich in cysteine and the basic amino acids.
- **Binding** of the hormone with the receptor **causes a conformational change in the receptor** and activates it.
- The **activated-receptor is**, thereafter, **translocated into the nucleus**.
- In the nucleus, activated-receptor **binds to the nuclear DNA**, upstream the specific hormone-response elements, and **activates the hormone-responsive genes**.
- This, in turn, **leads to the activation/repression of the transcription** of the genes.
- The nonactivated receptor cannot bind to DNA, because heteromeric heat-shock proteins (HSP) block its DNA-binding site (Fig. 23.1).

Mechanism of Action of Steroid Hormones

Steroids bring about their biological effects by binding to the steroid-specific hormone receptors.

- **Steroid hormones diffuse across the plasma membrane** and **bind to** their **receptors in the cytosol**.
- **Binding** of the hormone with the receptor **results in** a conformational change, that causes the **hormone-receptor complex** to **move into the nucleus** and **bind to the DNA at** a specific response element, called **steroid response element** (SRE) that may be present in the promoter or the enhancer region of the hormone-sensitive genes.
- The **interaction of the hormone-receptor complex with** the **SRE increase or decrease in the rate of gene transcription**.
- The **hormone-receptor complex binds to a receptor site on the regulatory region of one of the DNA strands,** associated with a particular gene. This region is known as the **hormone-response element** (HRE).

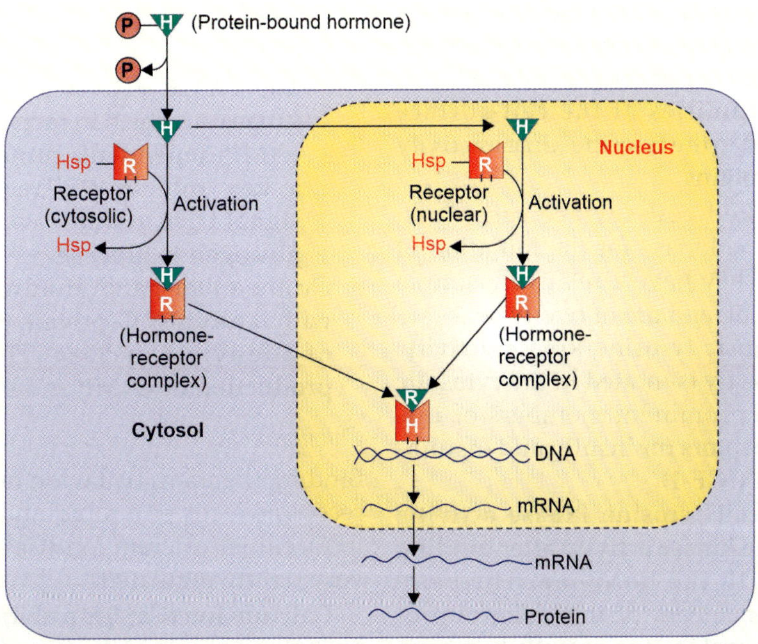

Fig. 23.1: Mechanism of action of hormones through intracellular receptors

- This, interaction, in turn, **influences the promoter region**, which then **permits DNA dependent-RNA polymerase to start transcription** of the triplet base code, by separation of the two strands of DNA to yield a specific mRNA.
- After post-transcriptional modifications, **mRNA comes out of the nucleus**.
- **After translation** of the message, on the ribosomes, attached to the endoplasmic reticulum, **proteins are formed**.
- Finally, modification of the protein occurs to give the **final gene product** (Fig. 23.1).

Extracellular Receptors

Water soluble hormones, such as the **pituitary-derived proteins and glycoproteins (being hydrophilic in nature) cannot cross the lipid barrier** in the **cytoplasmic membrane**. So, these hormones **interact with the receptors which are located on the cell surface**. These receptors are referred to as **membrane receptors or extracellular receptors**.

Interaction of the hormone with the extracellular receptors (also called cell-surface receptors or membrane receptors) **causes conformational change** in some **membrane proteins**. This, in turn, **activates enzymes inside the cell**, thereby, resulting in the **synthesis of the second messenger**, which activates the phosphorylating enzymes.

Extracellular receptors have three, clearly, identifiable **domains**, i.e.:

i. The **extracellular domain** or ectodomain (which binds the hormone with a high affinity),
ii. **Hydrophobic transmembrane domain** (the membrane spanning region which varies in structure), and
iii. The **cytosolic domain** (which initiates the intracellular signaling cascade). The **cytosolic domain** is the effector region of the receptor, which may be **linked with** another membrane protein system, a set of enzymes that are guanosine triphosphatases **(GTPases)**.

There are **two superfamilies of the cell-surface receptors**, one of it is **linked to the tyrosine kinase activity** and the other to the **G-proteins**.

- **Tyrosine kinase-linked cell-surface receptors:** They rely upon tyrosine kinase for the initiation of downstream signals. They have a relatively simple transmembrane segment, and are of two types:
  - **Receptor with intrinsic tyrosine kinase activity: Tyrosine kinase activity is located in the cytosolic domain**. The most prominent members of this subgroup are the **receptors for insulin and insulin-like growth factor-1 (IGF-1)**.
  - **Receptors that recruit tyrosine kinase activity:** They **recruit tyrosine kinase activity after binding of the receptor with the hormone.** The best-known endocrine members of this subgroup of receptors are the **receptors for growth hormone and prolactin**.
- **G-protein-linked receptors:** These receptors **interact with the membrane receptors** and cause conformational changes in the membrane proteins, such as **G-proteins** (guanine-proteins) which are associated with the inner surface of the cell membrane.

SECOND MESSENGERS

The most striking feature of the G-protein is the **generation of** some intracellular **molecule** which is referred to as **second messenger** such as cAMP, IP_3, etc.

These molecules are designated as second messengers since these are generated in response to the hormone (the first messenger). When a hormone binds to its receptor, the hormone-receptor complex, thereafter, triggers its action on the G-protein which in turn generates a second messenger, to exhibit various physiological actions of the hormone.

Various Second Messengers Include

Cyclic AMP

Cyclic AMP **(cAMP)** is a small molecule **derived from ATP** by the catalytic action of the signaling enzyme adenylate cyclase.

The catalytic action of the hormone receptor with the G-protein depends upon the type of the receptor **(β-adrenergic receptors or α-adrenergic receptors)** and the G-protein that may be **stimulatory (Gs)** or **inhibitory (Gi)**. The Gs causes activation of adenyl cyclase and production of cAMP. On the other hand, Gi causes inactivation of adenyl cyclase and inhibits the production of cAMP. For example:

- The **β-adrenergic receptors couple with** the **α-subunit of** the stimulatory **G-protein (Gsα)** and causes **activation of adenylate cyclase**.
  - The **Gsα** activates membrane-bound **adenylate cyclase**, which in turn catalyzes the **production of cAMP** (from ATP) that **acts as a second messenger**.
  - The **cAMP activates cAMP-dependent protein kinase A**, which in turn **modulates cell functions**.
  - **cAMP-dependent protein kinase A also has a key role in** the **regulation of intracellular signal translocation** leading to the **conversion of glycogen to glucose**.
- On the other hand, **α-adrenergic receptors couple with inhibitory G-protein (Gi)** and causes **inhibition of adenylate cyclase**. This in turn **inhibits the production of cAMP** and **exhibits opposite effects**.

Calcium ions

Binding (ligation) of a wide range of hormones with its receptors leads to a rapid and transient increase in the intracellular calcium ion **(Ca^{2+})** concentration which is very tightly regulated.

Calcium ion (Ca^{2+}) is a ubiquitous messenger and has an important role in the transduction of signals, leading to a **number of cellular responses, such as that:**

- Ca^{2+} **activates several enzymes**, including **protein kinases, calmodulin** and some isoforms of **protein kinase C**.
- It also **activates phospholipase A2** which liberates arachidonic acid from membrane phospholipids and, thereby, generates eicosanoids (precursors of important chemically related signal molecules) such as thromboxanes, leukotrienes, lipoxins and prostaglandins.
- Ca^{2+} also activates cytosolic guanylate cyclase and catalyzes the production of cGMP.

Inositol triphosphate

Some **hormones, such as epinephrine and norepinephrine** (through α-adrenergic receptors), **ADH** (via V1 receptor) and **angiotensin II**, after binding with their receptors, result in the **activation of phospholipase C**.

Phospholipase C, in turn, **catalyzes hydrolysis of** phosphatidylinositol-4,5-bisphosphate **(PIP_2)** leading to the **formation of** diacylglycerol **(DAG)** and inositol triphosphate (inositol-1,4,5-triphosphate or **IP_3**).

Both, DAG and IP_3 act as **second messengers**.

- **Diacylglycerol** (DAG) – DAG activates protein kinase C that, generally, phosphorylates a wide range of target signal-transduction proteins at several residues.
- **Inositol triphosphate** (IP_3) – IP_3 diffuses into the cytosol and thereafter, **causes the release of the intracellular Ca^{2+}** from Ca^{2+}-rich organelles, such as endoplasmic reticulum (ER). **Ca^{2+} interacts with the calcium-binding protein calmodulin** (CAM) and **forms Ca^{2+}-calmodulin complex** (Ca^{2+}.CAM) that in turn **activates calmodulin-specific kinases**.

Accordingly, protein kinase **C, Ca^{2+} ion and calmodulin-specific kinases** specifically **cause phosphorylation of the target protein**(s) to **exhibit hormone specific physiological actions** (Fig. 23.2).

Mechanism of Action of Epinephrine

Epinephrine acts through several distinct receptors on different cells. The **best studied** of these receptors **are α and β-adrenergic receptors**. They bind epinephrine with different affinities and work by different mechanisms.

In the liver

- Action of epinephrine on **hepatic glycogenolysis** is **via β-adrenergic receptors**, which is **similar to that for glucagon**. By this mechanism, epinephrine response **augments the effects of glucagon during severe hypoglycemia**.
- In the liver epinephrine also works, simultaneously, **through the α-receptors**, but by a different mechanism. The binding of epinephrine to the α-receptors **involves G-proteins**, which is specific for the **activation of an isoenzyme of phospholipase C**, that **cleaves phosphatidylinositol-bisphosphate** to diacylglycerol **(DAG)** and inositol-triphosphate **(IP3)**, both of which act as second messengers.
  - As discussed above, **DAG activates protein kinase C**, which **initiates a series of protein-phosphorylation reactions**.
  - **IP_3 promotes transport of Ca^{2+} into the cytosol.** Ca^{2+} **bind to** the cytoplasmic protein **calmodulin** and **activates phosphorylase kinase**, leading to phosphorylation and activation of phosphorylase, thereby providing glucose for blood.

  Ca^{2+}-calmodulin-dependent protein kinase and other enzymes are also activated either by phosphorylation or by association with the Ca^{2+}-calmodulin complex (Fig. 23.2).

In the muscle

In muscle, **glycogenolysis is activated** in response to epinephrine **through β-adrenergic receptor**, mediated **through cAMP**, providing supply of carbohydrate for the energy for muscle during prolonged exercise (Fig. 23.3).

Mechanism of Action of Glucagon

Glucagon promotes glycogenolysis **in the liver**, where its **mechanism of action is similar to that of epinephrine**

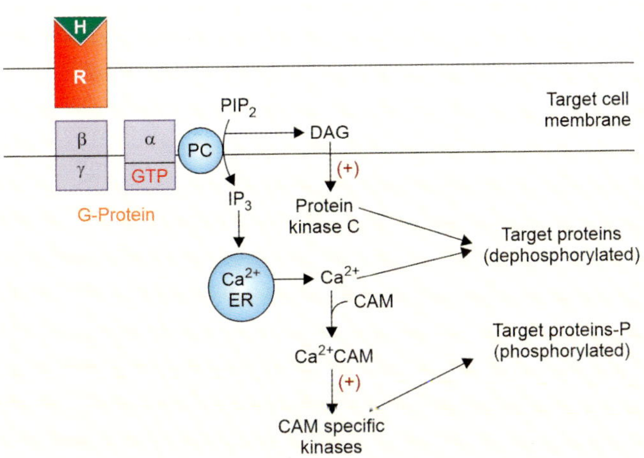

Fig. 23.2: Mechanism of action of epinephrine in the liver

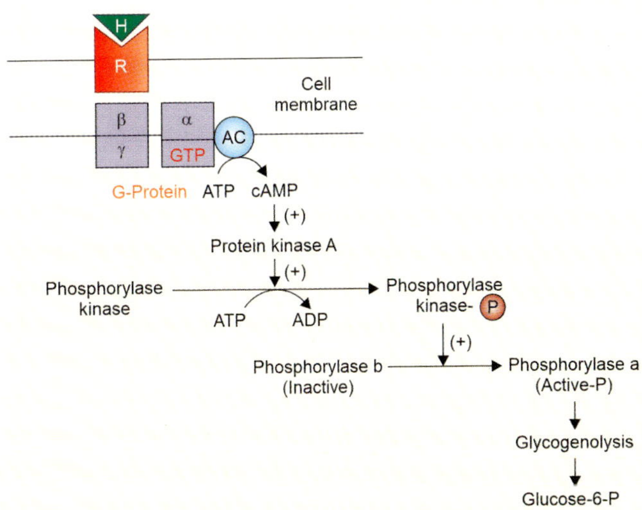

Fig. 23.3: Mechanism of action of epinephrine in muscle

in the muscle **through β-adrenergic receptor**, and is **mediated through cAMP**.

- Binding of the hormone **activates adenylate cyclase** on the inner surface of the membrane, leading to the **production of cAMP**.
- **cAMP**, in turn, **binds to the regulatory subunit of the cAMP-dependent protein kinase A**, which **phosphorylates phosphorylase kinase and glycogen synthase** (activation of phosphorylase kinase and inhibition of glycogen synthase).
- **Activated phosphorylase kinase,** in turn, **activates glycogen phosphorylase,** which **initiates glycogenolysis** leading to the production of the glucose-6-phosphate that is hydrolyzed to glucose and exported to blood (Fig. 23.3).

Mechanism of Action of Insulin

Insulin binds to its transmembrane receptors. This, in turn, **stimulates aggregation of receptors** and **promotes tyrosine kinase** activity in the intracellular domain of the receptor.

- The receptor kinase activity **auto-phosphorylates** its **tyrosine residues, enhancing its protein tyrosine kinase activity as** well as phosphorylating tyrosine residues of the other intracellular effector proteins, called **insulin receptor substrates** (IRS), mainly, IRS-1 and IRS-2.
- When phosphorylated, **these proteins interact with** another set of **proteins that contain two SH2 domains** (SH2 homology 2), which become activated upon binding to IRS.
- As a result of different signal proteins binding to the phosphorylated IRS, **several** separate **signaling pathways become activated**. These include kinases that phosphorylate serine and threonine residues on certain proteins, **such as GTPase, phosphodiesterase and phosphoprotein phosphatases**.
- Insulin-dependent activation of these proteins also **checks actions of glycogen**.
- One pathway may **stimulate DNA synthesis and cell division**, while other may **activate a transcription factor** that turns on the **expression of insulin specific genes**.
- In the muscle and adipose tissue, receptor tyrosine kinase activity **induces movement of glucose transporter-4** (GLUT-4) from the intracellular vacuoles to the cell surface, thereby increasing glucose transport into the cells (Fig. 23.4).

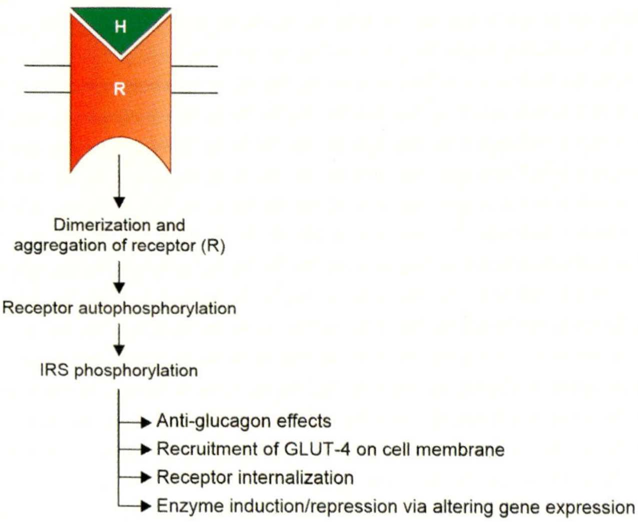

Fig. 23.4: Mechanism of action of insulin

- **Glucose is** then **used in muscle for the synthesis of glycogen**, and **in adipose tissue to produce glyceraldehyde-3-phosphate**, which is converted to glycerol-3-phosphate **for the synthesis of triacylglycerols**.
- Hormone-receptor complex **also** results in **internalization and degradation of receptor molecules.** The process of receptor internalization provides a means of regulating the effects of insulin and, effectively, **down regulates insulin receptors**.

Some Important Questions

1. Classify hormones. Discuss mechanism of action of steroid hormones.

2. What are hormone receptors? Classify them with examples.

3. Discuss:

i. Second messenger
ii. Mechanism of action of intracellular receptors
iii. Mechanism of action of membrane-bound receptors

4. Write notes on:

i. Hormone receptors
ii. Membrane-bound receptors
iii. Intracellular receptors

Unit VIII

Structural Components and Blood Proteins

Chapter 24

Connective Tissue

Connective tissue refers to the tissues which connect and support different tissues and organs of the body. Various types of connective tissues, including tendons, cartilage and the corneal stroma, contain extracellular matrix (ECM). Major components include proteins such as **collagens, elastin** and **glycosaminoglycans** (glycoproteins and proteoglycans) besides a variety of other proteins.

COLLAGENS

Collagens comprise a family of **fibrous glycoproteins** that are present only in extracellular matrices. Collagen is the most **abundant protein in the human body**. It has a **long rigid structure** in which three polypeptides, called α-chains, are wound around one another in a rope-like triple helix.

Collagens are **found throughout the body**. In some tissues collagen may **be dispersed as a gel** that gives support to the structure, e.g. in the extracellular matrix or the **vitreous humor of the eye**. In other tissues collagen may be **bundled in tight, parallel fibers** that provide great strength as **in tendons**.

Collagen is a **superfamily of proteins**, which include **27 distinct types**. Although there are many differences among the members of the collagen family, all share at least two important structural features, i.e. **all** the collagen molecules **are trimers** consisting of three polypeptide chains called α-chains and that the three polypeptide chains of a collagen molecule are **wound around each other to form** a unique, **rod-like triple helix**.

Organizational Classification of Collagens

Based on their location and functions in the body, **collagens are organized into three groups**:

- **Fibril-forming collagens:** These are **linear polymers of fibrils** with characteristic bonding patterns and have **rope-like triple-stranded helix**, e.g. type I, type II and type III.
  - **Type I collagen fibers are found in supporting elements** of high tensile strength, such as in **skin, bone, tendon, blood vessels and cornea**.
  - **Type II fibers are found in cartilaginous structures,** such as **cartilage, intervertebral disk and vitreous body**.
  - **Type III collagens occur in** more **distensible tissues**, such as **blood vessels and fetal skin.**
- **Network forming collagens:** They form a three-dimensional mesh, e.g. type IV and VII collagens.
  - **Type IV collagens are thin, sheet or mesh-like structures** that function as semipermeable basement membranes found **in the kidneys and the lungs.**
  - **Type VII collagens** are **found beneath stratified squamous epithelia.**
- **Fibril-associated collagens:** These collagens **link collagen fibrils to one another** as well as to other components in the extracellular matrix, e.g. type IX and type XII collagens.
- **Type IX collagens** are **found in cartilage**
- **Type XII collagen** occurs **in tendon and ligaments.**

Structure and Synthesis of Collagen

As discussed above, collagen is a **fibrous protein**, which has an **elongated triple-helical structure** (Fig. 24.1).

Collagens are **rich in proline and glycine. Glycine is found in every third position** of the polypeptide chain, **forming** part of a **repeating sequence of Gly-X-Y-**. The **X is frequently proline** while **Y may be proline or lysine**, which **gets hydroxylated** and occurs as hydroxyproline or hydroxylysine.

- Polypeptide **precursors** of collagens, called **pre-procollagens, are formed in the fibroblasts, osteoblasts** of bone and **chondroblasts** of cartilage.
- The **pro-α-chain is processed** by a number of enzymes. **Proline and lysine** residues, found in the Y-position, **are hydroxylated** by prolyl-hydroxylase and lysyl-hydroxylase, respectively. This is a **post-translational modification** and **requires vitamin C**.
- Some **hydroxylysine** residues **are** enzymatically **glycosylated.**
- **Procollagen molecules** are cleaved by the N- and C-procollagen peptidases, which remove the terminal propeptides, **releasing triple-helical molecules.**

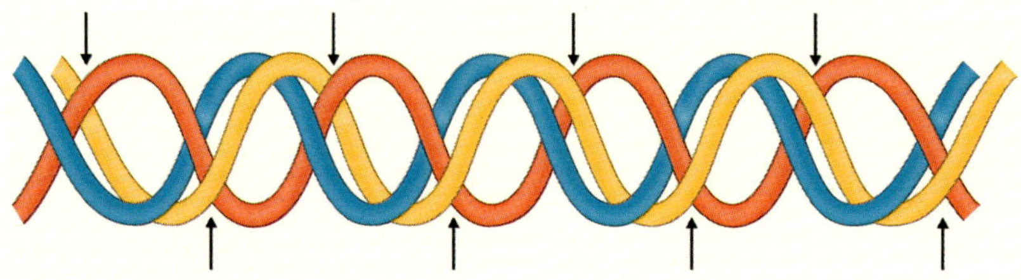

Fig. 24.1: Triple-helical structure of collagen, arrows indicate the sites where the three chains are very close to each other. Glycine is invariably present at these sites

- Individual **collagen molecules**, spontaneously, **associate to form fibrils.**
- **Lysyl-oxidase, deaminates** some of the **lysyl- and hydroxylysyl-** residues, resulting in the **formation of allysine and hydroxyallysine.**
- These reactive aldehydes condense with lysyl- and hydroxylysyl-residues, in the neighboring collagen molecules, to **form covalent cross-links of mature collagen**, called tropocollagen (Fig. 24.2).

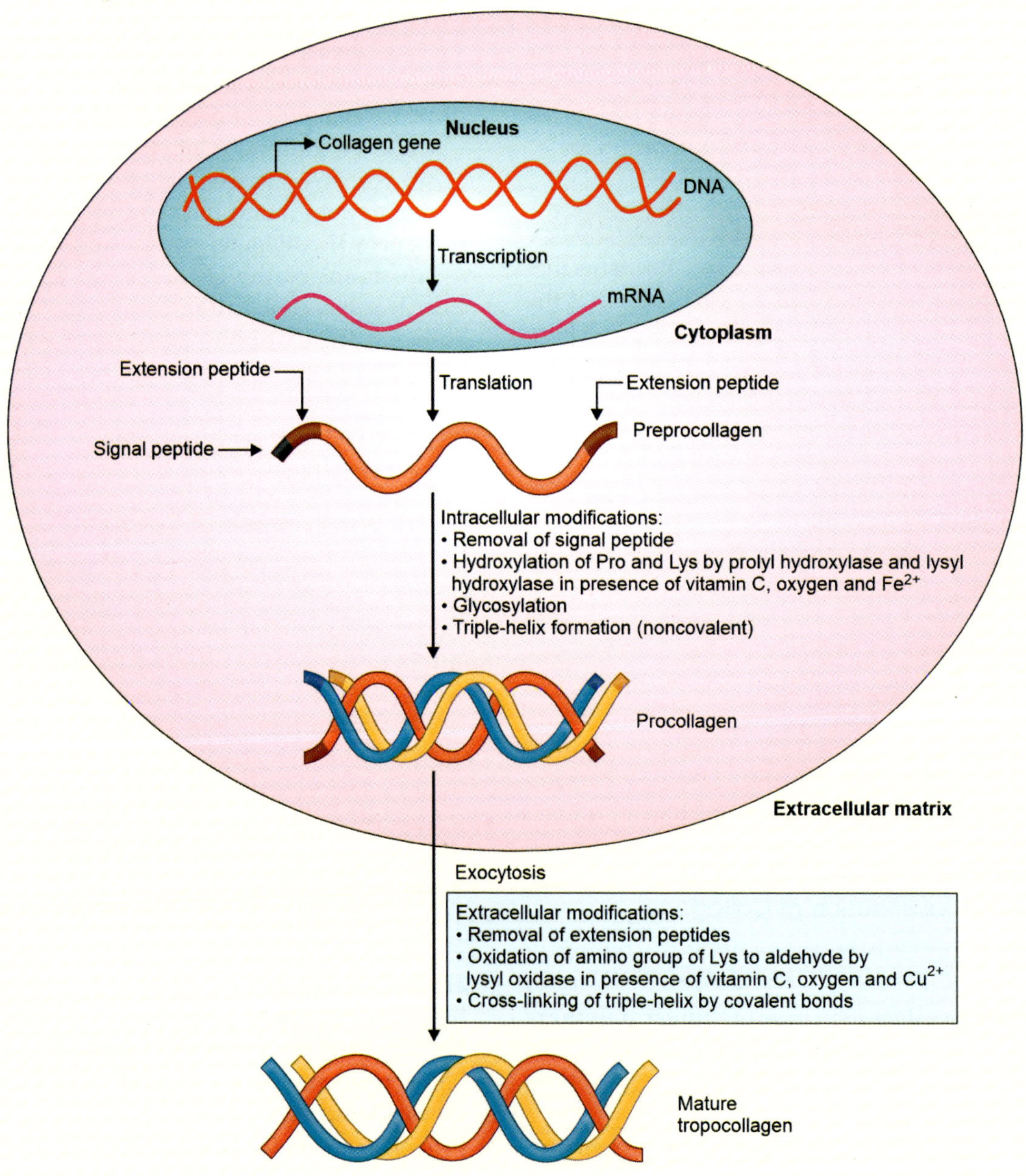

Fig. 24.2: Biosynthesis of collagen

It may here be mentioned that scurvy is caused by the **deficiency of vitamin C**, which is essentially **required for hydroxylation of proline and lysine** residues **by the enzyme prolyl-hydroxylase and lysyl-hydroxylase, during collagen synthesis and maturation.** As a result of vitamin C deficiency, collagen fibers cannot be cross-linked, thereby, decreasing the tensile strength of the assembled fiber. Scurvy is characterized by the inflamed gums and tooth loss, poor wound healing, brittle bones and weakening of the lining of blood vessels causing internal bleeding.

Degradation of Collagen

Collagen fibrils are broken down with the help of specific collagenases. These enzymes cleave the molecules into the smaller fragments, which are further degraded to the constituent amino acids by other matrix proteinases.

Disorders of Collagen Synthesis

- **Osteogenesis imperfecta:** Osteogenesis imperfecta (OI), also known as brittle bone disease, is a congenital bone disorder characterized by brittle bones that are prone to fracture. The majority of cases of OI are caused by a dominant mutation in a gene coding for type I collagen.
- **Ehlers-Danlos syndrome:** Ehlers-Danlos syndrome is due to the **deficiency of** any of the **collagen processing enzymes,** e.g. lysyl-hydroxylase or **procollagen peptidase, etc. Patients show defects in collagen type I and type III fibrils.** They **have hyper-flexible joints and highly extensible skin** (Fig. 24.3).

ELASTINS

Elastins give elasticity to tissues, allowing them to stretch, when needed and then return to their original state, e.g. blood vessels, lungs, skin and ligamentum nuchae.

Structure and Synthesis of Elastins

Elastins are **synthesized by fibroblasts** and smooth muscle cells. They are highly insoluble and are synthesized **from a precursor** called **tropo-elastin.**

- Some of **lysyl-side chains** of tropo-elastins **are oxidatively deaminated by lysyl-oxidase,** generating al-lysine in specific sequences.
- The reactive aldehyde of **al-lysine condenses with other al-lysine,** or with unmodified lysine, from the same or on different tropo-elastin polypeptide chains, to form desmosine cross-linked heterocyclic structures.
- As a result, elastin can stretch in any direction giving elasticity to the connective tissues.

Disorders of Elastin Metabolism

Marfan syndrome: It is due to mutations in the fibrillin gene. Patients have a typically tall stature, long arms and legs, and long spidery fingers (Fig. 24.4).

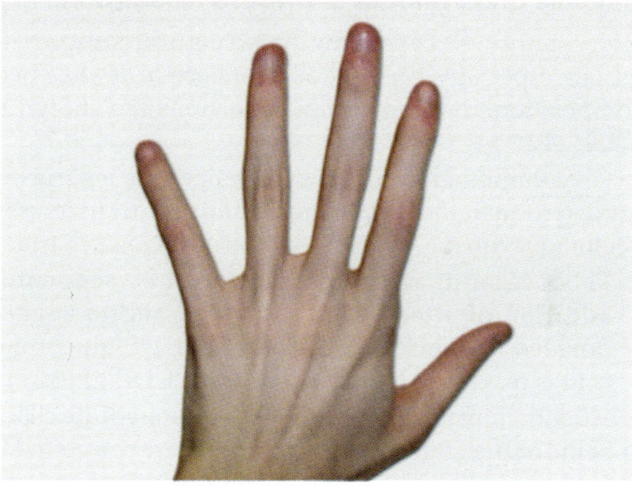

Fig. 24.4: Marfan syndrome: Arachnodactyly (long, slender, spidery fingers)

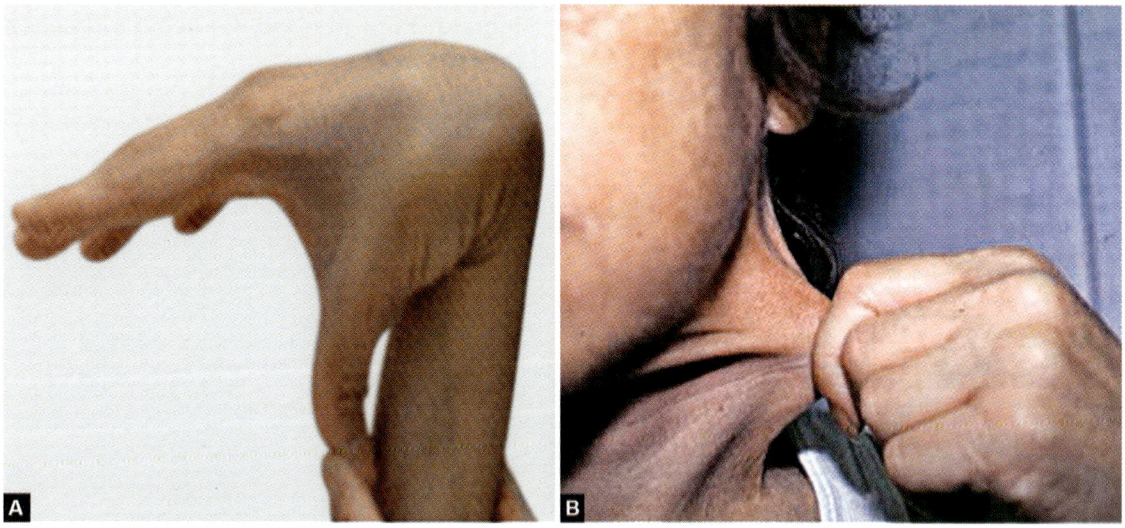

Fig. 24.3: Ehlers-Danlos syndrome. (A) Hypermobile joints; (B) Hyperextensible skin

The disease in a mild form causes loose joints, deformed spine, floppy mitral valves and lens dislocation. In severely affected individuals, the aortic wall is prone to rupture.

Emphysema: It is due to the **deficiency of α1-antitrypsin** (α1-AT), resulting from the destruction of the connective tissue of alveolar walls. The deficiency may be genetic (mutation in α1-AT gene) or acquired as a result of damage to α1-AT by reactive oxygen species present in tobacco smoke.

GLYCOSAMINOGLYCANS

Glycosaminoglycans **(GAGs)** are **unbranched polysaccharides** and consist of **alternating uronic acid and hexosamine residues**. Solutions of GAGs have slimy, mucus like consistency, due to their high viscosity and elasticity. Most important glycosaminoglycans are hyaluronic acid, chondroitin sulfates, heparin, etc. (*see* Chapter 1).

Structure and Synthesis of Glycosaminoglycans

Glycosaminoglycans provide structural support to tissues, especially, cartilage and connective tissue. There composition, distribution and functions are shown in Table 24.1.

Glycosaminoglycans are **synthesized by a series of glycosyltransferases, epimerases and sulf-transferases**, beginning with the synthesis of the core oligosaccharides.

- Polysaccharide **chains are elongated by sequential addition of alternating acidic and amino sugars**, donated by their UDP-derivatives (UDP-glucuronic acid is produced by the oxidation of UDP-glucose).
- After their incorporation into the carbohydrate chain, **some of the D-glucuronic acid units are converted to L-iduronic acid by** the enzyme **uronosyl-5-epimerase**.
- Sulfation of some the carbohydrate chains occur by active sulfate (Phosphoadenosyl-5′-phosphosulfate or PAPS) by sulf-transferases.

Degradation of Glycosaminoglycans

Glycosaminoglycans are **degraded by the sequential action of several lysosomal acid hydrolases**, including **exo-glycosidases and sulfatases**, beginning from the external end of the glycan chain. This may involve removal of the sulfate by a sulfatase, then removal of the terminal sugar by a specific glycosidase, and so on.

Disorders of Glycosaminoglycans Metabolism

If one of the enzymes involved in the stepwise degradation pathway is missing, the entire degradation process is stopped at that particular point only. As a result of it, the **undegraded GAG molecule accumulates in the lysosomes**, causing a number of disorders which are collectively referred to as lysosomal storage disorders.

LYSOSOMAL STORAGE DISORDERS

Lysosomes are responsible for the intracellular digestion of the extracellular and the intracellular substances and contain a number of hydrolyzing enzymes (hydrolases) for the hydrolysis of proteins, lipids, carbohydrates and nucleic acids. These hydrolases are most active at acidic pH and split complex molecules into simple low molecular weight compounds that can be reutilized. In lysosomal storage disorders, some of the lysosomal enzymes are missing, leading to the accumulation of the substrate of the missing enzyme. As a result of it, lysosomes become enlarged with undigested material, thereby interfering with the normal cell processes.

Lysosomal storage disorders include **muco-polysaccharidoses** and **sphingolipidoses**.

Mucopolysaccharidoses: This is a of lipid storage disorders **due to defects in glycosaminoglycans degradation**. Various **disorders** included in this group, **deficient enzymes** and the **products which accumulate in the lysosomes and are excreted in urine** are shown in Table 24.2.

Sphingolipidoses: This is a group of lipid storage diseases caused by the **deficiency of** the specific **lysosomal hydrolytic enzymes** that **cause defects in the degradation of sphingolipids**. These include **Niemann-Pick disease, Gaucher's disease** and **Tay-Sachs disease**.

- **Niemann-Pick disease:** It results from a **deficiency** of the enzyme **sphingomyelinase**, which leads to

Table 24.1: Composition and functions of glycosaminoglycans

Glycosaminoglycan	*Repeating disaccharide unit*	*Tissue location*	*Major functions*
Hyaluronic acid	[GlcUA-GlcNAc]	Joint and ocular fluids	Serves as excellent biological shock absorber and lubricant
Chondroitin sulfates	[GlcUA-GalNAc]	Cartilage, tendons, bone	Bind collagen and give it strength
Dermatan sulfate	[IdUA-GalNAc]	Skin, valves, blood vessels	Valve integrity
Heparan sulfate	[IdUA-GlcNAc]	Cell surfaces	Initiation of signaling processes
Heparin	[IdUA-GlcNAc]	Mast cells, liver	Serves as an anticoagulant
Keratan sulfates	[Gal-GlcNAc]	Cartilage, cornea	Corneal transparency

Table 24.2: Mucopolysaccharidoses

Syndrome	*Deficient enzyme*	*Degradation products which are accumulated in lysosomes and are excreted in urine*
Hunter syndrome	Iduronate sulfatase	Heparan sulfate and dermatan sulfate
Hurler syndrome	α-L-Iduronidase	–do–
Morquio syndromes		
A	Galactose-6-sulfatase	Keratan sulfate
B	β-Galactosidase	–do–
Sanfilippo syndrome		
A	Heparan sulfamidase	Heparan sulfate
B	N-Acetylglycosaminidase	–do–
C	Acetyl-CoA: Glucosaminide-N-acetyl-transferase	–do–
D	N-Acetylglucosamine-6-sulfate-sulfatase	–do–
Sly syndrome	β-Glucuronidase	Dermatan sulfate and heparan sulfate

accumulation of sphingomyelin in lysosomes. It is **characterized by hepatosplenomegaly**.

- **Gaucher's disease:** It is a lysosomal storage disease where the enzyme **glucocerebrosidase is missing**. It is characterized by **hepatomegaly, long-bone osteoporosis and neurodegeneration**.
- **Tay-Sachs disease:** It is due to **lack of** the enzyme **hexosaminidase.** It is the most common form of **GM_2 gangliosidosis**. Ganglion cells of the cerebral cortex are swollen due to the deposition of GM_2 gangliosides. The disease is characterized by **neurodegeneration, blindness, cherry-red macula, muscular weakness and seizures**.

Some Important Questions

1. **What are collagens? How these are synthesized? Describe some disorders of synthesis of collagens.**
2. **What are glycosaminoglycans? Describe various disorders of glycosaminoglycans metabolism.**
3. **Write notes on:**
   i. Collagens
   ii. Osteogenesis imperfecta
   iii. Ehlers-Danlos syndrome
   iv. Elastin
   v. Marfan syndrome
   vi. Glycosaminoglycans
   vii. Lysosomal storage disorders
   viii. Tay-Sachs disease
   ix. Emphysema

Chapter

25

Metabolism of Bone and Teeth

Bone is a tissue that is hard in structure like tooth but it differs from tooth in the way that bone **is regularly remodeled**.

Normal bone **metabolism** consists of **bone formation** and its **destruction**. The two processes are always **close to equilibrium**, though, bone formation is more than resorption during childhood whereas reverse happens in an elderly person.

BONE CELLS

Bone consists of two types of cells referred to as osteoblasts and osteoclasts.

Osteoblasts

Osteoblasts are **responsible for bone formation**; hence the process of bone formation **(mineralization)** is also referred to as **osteoblastogenesis**.

Osteoblasts are responsible for the **production of organic component of** the bone matrix, designated as **osteoid**.

Osteoid: It is the **unmineralized organic part of the bone.** After mineralization, osteoid is **converted to mature bone**. It is **composed of** the **fibrous tissue**, which primarily comprises **collagen**, and the ground substance that contains **osteocalcin** and a heteropolysaccharide called **chondroitin sulfate** (*see* Chapter 1).

- **Collagen:** Collagen (type I) is the main protein found in osteoids (*see* Chapter 24).
- **Osteocalcin:** Osteocalcin helps in calcification. It is a Gla-protein (γ-carboxy-glutamate-containing protein) which is formed with the help of vitamin K (*see* Chapter 9).
- **Osteonectin:** It is a **glycoprotein** which is **rich in cysteine**. Osteonectin is **secreted by the osteoblasts** during bone synthesis. It **has affinity for collagen** as well as calcium, and thus, **helps in calcification** and mineralization of bone.

Osteoclasts

Osteoclasts are **multinucleated cells** which are **large in size cells**. These are **derived in the bone marrow from the hematopoietic stem cells**.

- Osteoclasts secrete **H^+ ions, collagenase** and **other hydrolyzing enzymes**.
- Acidic pH and the hydrolytic enzymes, in turn, **cause demineralization (resorption)** of the calcified bone and play an **important role in bone remodeling**.
- After resorption of the bone, **osteoclasts undergo cell division** and are, **eventually, transformed to osteoblasts**.

BIOCHEMICAL COMPOSITION OF BONE

Bone comprises the organic matrix (mainly collagens) and the inorganic material consisting of, primarily, hydroxyapatite (Table 25.1).

Table 25.1: Biochemical composition of bone

Organic matrix
Collagen
Albumin
Osteocalcin
Glycoproteins
Gla-proteins
Sialoproteins
Inorganic material
• Crystalline hydroxyapatite
Ca^{+2}
P
Mg^{+2}
F
• Inter-crystalline fraction
Calcium carbonate
Calcium citrate
Calcium chloride
Calcium fluoride

1. Organic Matrix

- Organic matrix, mainly, consists of a **collagen-like protein**, referred to as **ossein**.
- Ossein is a **type I collagen** and comprises nearly, 90–95% of the organic matrix.
- Besides collagen, organic matrix also **contains** several other serum derived proteins such as **albumin, α2-HS glycoproteins, Gla-containing proteins (γ-carboxyglutamate-residues), osteocalcin** and **sialoproteins.**

  Some of these also **function in initiating mineralization** and/or help **binding of mineral phase to the matrix**.

2. Inorganic Material

Inorganic material, also referred to as **mineral structure** of the bone, consists of the **crystalline hydroxyapatite** and **inter-crystalline fraction**. Both of these **fractions differ from** each other in their composition and function. These include:

Crystalline hydroxyapatite: It is a crystalline fraction **(hydroxyapatite crystals)** which consists of mainly **calcium** (Ca^{+2}) and **phosphorus.** Its calcium/phosphorus ratio is less than that of the hydroxyapatite. It also contains small amount of Mg^{2+} and **fluoride**. Fluoride has bone-strengthening effect (Fig. 25.1).

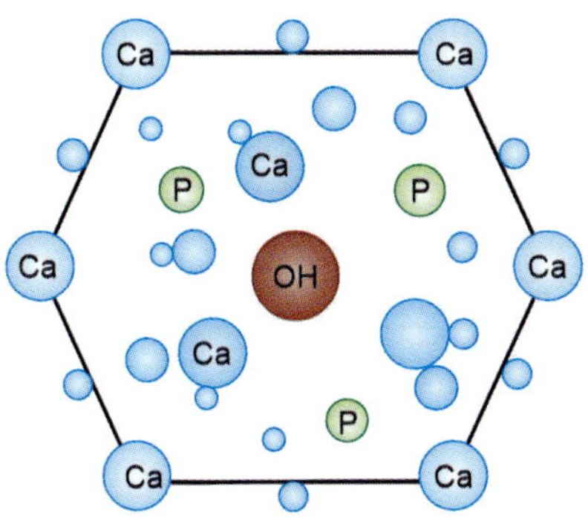

Fig. 25.1: Hydroxyapatite

Hydroxyapatite crystals are extremely small in size but have enormous surface area. These are relatively stable and not easily soluble in the aqueous fluid. Hydroxyapatite constitute nearly 70% weight of the bone.

Inter-crystalline fraction: Besides the crystalline fraction, bone also consists of the inter-crystalline fraction. Compared to the crystalline fraction, it is a **small** fraction and is **soluble** in nature. It comprises various calcium salts such as **calcium carbonate, calcium citrate, calcium chloride and calcium fluoride**, etc.

FUNCTIONS OF BONE

Bone performs, both structural as well as metabolic functions.

- **Structural functions:** Bone is important for the **structure of the body** and its different parts.
- **Metabolic functions:** Principal metabolic function of the bone, particularly the large bones, is in **calcium and phosphate homeostasis**.

BONE REMODELING

Bone remodeling **(metabolism)**, as mentioned above, consists of both, **bone** mineralization **(formation)** as well as its destruction **(resorption)**. Both the processes occur simultaneously.

Absorption of calcium by a bone or its release from the bone is regulated by several factors, which includes several hormones and the mechanical strain.

- **Calcitriol:** Calcitriol or **active vitamin D** (1,25-dihydroxy-cholecalciferol; *see* Chapter 9).
- **Parathyroid hormone:** Parathyroid hormone (PTH) is a large peptide **secreted by the parathyroid gland.** PTH, in turn, **increase serum calcium** concentration. It stimulates osteoblasts to secrete interleukins and cytokines which, in turn, activate osteoclasts for bone resorption and release of calcium.
- **Calcitonin:** It is a small peptide **secreted by the parafollicular cells of the thyroid gland**. It **inhibits** osteoclastic activity and thus, **bone resorption**.
- **Growth hormone:** Growth hormone (GH) has a direct effect on bone growth and is **essential**, particularly, **for the growth of long bones**.
- **Insulin-like growth factor 1 (IGF 1):** IGF1 acts like a paracrine hormone and **stimulate chondrocytes in the epiphyseal plate**. IGF1 also **stimulates the division of osteoblasts**.
- **Thyroid hormones:** Various bone cells, such as chondrocytes, bone marrow stromal cells, osteoblasts and osteoclast precursors, have been shown to express thyroid hormone receptors. Thus, thyroid hormones have been shown to play an important role in the regulation of bone metabolism.

  Besides thyroid hormones, it has been shown that thyroid stimulating hormone (**thyrotropin** or TSH) has **inhibitory effect on osteoclasts**.
- **Estrogens and androgens:** Receptors for both, estrogen as well as androgens have been shown to be expressed in bone cells. Accordingly,
  - **Estrogens** have been shown to **reduce bone resorption** and **stimulate bone formation** by reducing the number as well as activity of osteoclasts.
  - **Follicle stimulating hormone** (FSH)—**Osteoclast activity** has been shown to be **stimulated by FSH**.
  - It is known that there is **increased production of androgens and estrogens during puberty**. It is also the **period when growth spurt is seen**.
  - It is also known that **estrogen concentration is reduced during postmenopausal stage.** This is also the stage when **osteoporosis occurs**.

- **Glucocorticoids:** Glucocorticoids are also known to affect bone metabolism.
  - These have been shown to inhibit osteoblastic activity, reduce their function as well as life span.
  - Glucocorticoids have also been shown to promote osteoclasts activity and osteoporosis.
- **Mechanical strain:** Bodily **physical activities**, causing mechanical strain to bones, are **necessary for bone remodeling.** It is well known that physical inactivity, as seen in elderly persons and hospitalized patients, **lead to loss of bone strength.**

BONE DISORDERS

Osteoporosis

Osteoporosis means abnormally porous bone that is compressible like a sponge. It is characterized by decrease in bone density and strength, thereby, resulting in fragile bones and frequent fractures (Fig. 25.2).

In postmenopausal woman, decreased calcium intake, particularly, during menopause leads to **increased fragility** and **fractures of bones,** mainly of the extremities and the pelvis (*see* Chapter 10).

Osteoporosis **can be retarded by the increased supply of calcium** in food **along with the estrogen therapy**.

Besides calcium, various other **dietary micronutrients are essential to prevent osteoporosis**. These include:

Vitamin D: It is essential for the absorption and utilization of calcium.

Vitamin C: It is required for the formation of bone matrix.

Magnesium, phosphorus, copper, zinc, manganese and boron: These minerals form essential part of the bone structure.

Vitamin K: It is essential for γ-carboxylation, which is needed for the synthesis of Gla-proteins and thus, is important in bone formation.

Therefore, **a well-balanced diet which supplies** all the nutrients and a regular exercise is necessary for the prevention of osteoporosis.

Rickets and Osteomalacia

As discussed in Chapter 9, both rickets and osteomalacia are the result of lack of vitamin D. In these conditions, though the organic matrix is synthesized but due to the **deficiency of vitamin D** which plays an important role in calcium homeostasis, the organic matrix **lack mineralization** resulting in **weak bones.**

Rickets is characterized by bowed-legs and knock-knees (Fig. 9.4).

Osteomalacia, also called adult rickets, is characterized by weakness, bone pain and delayed parturition due to pelvic bone deformities, in females.

Both, the conditions can be prevented by vitamin D and Ca^{2+} supplementation.

Biochemically, there is **decrease** in **serum calcium** and **phosphorus** along with an **increase in serum alkaline phosphatase**. There also occurs **increased excretion of phosphorus** in urine.

Product of serum calcium and phosphorus, which is normally 40 (10 mg calcium × 4 mg phosphorus), is decreased to below 30, in such patients.

Fluorosis

Large doses of fluoride may be toxic and leads to an important public health problem, in many parts of the world, referred to as **fluorosis**. It may affect teeth **(dental fluorosis)** and bones (**skeletal fluorosis;** *see* Chapter 10).

Clinical features of **skeletal fluorosis** include **pain, inflammation and restricted movement of joints** besides **stiffness of the spine**.

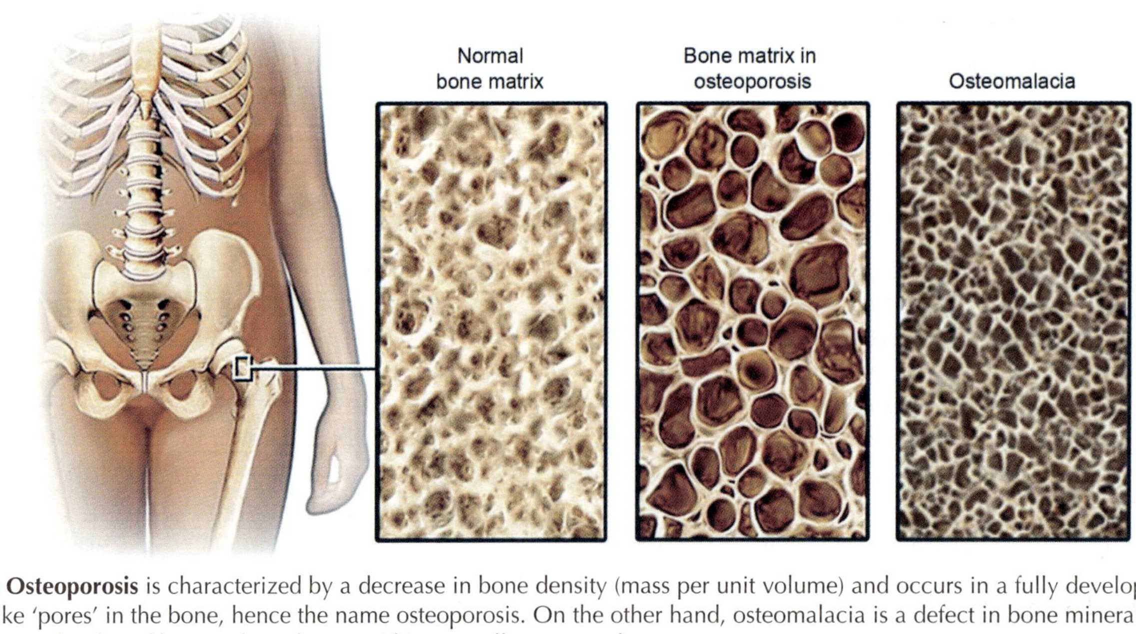

Fig. 25.2: Osteoporosis is characterized by a decrease in bone density (mass per unit volume) and occurs in a fully developed bone. It appears like 'pores' in the bone, hence the name osteoporosis. On the other hand, osteomalacia is a defect in bone mineralization in a developing or developed bone, where the osteoid is generally preserved

Further, significantly higher intake of fluoride (more than 3 mg/L, in drinking water, results in a variant of severe form of the skeletal fluorosis referred to as **genu valgum** (knock-knee; Fig. 10.8).

METABOLISM OF TEETH

Teeth are the major components of oral cavity. These are essential for start of digestion of carbohydrates and play an important role in mastication of food. Teeth are also important components of our facial skeleton and add to the aesthetics, phonation and speech.

Components of a Tooth

A tooth is made up of specialized tissues called enamel, dentin, cementum and pulp (Table 25.2).

Table 25.2: Composition of a tooth

Part of tooth	*Composition*
Enamel	Hydroxyapatite Amelogenins Enamelins Ameloblastins Tuftelins Alkaline phosphatase
Dentin	Hydroxyapatite Collagens Phosphoproteins Sialoproteins Glycosaminoglycans Alkaline phosphatase Gla-proteins
Cementum	Hydroxyapatite Collagens Proteoglycans Mitochondrial-DNA
Pulp	Connective tissue Macrophages Fibroblasts T lymphocytes

Enamel

It is one of the four major tissues which along with dentin, cementum and pulp make a tooth. Enamel is **avascular** and has no nerve supply.

Biochemically, nearly 96% of the enamel is **hydroxyapatite** (crystalline calcium phosphate) while the remaining of it is **organic material and water**.

The process of enamel formation is referred to as **amelogenesis**. It **occurs via ameloblasts** in two stages:

- **Stage I:** It is called the **secretory stage**, where **protein synthesis** occurs in the rough endoplasmic reticulum of the ameloblasts and the synthesized protein is released into the surroundings. There also occurs **synthesis of the organic matrix** with the partially mineralized enamel by **alkaline phosphatase**.
- **Stage II:** The second stage of amelogenesis is designated as the **maturation stage** where the process of **mineralization** is completed **by enamel proteins**, mainly, **amelogenins and enamelins**.

  Besides amilogenins and enamelins, enamel also contains **ameloblastins** and **tuftelins**, but does **not** contain **collagen**.

Dentin

Dentin or **dentine** is present between the enamel and the cementum and pulp chamber. The **process of dentin synthesis** is referred to as **dentinogenesis**. The process of dentinogenesis is **initiated by odontoblasts** form **pre-dentin**.

Pre-dentin: Pre-dentin is the unmineralized component. It is an organic matrix, which comprises about 90% of the **type I collagen**. The remaining **10%** of it consists of **non-collagen proteins** comprising of some **phosphoproteins** which are rich in aspartate and serine, **sialoproteins (proteoglycans), glycosaminoglycans** (GAG), **several growth factors,** various phosphatases (predominantly **alkaline phosphatase**) and **Gla-proteins** (γ-carboxy-glutamate containing proteins) which help in the binding of calcium.

Pre-dentin is **mineralized** and form dentin, which is a calcified tissue (bone like matrix) of the body of the tooth. It is **made up of 70% of the inorganic material** (a mineralized connective tissue). Besides, it contains **20% of organic materials** and **10% of water**.

- The principal inorganic material is hydroxyapatite $[Ca_{10}(PO_4)6{\cdot}(OH)_2]$.
- The **organic material** present in dentin is mainly a **type I collagen** (nearly 90%) with small amount (about 10%) of the non-collagen matrix.
- The **non-collagen material** includes various substances present in pre-dentin.

Cementum

It is **acellular**, bone like substance covering root of the tooth. Cementum has **45–50% inorganic material** (mainly **hydroxyapatite**), **30–35% organic matter** (comprising of **collagen** and **proteoglycans**) and **20–25% water**. It has **highest content of fluoride** compare to all the other mineralized tissues.

Cementum has been shown to contain large amount of the **mitochondrial DNA (mt DNA)**.

Dental Pulp

It is the central part (the inner most layer) of tooth and is also referred to as **nerve of the tooth**. It has the **connective tissue, nerve, blood vessels** and number of cells including **fibroblasts, predontoblasts, macrophages** and **T lymphocytes**.

Pulp has two types of sensory nerve fibres:

- **Myelinated nerve fibres** (A-fibres), and
- **Unmyelinated fibers** (C-fibres)

The main function of dental pulp is the **formation of dentin.** Besides, it also has nutritive function and provides nutrients and moisture to the organic components.

TOOTH DISORDERS

Dental Caries

Dental caries, **caries** or **decay** also referred to as **cavity formation** is characterized by destruction of the tooth enamel due to the action of microorganisms (which are normally present in the oral cavity) on carbohydrates, particularly, during the formation of teeth. Acid-producing bacteria utilize carbohydrates (mainly sucrose) for energy and **produce acids** (lactic, propionic, and acetic acids) by fermentation. These acids **bring about demineralization of the enamel** (Fig. 10.6).

Dental Fluorosis

It occurs, mainly, in children, who are exposed to high fluoride intake, before the completion of mineralization of the tooth enamel. Their teeth exhibit mottled enamel. **Mottling** is confined to the permanent teeth and is **characterized by multiple, minute white flecks and yellow/brown spots,** which are **scattered irregularly over the tooth surface** (Fig. 10.7).

Some Important Questions

1. **Describe various components of bone.**
2. **Describe various components of tooth.**
3. **Write notes on:**
   i. Bone remodelling
   ii. Osteoporosis
   iii. Biochemical composition of bone
   iv. Osteomalacia
   v. Dental caries
   vi. Dental fluorosis

Chapter
26

Biological Membranes

All living cells are surrounded by a highly viscous and flexible structure called **cell membrane**, which, in animal cells, is also called **plasma membrane**. Structure and function of cells are, primarily, dependent on the membranes. Cell membrane clearly **separates the interior of the cell from its exterior**. In addition, **membranes in the eukaryotic cells also define their internal compartments,** such as **nucleus, mitochondria, lysosomes**, etc. Accordingly, all these membranes are collectively referred to as **biological membranes**.

STRUCTURE OF A BIOLOGICAL MEMBRANE

All biological membranes are the bilayers of phospholipids that are associated with proteins. Structurally, **formation of biological membranes is based on the properties** of lipids, especially the **phospholipids,** which are the fundamental building block of all the membranes.

- **Phospholipids are amphipathic molecules,** consisting of two hydrophobic (nonpolar) fatty acyl chains, which are linked to a phosphate-containing hydrophilic (polar) head group. The fatty acyl chain may be saturated or unsaturated. **Due to presence of the cis-double bond, unsaturated fatty** acyl chains **form kink** (Fig. 26.1).

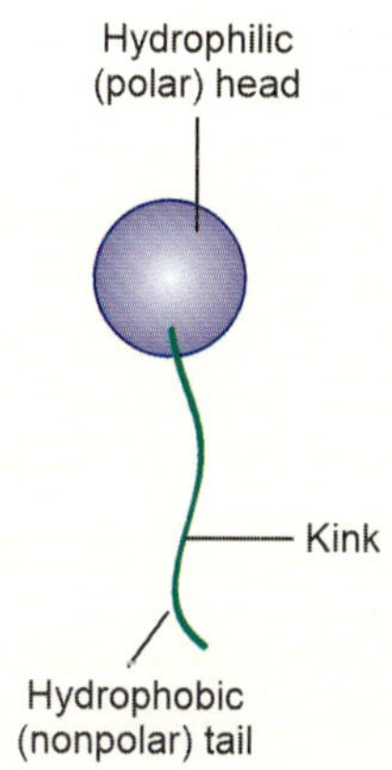

Fig. 26.1: A phospholipid

- Various phospholipids, spontaneously, form bilayers (lipid bilayer) in aqueous solutions, where the hydrophobic tails are buried in the interior of the membrane while the hydrophilic head groups are exposed on both sides, and are in contact with the aqueous environment (Fig. 26.2).

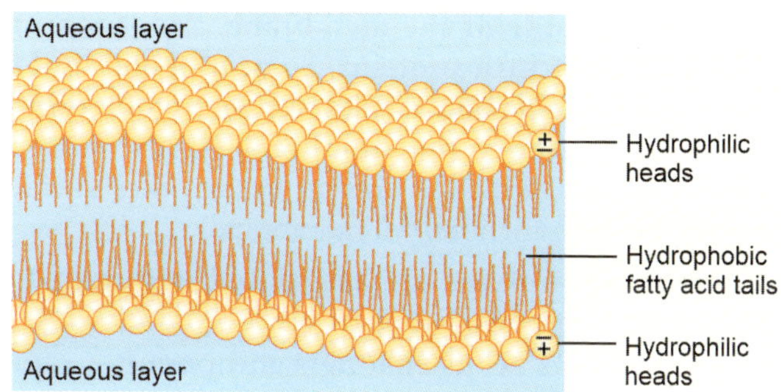

Fig. 26.2: A lipid bilayer

Fluid-mosaic Model of a Biological Membrane Structure

Bilayer of phospholipids associated with proteins is referred to as **fluid-mosaic model of biological membrane,** since a membrane is fluid in consistency consisting of the **mosaic of proteins and lipids** (Fig. 26.3).

According to their mode of interaction with the lipid bilayer, membrane proteins are divided into two groups, as **integral proteins** and **peripheral proteins.**

- **Integral membrane proteins:** These proteins **span the lipid bilayer** from one side to the other and, thus, are also called **transmembrane proteins** or **intrinsic proteins**. The transmembrane protein **has three domains**, i.e. a **sequence exterior to the cell** (containing the amino-terminal end), **transmembrane sequence** and the **sequence extending into the cell** (with the carboxy-terminal end), e.g. glycophorin A, the protein which spans the erythrocyte membrane.
- **Peripheral membrane proteins:** These proteins are **immersed only partially**, i.e. they are **embedded**

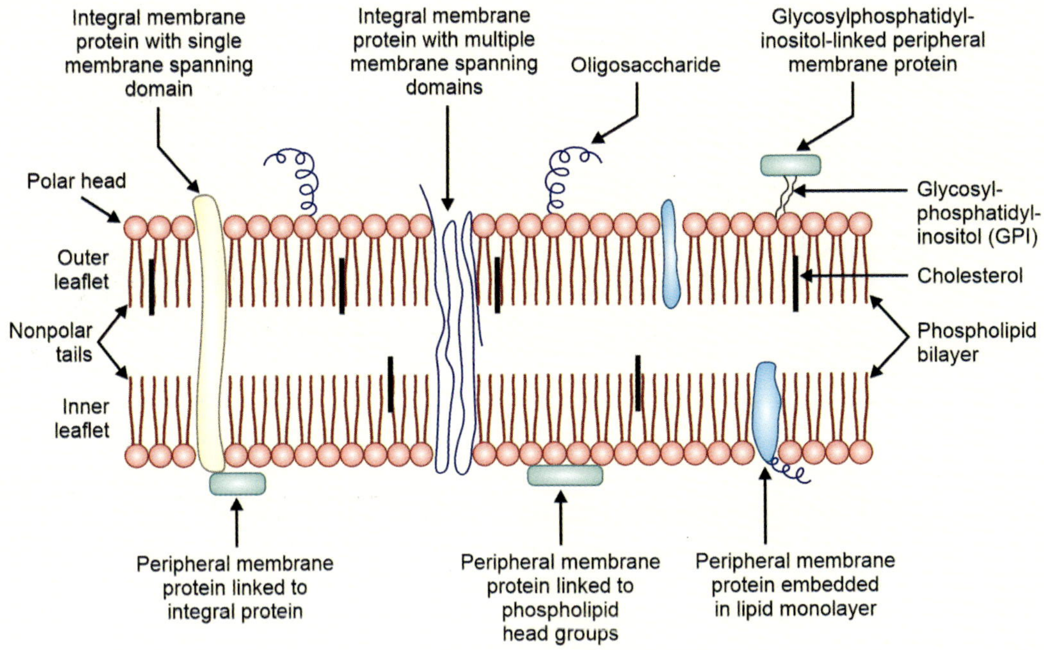

Fig. 26.3: Fluid-mosaic model of biological membrane

on any one side of the membrane, and, thus, are also called **extrinsic proteins. Some of them bind to integral proteins** (such as an antigen) while **others** serve **as anchor in the membrane lipids** (such as cytochrome c, which is present in the outer surface of the inner mitochondrial membrane).

Membrane proteins are associated with various specialized functions. For example:

- Some **proteins act as channels** and **permit a rapid movement of specific ions or molecules** from one side of membrane to the other
- Some of the **proteins act as receptors** and work as **recognition sites** (such as **hormone receptors** for insulin or glucagon, or **immunoreceptors** present on B lymphocytes for the recognition and response to foreign antigens, etc.) and allow the cell to respond to external signals.
- Some of the **proteins act as enzymes** which are **located either within the cell or on the cell membrane** (e.g. the inner mitochondrial membrane proteins which act as enzymes and participate in electron transport and oxidative phosphorylation. Some membrane proteins also control interactions between cells of multicellular organisms.

Functions of a Cell Membrane

- Cell membrane **provides shape, protection, support and movement** for the cell.
- **Regulate transfer (transport or translocation) of molecules,** such as amino acids, glucose and various ions, etc. **into and from the cell** to maintain their concentrations and homeostasis.

MEMBRANE ASSOCIATED PROCESSES

Most important membrane associated process is the translocation (transport) of the substances into and from the cell, **to maintain their concentrations and homeostasis.**

TRANSPORT OF SUBSTANCES ACROSS THE MEMBRANE

The translocation may or may not require the formation of a membrane-bound vesicle; accordingly, the translocation may be **non-vesicular or vesicular.**

Non-vesicular Translocation Systems

Non-vesicular translocation systems are of two types, i.e. **non-mediated translocation** and **carrier-mediated translocation,** which includes passive transport (passive mediated transport or facilitated diffusion) and active transport (Fig. 26.4).

Non-mediated Translocation (Diffusion)

Some solutes, such as O_2, N_2, CO_2, NO, urea, etc. **move across the cell membrane by diffusing down an electrochemical gradient and do not require metabolic energy.** This, **passive non-mediated translocation** is called **diffusion** or **passive diffusion**. The direction of flow is always from a higher to a lower concentration and the net movement of a molecule from one side to the other continues until concentration on each side is at chemical equilibrium.

Diffusion of a substance may also occur through membrane channels or pores.

- **Channels:** Channels are **pore-like structures**, which are **formed by the integral membrane proteins.**

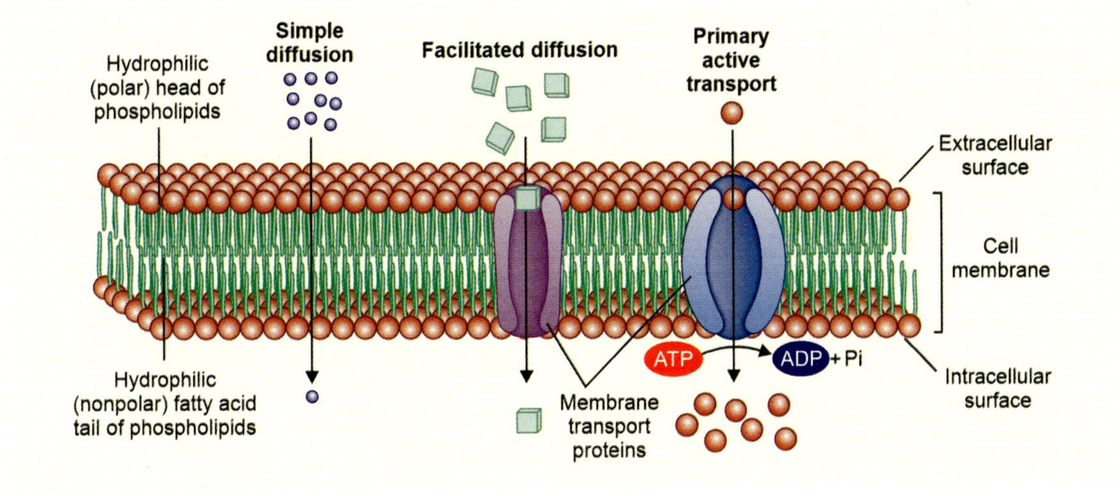

Fig. 26.4: Transport systems

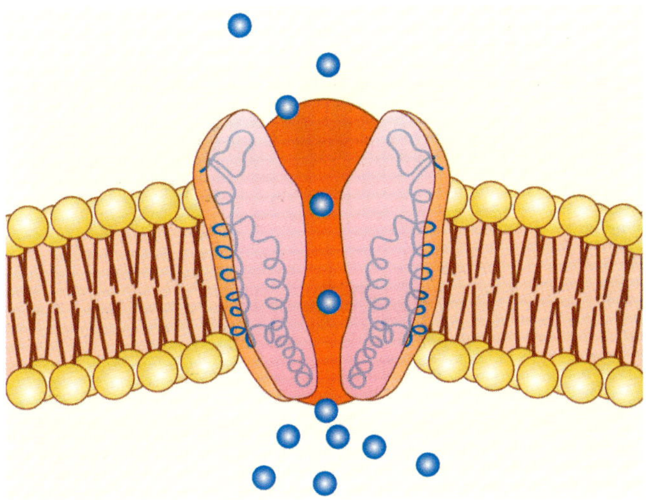

Fig. 26.5: Channel

Channels **permit rapid movement of specific ions or molecules from one side of membrane to the other** (Fig. 26.5).

Channels are **opened transiently**, i.e. they are gated. The channel opening and closing involves a change in the voltage/membrane potential **(voltage-gated channel)** or the binding of a chemical agent **(ligand-gated channel)**.

CHANNELOPATHIES

Mutations in genes encoding polypeptide constituents of ion channel may lead to certain diseases termed **channelopathies**, e.g. myasthenia gravis and cystic fibrosis.

Myasthenia gravis: Myasthenia gravis is an **acquired autoimmune disease** characterized by muscle weakness due to decreased neuromuscular signal transmission. Autoantibodies against acetylcholine receptors accelerate their turnover and reduce their number. Acetylcholinesterase inhibitor drugs are given to enhance the stay of acetylcholine at the neuromuscular junction.

Cystic fibrosis: Cystic fibrosis is a multiorgan disease. Its gene product is a **cystic fibrosis transmembrane conductance regulator** (**CFTR** protein), which is a **cAMP-dependent Cl^- channel**. Patients have reduced membrane permeability which impairs fluid and electrolyte secretion, and leads to luminal dehydration.

Aquaporins (AQP): Some specific integral membrane proteins function as **water channels**. They allow rapid movement of water across the plasma membrane and are known as aquaporins (AQP). Many forms of AQP have been discovered. So far, at least six forms of AQP have been shown to be expressed in cells in the kidneys and seven in the gastrointestinal tract, the tissues in which water movement across plasma membranes is particularly rapid.

Carrier-mediated Transport

Molecules that cannot freely diffuse through the membrane by themselves, need to be **transported in association with** some specific carrier molecule or transport protein, which may be designated as **carrier, permease, porter,** translocase or transporter. Carrier-mediated transport includes passive transport (passive-mediated transport or facilitated diffusion) and active transport.

- **Facilitated diffusion:** Facilitated diffusion, also referred to as passive mediated transport, leads to the **translocation of solutes through membrane transport proteins,** but **without the expenditure of metabolic energy.** The process can operate either **unidirectionally** (uniport) or **bidirectionally** (cotransport).

UNIPORT AND COTRANSPORT

Uniport: Uniport refers to the transport (movement or transfer) of one type of ions or molecules only in one direction by the membrane, e.g. uptake of glucose by the erythrocytes.

Cotransport: Cotransport refers to the transport of two types of ions or molecules, where the transfer of one depends upon the simultaneous or sequential transfer of the other. It may be:

- **Symport:** Symport refers to the transport of two types of molecules in the same direction, such as Na^+-glucose transporter-1 (SGLT1), Na^+-amino acid transporters, etc.
- **Antiport:** Antiport refers to the transport of two types of molecules but in opposite directions, e.g. Na^+, K^+-pump, Cl^--HCO_3^- transporter, etc.

The net flux across the membrane occurs down a concentration gradient, i.e. the molecules flow from a higher to the lower concentration (Fig. 26.6).

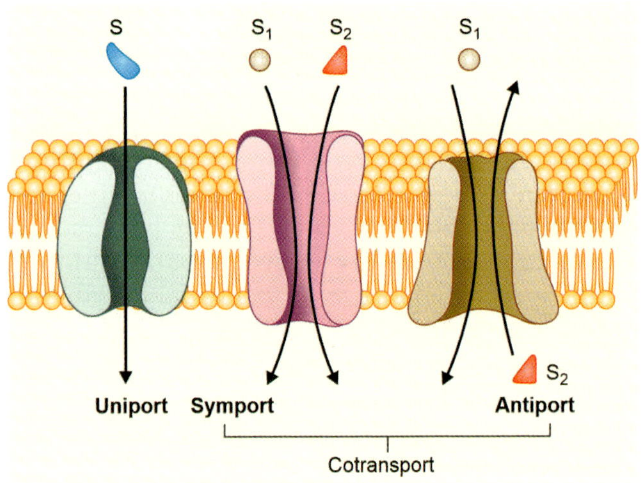

Fig. 26.6: Transport of substances with respect to the number of molecules and the direction of movement

Some of the examples of transport proteins, which mediate facilitated diffusion, include:

1. **Glucose transporters (GLUT):** A group of transport proteins present in the plasma membrane of mammalian cells for the transport of D-glucose, e.g. GLUT1, GLUT2, etc. They translocate several D-sugars by a uniport mechanism and are also referred to as glucose permeases.
2. **Cl^-/HCO_3^--exchanger:** Chloride-bicarbonate exchanger is an anion exchanger protein for the antiport movement of Cl^- and HCO_3^- in RBC membrane.
3. **ATP-ADP translocase:** ATP-ADP translocase is an antiport for the exchange of anions (ADP^{3-} and ATP^{4-}) between the cytosol and the mitochondrial matrix. It is located in the inner mitochondrial membrane.

Active transport: Active transport refers to the process in which the transport protein (transporter) moves a specific molecule against the concentration gradient, i.e. from the lower concentration to the higher concentration, and requires energy (which in most cases is coupled with the hydrolysis of ATP). The active transport can be grouped as primary active transport and secondary active transport.

a. Primary active transport: It is a process that requires energy which is provided by the direct hydrolysis of ATP. Primary active transporters consume nearly one-third of the total energy expenditure of a cell. Examples of primary active transport systems include Na^+/K^+-ATPase, Ca^{2+}-ATPase, H^+/K^+-ATPase, etc.

- **Na^+/K^+-ATPase:** Na^+/K^+-ATPase, also referred to as Na^+/K^+-pump, is an antiport that moves three Na^+ ions out of the cell, in exchange of two K^+ ions into the cell, with the concomitant hydrolysis of intracellular ATP. Na^+/K^+-pump is an integral part of the membrane and has binding sites for, both ATP and Na^+ on the cytoplasmic side, and K^+ on the extracellular side of the membrane (Fig. 26.7).

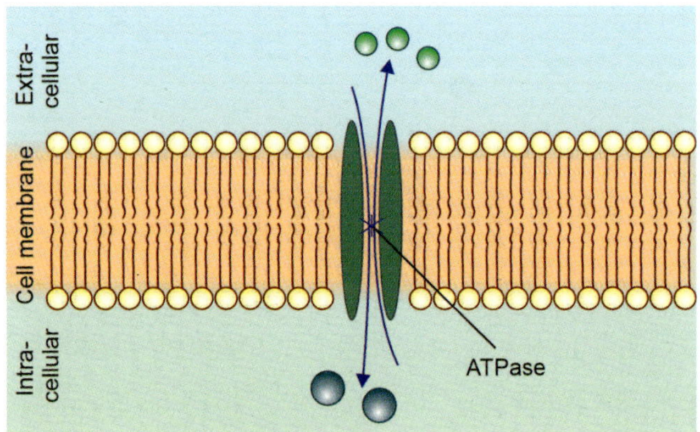

Fig. 26.7: Na^+-K^+ pump

Cardiac glycosides (digitalis, i.e. the drugs such as digoxin and ouabain that inhibit the Na^+/K^+-pump are of clinical importance.

Na^+/K^+-pump and cardiac glycosides

The cell membrane of cardiomyocytes (cells of the myocardium) contains, both Na^+/K^+-pump and Na^+/Ca^{2+} exchanger. Whereas, Na^+/K^+-ATPase removes Na^+ and serves its usual function of maintaining low intracellular Na^+-concentrations, Na^+/Ca^{2+} exchanger, depending on the Na^+-gradient, extrudes Ca^{2+} out of the cell.

Cardiac glycosides (digitalis), such as digoxin and ouabain, inhibit Na^+/K^+-ATPase. As a result of it, intracellular Na^+-concentration is increased, which slows the removal of Ca^{2+} by the Na^+/Ca^{2+} exchanger. This, in turn, increases Ca^{2+}-concentration and the force of contraction. Thus, these drugs are useful in the management of cardiac failure (Fig. 26.8).

- **Ca^{2+}-ATPase:** Ca^{2+}-ATPase, also called Ca^{2+}-pump, actively pumps two Ca^{2+} ions out of the cytosol at the expense of ATP. Mechanism of Ca^{2+}-ATPase resembles that of the Na^+/K^+-ATPase. Ca^{2+} ions act as an important intracellular messenger (also referred to as second messenger) and regulate various cellular processes, such as muscle contraction, release of neurotransmitters, and glycogen breakdown.

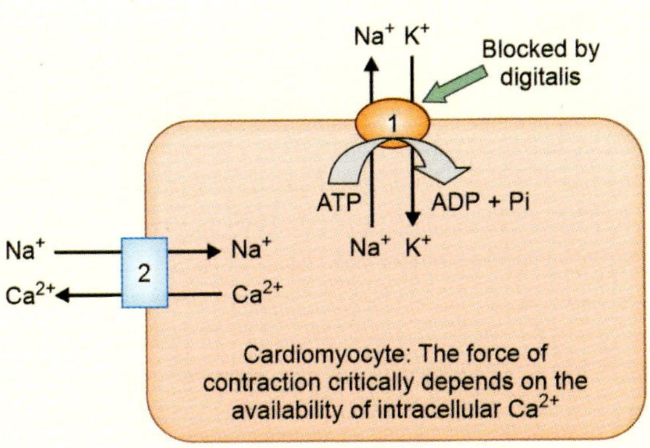

Fig. 26.8: Role of digitalis in heart failure: Normally, the Na^+-K^+-ATPase (1) in the cardiomyocyte membrane moves Na^+ out of the cell in exchange for K^+. The low cytosolic Na^+ maintains the Na^+ gradient for the functioning of the Na^+-Ca^{2+} exchanger (2), so that low cytosolic Ca^{2+} levels are maintained. (In a failing heart, the aim of treatment is to make the myocardium contract with greater force. This is achieved with digitalis, which, by inhibiting Na^+-K^+-ATPase, abolishes the Na^+-gradient. Consequently, Ca^{2+} cannot exit the cell and attains sufficiently high intracellular levels to mediate excitation-contraction coupling and generate greater contractile force. As more blood is pumped out, the symptoms of heart failure are alleviated)

Ca^{2+} ions are also important activator of oxidative metabolism.

- **H^+/K^+-ATPase:** H^+/K^+-ATPase, also called proton pump, is an antiporter. It is important in the secretion of H^+ ions in the luminal membrane. As H^+ ions are pumped out, K^+ ions, which enter the cells, are subsequently externalized. Since chloride channels secrete Cl^- ions into the lumen, the overall product, i.e. HCl is secreted by the parietal cells in the gastric mucosa. Excess production of HC1 can damage gastric mucosa and may lead to peptic ulcer. Drugs such as omeprazole act as proton pump inhibitors and are used clinically.

b. Secondary active transport: In secondary active transport, also called ion gradient-driven active transport, free energy of the electrochemical gradient (which is generated by an ion pumping ATPase) drives the transport of a substance, such as sugar or amino acid against its concentration gradient. Examples of secondary active transport systems include Na^+-glucose transport system, amino acid transport systems, etc.

- **Na^+-Glucose transport system: Plasma membrane of the epithelial cells** lining small intestine and renal tubules **has** two distinct regions, which are referred to as the **apical membrane** (facing the lumen) and the **basolateral membrane** (facing the blood supply). The **polarized organization of the cells is maintained by the presence of tight junctions** at the areas of contact between adjacent cells. These tight junctions **prevent proteins on the apical membrane from migrating** to the basolateral membrane and vice versa. Thus, the entry and exit steps for solutes can be localized to opposite sides of the cell (Fig. 26.9).

Accordingly, transport of glucose in the apical membrane is an example of Na^+-glucose secondary active transport system. In this process:

- **Na^+/ K^+-ATPase,** which is located in the basolateral membrane, pumps **Na^+** out, via primary active transport.
- Na^+-gradient, generated by the primary active transport, facilitates the **transport of Na^+ and glucose** (symport), **via secondary active transport,** thru **SGLT-1** (sodium-glucose transporter-1) which is located in the apical membrane.

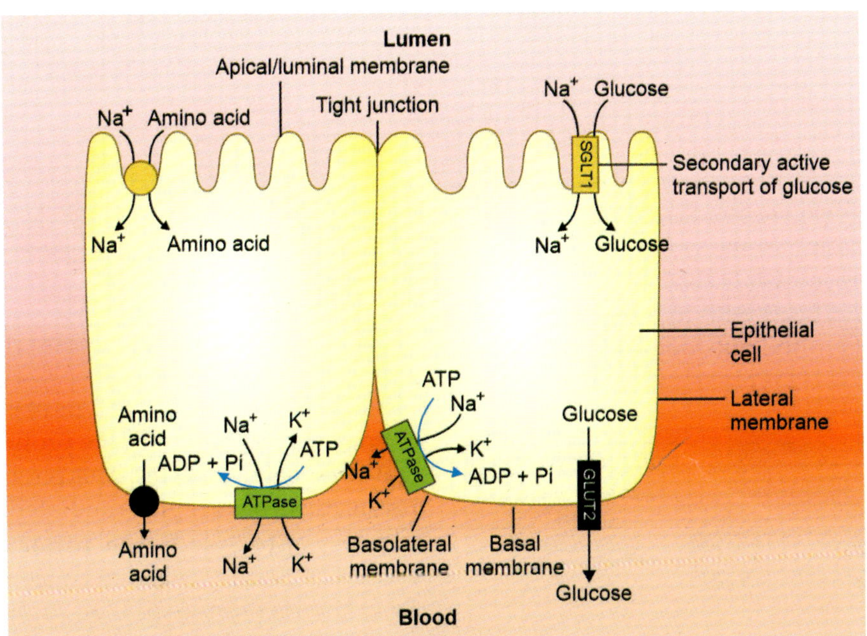

Fig. 26.9: Secondary active transport of glucose in the apical membrane

- **Glucose is passively transported out of the cell** in the basolateral membrane, via GLUT2 (a sodium-independent glucose transporter that moves glucose down its concentration gradient), by facilitated diffusion.

Thus, **uptake of glucose and sodium** (symport) is **secondarily dependent on the Na^+ gradient,** which is **maintained by the primary active transporter, Na^+/K^+-ATPase.** This is also the basis of the oral rehydration therapy using oral rehydration solution (ORS).

ORAL REHYDRATION SOLUTION

Ingredients of the oral rehydration solution (ORS) include glucose, NaCl or $NaHCO_3$, KCl and water. When administered, glucose and Na^+ are reabsorbed in the apical membrane of the enterocytes by sodium-glucose transporter-1 (SGLT1). Transfer of solutes on the basolateral site of the enterocytes increases osmolarity, thereby, favoring osmotic absorption of water. Thus, absorption of glucose accompanied by the obligatory increase in the absorption of NaCl and water, helps to compensate for the diarrheal losses of water as well as solutes to treat dehydration.

Amino acid transport systems: Amino acids are transported by the luminal epithelial cells of the intestine by the Na^+-dependent pathway, similar to the Na^+-dependent glucose transport system. Several brush-border specific transport systems have been identified for the uptake of different groups of amino acids in the luminal membrane (*see* Chapter 8).

Vesicular Translocation Systems

Translocation of some of the macromolecules, such as proteins, across the plasma membrane involves vesicle formation with, or from the plasma membrane, by the processes referred to as exocytosis and endocytosis.

Exocytosis

Exocytosis is a process for the translocation of large molecules, such as proteins, out of the cell. It involves contact of two inside surface monolayers, from the cytosolic side, and release of the macromolecules to the exterior of a cell. In this process, a secretory vesicle in the cytoplasm, originating in the Golgi complex or the endoplasmic reticulum, moves to the inner surface of the plasma membrane and fuses with it, thereby, releasing the vesicular contents to the outside of the membrane (Fig. 26.10).

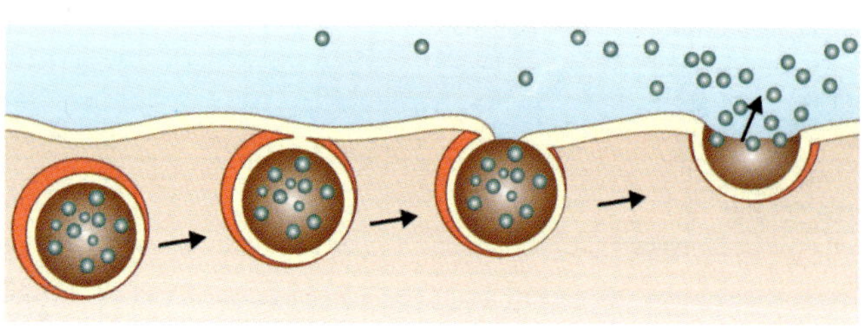

Fig. 26.10: Exocytosis

Endocytosis

Endocytosis is a process of the uptake of large molecules, such as polysaccharides, proteins or polynucleotides, into the cytoplasm. In this process, a region of the plasma membrane invaginates, enclosing a small volume of the extracellular fluid and its contents within a bud, and generates endocytotic vesicles. These vesicles pinch off, as fusion of the plasma membrane seals the neck of the vesicle at the original site of invagination. The resulting small vesicle, called **endosome,** moves into interior of the cell and delivers its contents to some other organelle, which is bound by a single membrane (e.g. lysosome), by fusion of the two membranes forming a secondary lysosome. Due to presence of the hydrolytic enzymes, macromolecular contents are hydrolyzed to their monomers, such as amino acids, simple sugars or nucleotides, which diffuse out of the vesicle and are released into cytoplasm. Endocytosis includes phagocytosis and pinocytosis.

- **Phagocytosis (cell-eating):** Phagocytosis occurs in specialized cells like macrophages and granulocytes, for the ingestion of large particles such as bacteria, viruses, etc.
- **Pinocytosis (cell-drinking):** Pinocytosis (simple pinocytosis) refers to the process of the cellular uptake of fluid and its contents, as a result of invagination of the plasma membrane (Fig. 26.11).

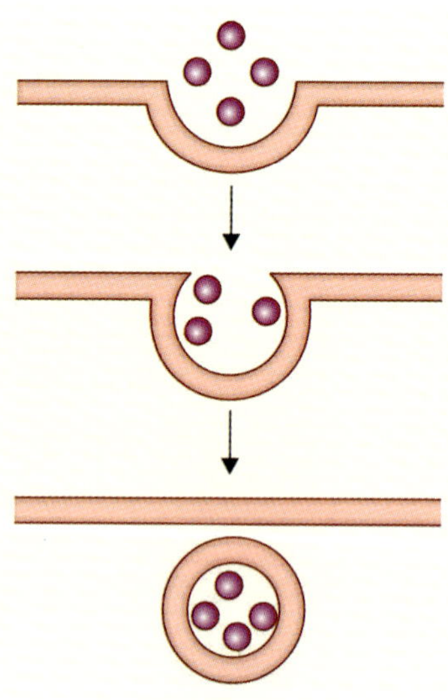

Fig. 26.11: Endocytosis

There is a very selective type of pinocytosis that occurs in coated-pits lined with the protein **clathrin** and forms **clathrin-coated vesicles.** This is referred to as **absorptive pinocytosis** or **receptor-mediated pinocytosis.**

In **receptor-mediated pinocytosis,** high affinity receptors permit selective concentration of the ligand from the medium (e.g. LDL, transferrin, etc.), and the receptors are subsequently internalized by means of the coated pits containing the receptors. These coated vesicle fuse with the lysosomes, their contents are digested and clathrin is recycled back to the membrane (Fig. 26.12).

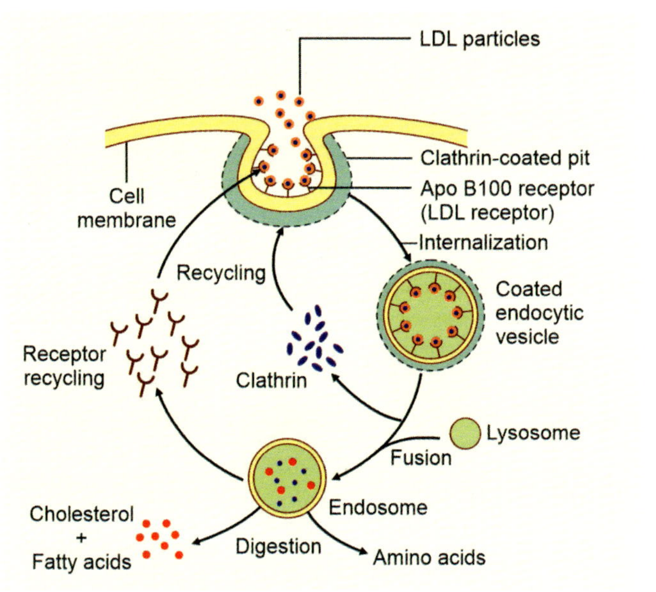

Fig. 26.12: Receptor-mediated pinocytosis

Sometimes (such as in case of some of the hormones), clathrin is not required for receptor-mediated pinocytosis, but the internalized vesicle fuses with the other organelle such as Golgi complex, and secondary lysosomes are not formed. This process is known as adsorptive pinocytosis.

MEMBRANE ASSOCIATED OTHER PROCESSES

Besides translocation (transport) of substances across the biological membrane, there are also some other processes that are associated with membranes, e.g. osmosis, dialysis, etc. These membrane-associated processes are used to separate components from a solution, based on their properties.

Osmosis

Osmosis refers to spontaneous, net movement of solvent molecules through a semipermeable membrane (a membrane which is permeable to solvent but not the solute) into a region of higher solute concentration, in the direction that tends to equalize the solute concentration on the two sides (Fig. 26.13).

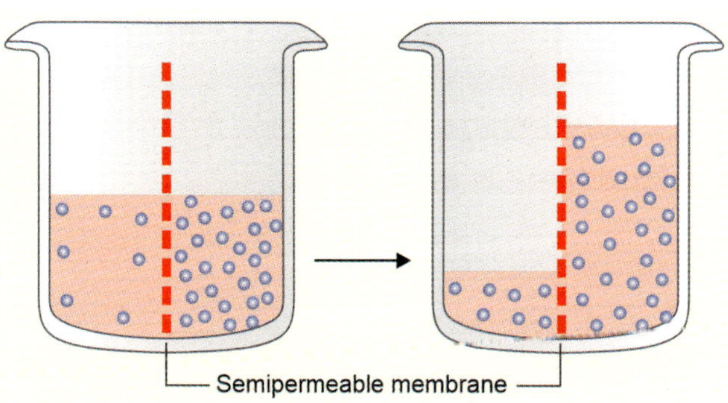

Fig. 26.13: Osmosis

Osmosis is a vital process in biological systems, as biological membranes are semipermeable in nature. For example, when an animal cell is placed in a solution of sugar or salt in water, the cell is submerged in water and the water molecules pass through the cell membrane, from an area of low solute concentration to high solute concentration. Accordingly, if the medium is **hypotonic**, the cell will gain water, meaning that it will swell, and may even burst. On the other hand, if the medium is **hypertonic**, the cell will lose water, meaning thereby that it will shrink.

In an isotonic solution, there will be no net movement of water across the cell membrane.

The process of filtering, commonly used to purify water, is based on the principle of osmotic pressure and is referred to as r**everse osmosis**. In this process, water (to be purified) is placed in a chamber and put under an amount of pressure greater than the osmotic pressure exerted by water and the solutes dissolved in it. A part of the chamber opens to a differentially permeable membrane that allows water molecules to pass thru but not the solute particles.

Dialysis

Dialysis is the process of separating molecules in solution by the differences in their rate of diffusion through a semipermeable membrane (such as a dialysis tube). General principle of dialysis is that when a solution containing several types of molecules (e.g. a colloidal solution, which is made of small sized particles that may not settle down under force of gravity and have much slower rate of diffusion, such as impurities of electrolytes and other soluble substances) is placed in a semipermeable dialysis bag (such as a cellulose membrane with pores). After the bag is sealed and placed in a container of a different solution (or pure water), the molecules which are small enough to pass through the tube (like water, salts, etc.) will move into or out of the dialysis bag, in the direction of decreasing concentration. On the other hand, the larger molecules (proteins, DNA or poly saccharides) that have dimensions significantly greater than the pore diameter are retained inside the dialysis bag.

USE OF DIALYSIS IN MEDICINE

In medicine, dialysis is used for removing waste and excess water from blood as an artificial replacement for the lost kidney, in people with renal failure, by using a special fluid called dialysate (a mixture of water and certain chemicals). The dialysate is carefully controlled to remove waste products from blood, without removing the useful substances from the body. A semipermeable membrane is used that separates blood from the dialysate and removes the waste products and fluid flow into the dialysate. There are two main types of kidney dialysis processes, referred to as hemodialysis and peritoneal dialysis.

Hemodialysis: In hemodialysis, blood from a peripheral artery of the patient is allowed to flow on one side of a semipermeable membrane while an artificially prepared fluid of known solute concentration (dialysate), flows from the other side, but in opposite direction. The purified blood is returned through a peripheral vein Solute concentration of the dialysate is designed in the way that it maximizes the diffusion of water and solutes across the membrane. Net effect of the process is to decrease toxic molecules in the blood while improving the levels of the essential ones (Fig. 26.14).

Peritoneal Dialysis: In peritoneal dialysis the dialysate is run through a tube into the peritoneal cavity and the peritoneal membrane itself serves as the semipermeable membrane. The dialysate is retained for some time and eventually drained out through the tube, removing the excess of water and the waste products.

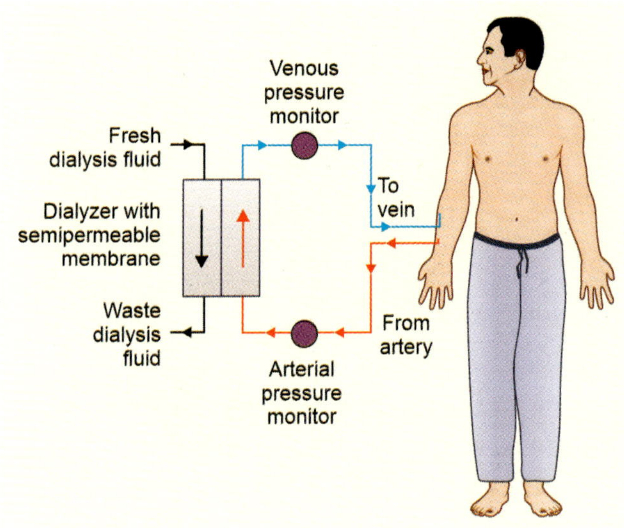

Fig. 26.14: Hemodialysis

Some Important Questions

1. **Describe:**
   i. Fluid mosaic structure of membrane
   ii. Important functions of membranes
   iii. Lipid bilayer
   iv. Membrane proteins
2. **Write notes on:**
   i. Channels
   ii. Channelopathies
   iii. Membrane associated processes
   iv. Facilitated diffusion
   v. Osmosis
   vi. Aquaporins
   vii. Na^+, K^+-pump
   viii. Active transport
   ix. Dialysis
   x. Exocytosis
   xi. Endocytosis

Chapter 27

Cytoskeleton

Cytoskeleton is a **system of protein fibers** that pervades cytoplasm. It **performs several functions**.

Functions of Cytoskeleton

- Cytoskeleton **provides structural support** that **determines shape of the cell** and resists forces that tend to deform it.
- It also **functions as an internal framework** that is **responsible for positioning various organelles within** interior of **the cell**.
- Cytoskeleton also **provides a network that directs movement of the materials and organelles** within the cells, e.g. delivery of mRNA to the specific parts of the cell, movement of membranous carriers from endoplasmic reticulum to the Golgi complex, etc.
- It also functions as the **force-generating apparatus that moves cells from one place to another**, e.g. locomotion of sperm, white blood cells, fibroblasts, etc.
- Cytoskeletal elements also **make up an apparatus** that is **responsible for separating chromosomes during mitosis** and meiosis, and for splitting a parent cell into two daughter cells during cytokinesis.

COMPOSITION OF CYTOSKELETON

Cytoskeleton is composed of three distinct types of fibrous structures, which are referred to as **microtubules, intermediate filaments** and **microfilaments**.

These are the **polymers of protein subunits**, which are held together by weak, non-covalent bonds. Each cytoskeletal element, of different non-muscle cells (such as an epithelial cell, a nerve cell and a dividing cell), has **distinct properties** and **perform distinct functions** (Table 27.1).

MICROTUBULES

Microtubules are **stiff, hollow, tubular structures** which are, approximately, **25 nm in diameter**. Microtubules are **assembled from protein tubulins** that are **arranged in longitudinal rows**, called **protofilaments**.

Assembly of the microtubule

Assembly of the microtubules (from αβ-tubulin dimers) **takes place in two distinct phases. These include** a slow phase of **nucleation** (in which a small portion of the microtubule is initially formed) and a rapid phase of **elongation**.

Table 27.1: Properties of different cytoskeletal elements

Properties	*Cytoskeletal elements*		
	Microtubules	*Intermediate filaments*	*Microfilaments (Actin filaments)*
Structure	Stiff, hollow tube	Tough, ropelike fibers	Flexible, helical filament
Dimensions (diameter)	25 nm (outer)	10 nm	8 nm
Subunits	GTP-tubulin heterodimer	Globular proteins	ATP-actin monomers
Enzyme activity	GTPase	—	ATPase
Major group of associated proteins	Microtubule associated proteins	Plectin	Actin-binding proteins
Motor proteins	Kinesins, dyneins	—	Myosins
Primary functions	Support, intracellular transport, cell organization	Structural support	Motility, contractility

Nucleation is controlled by the specialized structures called **microtubules-organizing centers**, which govern the number of microtubules, their polarity, and the number of protofilaments that make up their walls as well as the time and location of the assembly. Some external factors (e.g. cold temperature, increased Ca^{2+} concentration, and drugs like colchicine and vincristine) interfere with the functions of microtubules, since these factors promote disassembly of the microtubules.

- **Colchicine** is very beneficial in acute attacks of gout involving joints, because it binds to the protein tubulin, and rapidly leads to the disassembly of microtubules.
- **Vincristine** is an alkaloid. It binds to tubulin dimers, thus, inhibiting the assembly of microtubules. This, in turn, arrests mitosis (in metaphase) and is, therefore, useful as an anticancer drug.

Microtubule dimers (that are polymerized into a microtubule) **contain GTP** that is hydrolyzed soon after its incorporation into the polymer. Microtubules of the **epithelial and the nerve cells** functions, primarily, in **support and organelle transport**, whereas microtubules of the **dividing cell form mitotic spindle** that is required for chromosome segregation.

Functions of Microtubules

- Microtubules **provide structural support, determine cell shape** and resist forces that tend to deform it.
- These structures also provide **internal framework** that is responsible **for positioning various organelles**.
- Microtubules also provide a network of tracks that **direct movement of materials and organelles within the cell,** e.g. delivery of mRNA from the nucleus to the ribosomes, movement of molecules destined for exocytose, etc.
- These structures also **form a part of the locomotor machinery** for the movement of cell as a whole, e.g. spermatozoa, WBC, fibroblasts, etc.
- Microtubules also **help in spindle formation during chromosome segregation** and **cell division**.
- Certain accessory proteins are required for the proper functioning of microtubules. These include:
  - **Microtubule associated proteins (MAP)**, e.g. **tau protein**. Tau proteins **influence many properties of the microtubules**, including their **flexibility and stability**.

    Abnormally high level of phosphorylation of tau protein has been implicated in several neurodegenerative disorders, e.g. Alzheimer's disease.
  - **Motor proteins**, such as **kinesins** and **dyneins**. Motor proteins **generate forces** that are **required for the intracellular movement** as well as movement of the entire cell. To achieve this, motor proteins convert chemical energy (of ATP) into the mechanical energy.

INTERMEDIATE FILAMENTS

Intermediate filaments are **strong rope-like fibers** which are, approximately, **10 nm in diameter**.

- Depending on the cell type, intermediate filaments are **composed of a variety of globular protein subunits**, which are capable of assembling into similar types of filaments.
- The **basic unit** of an intermediate filament **is a tetramer** (formed by two dimers, which may be homodimers or heterodimers).
- Intermediate filaments **provide mechanical stability to the cell** that may be required for the specialized tissue-specific functions.
- These are **often connected by** long wispy cross-bridges consisting of **fibrous protein** called **plectin**.
- Intermediate filaments **have tissue specific functions**, which are more important in some cells than in others.
- Intermediate filaments include **keratin filaments** and **neurofilaments**:
  - **Keratin filaments constitute primary structural proteins of epithelial cells**, including epidermal cells, liver hepatocytes and pancreatic acinar cells.
  - **Neurofilaments** are **present in the cytoplasm of neurons** as loosely packed bundles, whose long axis is oriented parallel to that of the nerve cell axon.

MICROFILAMENTS

Microfilaments are, approximately, **8 nm in diameter**. These are **composed of a double helical polymer of** the protein actin, which is one of the **major contractile proteins of the muscle cells**.

- In the presence of ATP, actin monomers polymerize to form a flexible, helical filament, called **actin filament** or **F-actin**.
- Before being incorporated into a filament, an actin monomer binds to a molecule of ATP, and as the actin filament grows (due to the ATPase activity of the actin), ATP is hydrolyzed to ADP. Thus, bulk of an actin filament consists of ADP-actin subunits.
- **F-actin plays a key role in**, virtually, **all types of contractility and motility, within the cell**.
- Depending upon the type of the cell and the activity, actin filaments can be organized into highly ordered arrays, loose ill-defined networks or tightly held bundles.
- The molecular motors of actin filaments are the **myosin** family of proteins, which are, generally, divided into two groups:

- **Type I (unconventional myosins)** which have a single globular head and a variable tail length. These are implicated in cell motility and organelle transport.
- **Type II (conventional myosins)**, which were first identified in muscles. These contain a long, rod-shaped tail that is attached at one end, to two globular heads. Its head binds the actin filament, hydrolyzes ATP and undergoes conformational changes, required for generating the force during muscle contraction as well some non-muscle activities, like cytokinesis.

Some Important Questions

1. **What is cytoskeleton? Name various cytoskeletal elements.**
2. **Briefly discuss various types of cytoskeletal elements.**
3. **Write note on:**
   i. Microtubule assembly
   ii. Microfilaments

Chapter

28

Muscle Contraction

Muscles are the **multicellular units** and are **classified into three different groups**, which include skeletal muscle, cardiac muscle and smooth muscle.

- **Skeletal muscle: Voluntary muscles**, which include skeletal muscle, **have a striated (stripped) appearance**. Such muscles **consist of long, thin, multinucleated cells**, known as **muscle fibers** that run along the length of the muscle.
- **Cardiac muscle:** Cardiac muscles **consist of** a large number of **smaller cells**, referred to as **cardiomyocytes** that run, in series, along the length of the muscle.
- **Smooth muscle:** Smooth muscle **consists of several spindle-shaped cells**. They **surround internal organs and blood vessels**.

Muscles form a large proportion of the active tissues of the body. In a normal adult, though **muscle mass is, nearly, 40% of the body weight, metabolically** it is a **highly active tissue**, and performs more than 50% of the total metabolic activities.

BIOCHEMICAL COMPOSITION OF MUSCLE

- Adult muscle is **70–80% water**.
- Besides, it also contains, nearly, **20% proteins** and **3% lipids** (with variable amounts of triacylglycerols, cholesterol and phospholipids).
- Muscle also contains **0.5–1.0% glycogen**, which, in turn, serves as a source of ATP (via anaerobic glycolysis).
- It also contains several other substances, such as **inositol** (predominantly myoinositol), **carnitine, free amino acids, various enzymes** and several **cations** (K^+, Na^+ and Mg^{2+}) as well as **anions** (phosphates, sulphates and bicarbonates; Table 28.1).

Table 28.1: Biochemical composition of skeletal muscle

Ingredients	*Percentage of total muscle mass*
• **Water** • **Proteins** – Myosin – Actin cross-linking proteins – Tropomyosin – Troponin – Myoglobin	70–80% 20%
Lipids • Triacylglycerols • Cholesterol • Phospholipids	3%
• **Glycogen** • **Other substances** – Inositol (Myoinositol) – Creatine phosphate – Oligopeptides (Carnosine, anserine and glutathione) – Free amino acids – Enzymes – Carnitine	0.5–1.0% Traces
Inorganic ions • Cations (Na^+, K^+, Mg^{2+}) • Anions (Phosphates, sulphates and bicarbonates)	Traces

CONTRACTILE ELEMENTS IN SKELETAL MUSCLES

Muscle Fibers

Muscle fibers are, nearly, **0.01–0.1 nm in diameter** and **1.0–40 nm in length**. A large number of these fibers are **bound together by the areolar connective tissue** and are **attached, via tendons, to the bone or other structures**, whose movement they control.

Muscle fibers are **packed in** an elastic sheet, known as **sarcolemma**, which also **has several nuclei and mitochondria**.

- Sarcolemma **contains** a large number of transport ducts called **sarcotubules**.
- It also contains **sarcoplasmic reticulum**, similar in structure and functions to the endoplasmic reticulum, found in other cells.
- Bundles of muscle fibers are surrounded by the **sarcoplasm**, which may be **called muscle plasma**.

Myofibrils

Myofibrils are the **structural component of the muscle. Muscle fibers contain parallel bundles of myofibrils** (Greek, *myos* means muscle).

Major features of the myofibril are as follows:

- It has a **light band, called** the isotropic band or **I-band**, which **contains thin filaments**, and
- A **dark band**, designated as anisotropic band or **A-band**, which **has a central H-zone containing thick filaments**, and an outer segment with the **overlapping thick and thin filaments**.
- The **I-band is bisected by** a dark zone (present in the center of I-band) called **Z-line**.

Functional unit of a myofibril: Functional unit of a myofibril is known as **sarcomere** (Greek, *sarkos* means flesh).

- Sarcomere is a **region between two successive Z-lines** (present at the center of each I-band), i.e. the region **comprising of one-half of the I-band, the A-band and one half of the next I-band**.
- The **A-band is formed of a large number of thick filaments**, whereas **I-band** is composed of a comparable number of **thin filaments**, which are interspaced between the thick filaments.
- Two sets of the filaments, in turn, are linked by cross-bridges in the area where they overlap (Fig. 28.1).
- **Thin filaments slide over the thick filaments.** As a result, muscle contraction leads to **decrease in length of the sarcomere**, which is caused by a reduction in distance between the I-band and the H-zone.
- The **lengths of the thick filaments and the thin filaments, however, remain constant.**
- A contracted muscle is reduced to nearly two-thirds of its fully extended length.

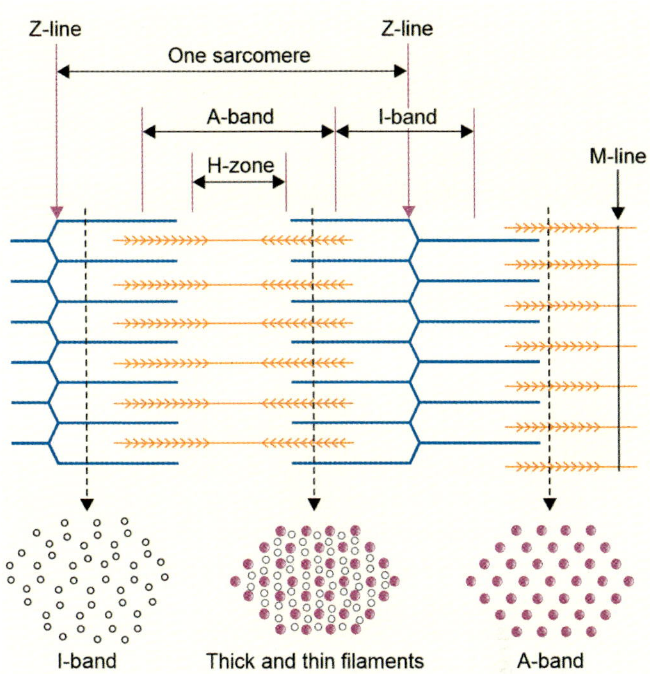

Fig. 28.1: Structure of myofibril

CONTRACTILE PROTEINS

More than half of the total proteins present in skeletal muscle are **structural proteins**, which include **myosin, actin, actin cross-linking proteins, tropomyosin and troponin**. Myosin and actin together, account for more than two-thirds of total muscle proteins. Besides, **muscle also contains myoglobin, several enzymes, collagen and some proteins of the connective tissue**.

Myosin is a contractile protein of thick filaments. On the other hand, **thin filaments consist of** chains of the actin molecules with the associated **tropomyosin and troponin** molecules (Fig. 28.2).

Myosin

Myosin is **present in thick filaments**, which are placed end-to-end with the light chains striking out in the form

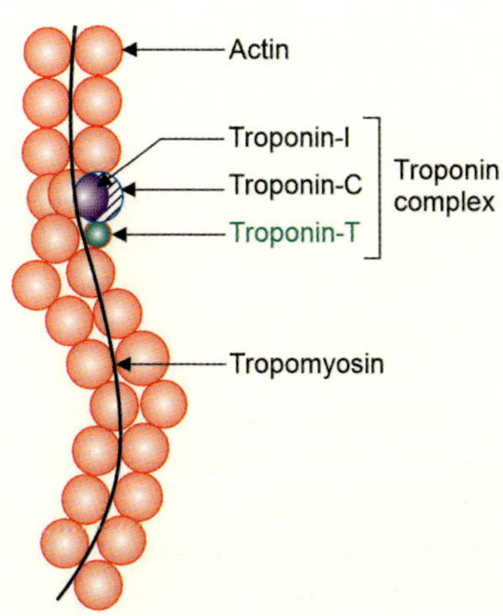

Fig. 28.2: Structure of thin filament

of double heads. It **consists of six polypeptide chains,** which include **two identical heavy chains and two pairs of two different types of the light chains.**

- Two types of the **light chains** are described **as regulatory light chains and essential light chains.**
- **Each myosin head associates with an essential light chain and a regulatory light chain.**
- **Regulatory light chains play a role in the control of muscle contraction** by Ca^{2+} ions, whereas the **essential light chains are required for ATPase activity of the myosin head.**
- Thus, **both types of light chains are involved in the regulation of muscle contraction.**
- The **N-terminal half of each of the heavy chain forms an elongated globular head** to which one subunit, each of the two light chains, binds.
- The **C-terminal half of the heavy chain forms a long fibrous α-helical tail,** two of which associate to form a left-handed coil.
- Taken together, a molecule of **myosin,** thus, **consists of a long rod-like segment with two globular heads** (Fig. 28.3).

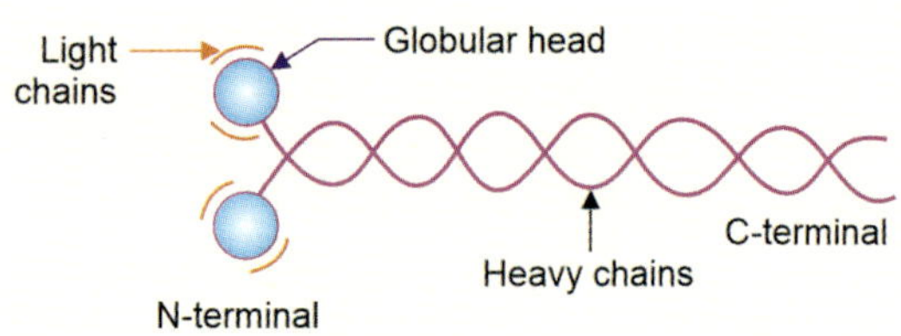

Fig. 28.3: Structure of myosin

Actin

Actin is a **globulin.** It is a **most abundant cytoplasmic protein in eukaryotic cells,** accounting for 5–10% of the total protein.

- Actin is a **major constituent of thin filament of the sarcomere.**
- It **exists in two forms,** i.e. as G-actin and F-actin (filament-actin).
- **G-actin is a low molecular weight monomeric protein** with a **globular** configuration.
  - **G-actin monomers** readily **form** large, elongated actin filament polymers called **F-actin.**
  - **Mg^{2+} ions are** essentially **required for assembly of** the **G-actin** monomeric units **into a polymeric F-actin.**
  - Besides, **monomeric G-actin** units are oriented in such a way that they **acquire a pointed-region** (pointed-end) and **a barbed-region** (barbed-end).
  - **Assembly** of the monomeric units **occurs at the barbed-end.**
- **F-actin contains,** nearly, **1000 monomeric units,** which are **organized as a string of beads.** F-actin filaments are **made up of two strings of the G-actin monomers** (Fig. 28.4).

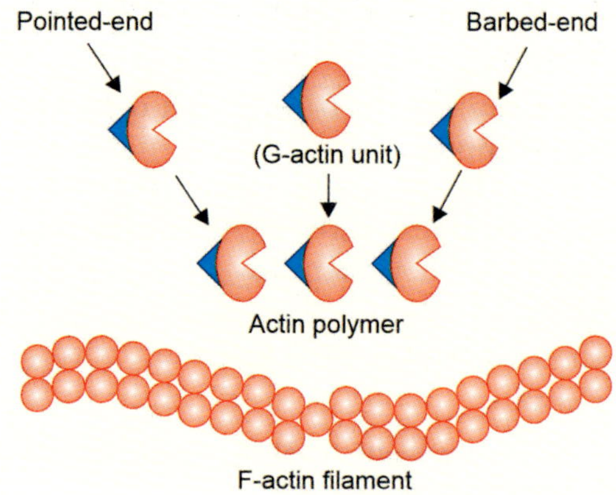

Fig. 28.4: Structure of F-actin

Some proteins like **filamin, α-actinin and β-actinin cross-link and stabilize actin chains.**

Tropomyosin

Tropomyosin is a **double-stranded, α-helical protein.** It is **intervened between the two helical strands of F-actin,** i.e. tropomyosin molecules attach end to end and form a thin filament on each strand of the actin molecule. One tropomyosin molecule extends over seven actin molecules, whereas 300–400 actin molecules are contained in each filament of the skeletal muscle (which is about 1 μm in length).

Troponins

Troponin is a **spherical molecule,** with a molecular weight of about 70 kD. It is **placed at regular intervals along the actin filaments.** Troponin is **composed of three different types of subunits, referred to as** troponin-T, troponin-I and troponin-C:

- **Troponin-T:** It **binds the other two subunits to the tropomyosin molecules,** noncovalently. **Tropomyosin-troponin complex,** in turn, **regulates muscle contraction,** by controlling access of the myosin heads on the thick filaments to their binding sites on the actin.
- **Troponin-I:** It is the **inhibitory subunit.** Its function is to **inhibit the interaction of the head of myosin with actin,** thereby, **preventing contraction of myofibrils.**
- **Troponin-C:** It is a **Ca^{2+}-binding protein,** and is rich in aspartate and glutamate.

Titin

Titin, also referred to as **connectin,** is the **largest known single polypeptide,** which **participates in muscle contraction.** Mutations in titin are associated with familial hypertrophic cardiomyopathy and tibial muscular dystrophy. Autoantibodies to titin are found in scleroderma.

Dystrophin

Dystrophin is **localized to the inner surface of the sarcolemma of the muscle fiber.** Actually, dystrophin itself is only a **part of a more elaborate system of proteins bridging the cytoskeleton (actin filaments) and the extracellular matrix, via a matrix protein laminin.**

Dystrophin-anchored complex serves following functions:

- The complex **stabilizes sarcolemma membrane** during contraction/relaxation cycles.
- It also **links contractile force,** generated in the muscle fiber, **with the extracellular environment.**
- The complex also **maintains local organization of key membrane proteins,** called dystroglycans and sarcoglycans.
- **Abnormal dystrophin results in** a disorder referred to as **Duchenne muscular dystrophy** (DMD).

Duchenne Muscular Dystrophy

Duchenne muscular dystrophy (DMD) is an **X-linked recessive disorder caused by a mutation in the dystrophin gene.** It is a **group of congenital diseases** involving muscles, **characterized by a progressive course in children and death by adolescence.** Children present with **delayed walking, difficulty in climbing stairs and bulky calf muscles.** A **common cause of death is lower respiratory tract infections,** due to **non-functioning of respiratory muscles.**

MECHANISM OF MUSCLE CONTRACTION

- **Impulses transmitted via motor nerve** (across the neuromuscular junction to the sarcolemma of the muscle fiber), **initiate contraction of the myofibrils.**
- This, in turn, **stimulates release of Ca^{2+},** which **bind to troponin C** of the thin actin filament and **produce a conformational change** in it, followed by the **shift of tropomyosin** and **attachment of cross bridges of the thick myosin filament to the thin actin filaments.**
- **ATP binds to specific sites on the surface of myosin.** The tendency for ATP to bind is so efficient that normally almost every myosin head is bound to ATP.
- Formation of the charged **myosin. ATP-complex** alters conformation of the protein in a manner that the charged complex shows a greater tendency to **bind to an actin molecule.**
- After myosin ATP-complex binds to actin, ATP binds to the myosin head (whose ATPase action causes **hydrolysis of ATP**). This puts the **myosin head into a high-energy conformation.**
- The myosin head is now weak to bind to actin monomer that is closer to the Z-line. This results in the **release of inorganic phosphate** (Pi), which further causes a conformational shift and **increases affinity of myosin for actin.**
- The resulting transient state is immediately followed by power stroke, causing a further conformational shift that **sweeps myosin head's C-terminal tail toward the Z-line.**
- **ADP is** then **released,** thereby, **completing the cycle** (Fig. 28.5).
- **Myosin heads walk** or row-up **the adjacent thin filaments toward the Z-line, with the concomitant contraction of the muscle,** i.e. the actin filaments slide

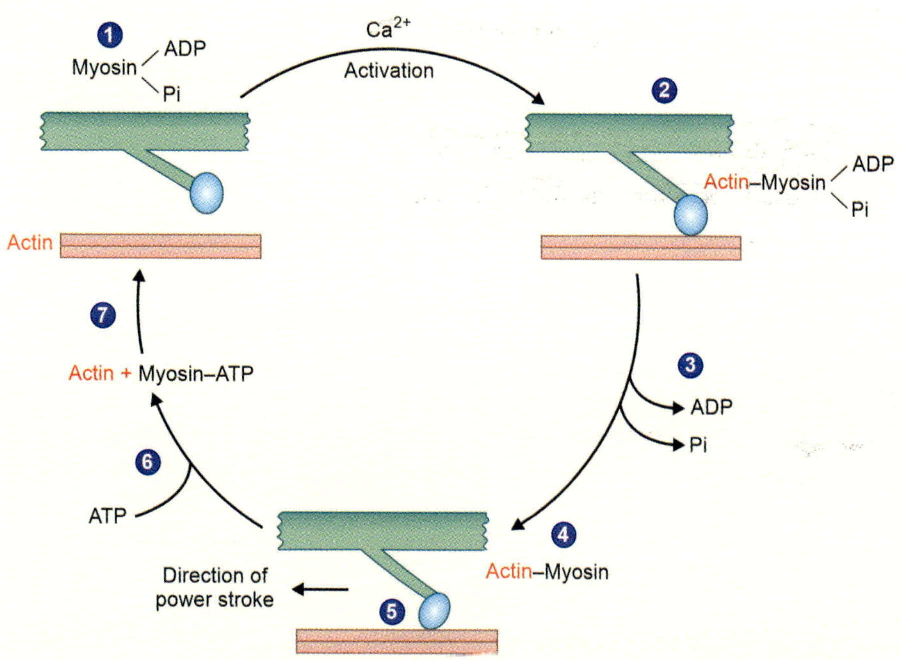

Fig. 28.5: Biochemical changes during muscle contraction. 1. Resting state: Myosin not interacting with actin, hence energy at ATP hydrolysis not released; 2. Activated state: Mysoin interacting with actin; 3. Release of products of ATP hydrolysis; 4. Power stroke; 5. Rigor state; 6. Detachment of actin accompained by binding of new ATP molecule; 7. ATP hydrolysis and return to resting state

along the thick myosin filaments (which otherwise were stationary) toward the center of the sarcomere, thereby, **shortening its size**.

- These events occur so rapidly that the **whole process of muscle contraction takes only 10–20 milliseconds**.
- At the end, **Ca^{2+} are taken-up into the sarcoplasmic reticulum** network and cross-bridges of the myosin retract. As a result, the **sarcomeres and the muscle fibers relax** and return to the resting state.
- In the low-energy state, the **complex remains intact until a new molecule of ATP is bound**, usually, within a very short time (about 1 millisecond).
- The **sequence continues depending upon the supply of ATP** and other components essential for the muscle contraction.

ENERGY METABOLISM DURING MUSCLE CONTRACTION

Energy for muscle contraction, as discussed above, is **provided by ATP**, which is hydrolyzed to ADP and Pi. **ATP**, in turn, **is regenerated** in the muscle, **by several routes** (Fig. 28.6).

- **By utilizing creatine-phosphate:** ATP (used in muscle contraction) **can be regenerated by utilizing high-energy phosphate compound creatine phosphate**. This reaction is catalyzed by creatine kinase (creatine phosphokinase or CPK) and is called Lohmann reaction.
- **By the adenylate kinase reaction:** ATP can also be regenerated from ADP by the enzyme adenylate kinase, also referred to as myokinase.
- **From anaerobic glycolysis:** Muscles possess capacity to synthesize ATP **under anaerobic conditions by utilizing its glycogen stores**. A limited supply of oxygen as may occur during a short period of strenuous exercise, results in the accumulation of lactate in the blood.
- **By oxidative processes:** Prolonged exercise, gradually, increases oxygenation of the muscle to a maximum. Thus, ATP may also be produced by various oxidative processes, such as from **aerobic glycolysis** followed by the **citric acid cycle** and from **β-oxidation of fatty acids**.

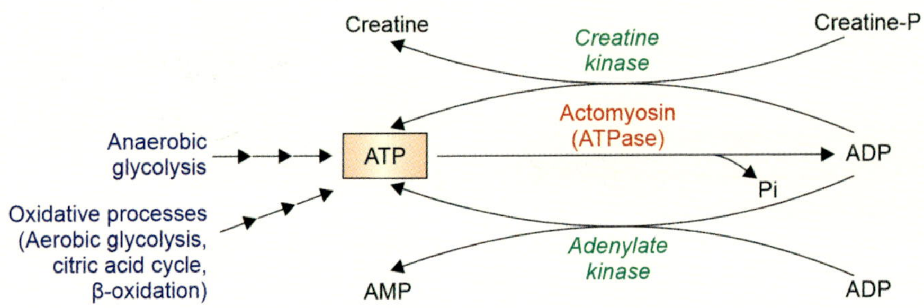

Fig. 28.6: Processes of regeneration of ATP in muscles

Some Important Questions

1. **Describe structure and composition of skeletal muscle.**
2. **Describe various contractile proteins and their functions.**
3. **Describe:**
   i. Events during muscle contraction
   ii. Types of muscle fibers
   iii. Regeneration of ATP in muscle
4. **Write notes on:**
   i. Contractile proteins
   ii. Actin
   iii. Myosin
   iv. Troponins
   v. Duchenne muscular dystrophy
   vi. Titin

Chapter

29

Hemoglobin Metabolism

Hemoglobin is a **metalloprotein** that **has heme as a prosthetic group**, which is **attached to globin protein chains**. Hemoglobin has a quaternary structure, i.e. it is a tetramer **having four** protein subunits **(globin chains)**.

Normal adult hemoglobin, i.e. the hemoglobin found in normal adult human beings, also referred to as **HbA** or HbA_1, **has two alpha chains and two beta chains** ($\alpha_2\beta_2$). It is a globular protein, **present in high concentration in red blood cells** (RBC).

HEMOGLOBIN VARIANTS

Any **change in its structure**, i.e. the **type of the globin chain** and/or its **size**, results in a variant of normal adult hemoglobin, which, in turn, **may result in a group of pathological disorders** referred to as **hemoglobinopathies**.

Several variants of normal adult hemoglobin are known to occur at different developmental stages in human beings. These include:

- **Embryonic hemoglobin:** Embryonic hemoglobin **contains two zeta chains** along **with either two epsilon chains** (as $\zeta_2\varepsilon_2$) **or two gamma chains** (as $\zeta_2\Upsilon_2$). Accordingly, these are referred to as **Hb Gower-1 and Hb Portland,** respectively. Embryonic hemoglobin is **found in the embryonic stage**, i.e. in the **first month after conception**.
- **Fetal hemoglobin:** Fetal hemoglobin (HbF) **contains two α chains along with two γ chains** ($\alpha_2\gamma_2$). HbF predominates **in the blood of human fetus**. After birth, fetal hemoglobin is rapidly replaced with the adult hemoglobin (HbA_1), whose synthesis actually starts in the late fetal life. HbF comprises only about 0.5% of the total hemoglobin in adults.
- **Minor adult hemoglobin:** Minor adult hemoglobin, also referred to as HbA_2, consists of **two α chains and two δ chains** ($\alpha_2\delta_2$). It comprises only about 2.5% of the normal adult hemoglobin (HbA_1). Compared to HbA_1, HbA_2 has a reduced efficiency to transport oxygen.

FUNCTIONS OF HEMOGLOBIN

The main physiological function of hemoglobin is to transport gases, for example:

- Hemoglobin **binds oxygen in the lungs** (oxygenation) and **transports it to cells** (deoxygenation). Further, it **also transports CO_2 and H^+ from tissues to the lungs.**

  When blood cells pass through the lungs, they bind up as much oxygen as the iron in the heme can handle. The blood cells then travel to various parts of the body, such as the muscles. These cells are actively using up oxygen and releasing carbon dioxide as a by-product. Carbon dioxide forms an acid in the blood plasma, lowering the pH of the blood. Like all proteins, hemoglobin reacts to change in pH, by changing shape. This change in shape forces the oxygen off the heme complex, releasing the oxygen into the blood plasma. The oxygen diffuses into the muscle cells, where it is bound by myoglobin and transported to the mitochondria and is used.
- Hemoglobin **also carries and releases NO** in the blood vessels of the tissues.

HEME SYNTHESIS

Heme is an organic, ring-shaped molecule that forms a prosthetic group of hemoproteins. Red color of blood is produced by heme. Heme is **made from 4 pyrroles,** which are small pentagon-shaped molecules. Each pyrrole ring contains 4 carbons and 1 nitrogen (Fig. 29.1).

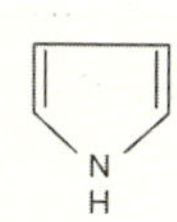

Fig. 29.1: A pyrrole ring

Four pyrroles, together, form a tetrapyrrole. When the **tetrapyrrole has substitutions on the side chains,** which allow it **to hold a metal ion,** it is **called a porphyrin.**

Heme consists of one atom of ferrous ion (Fe^{2+}) **and a tetrapyrrole ring,** called **protoporphyrin IX** (Fig. 29.2).

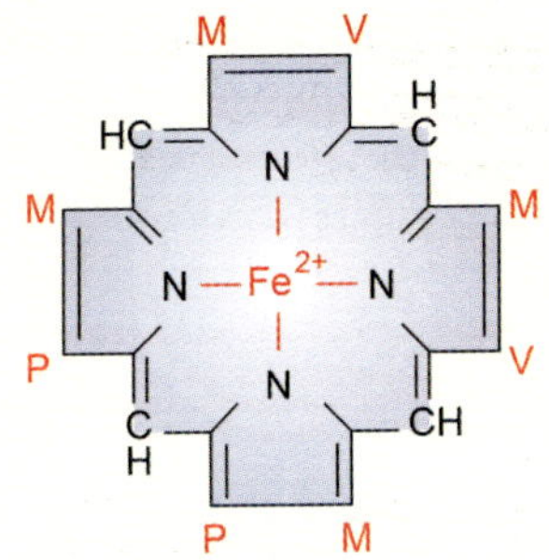

Fig. 29.2: Heme

In the biosynthesis of heme, **firstly** four **pyrrole rings are formed from** eight molecules, each of **glycine and succinyl CoA**. During the process of heme biosynthesis, some of the reactions occur in mitochondria while others (the intermediate steps) in cytosol (Fig. 29.3).

1. In the first step, **succinyl-CoA** (an intermediate of the Krebs cycle) **condenses with glycine** and forms **δ-aminolevulinic acid (ALA)**, in the mitochondria. This reaction is catalyzed **by δ-aminolevulinic acid synthase (ALA-synthase or E1)**, which requires

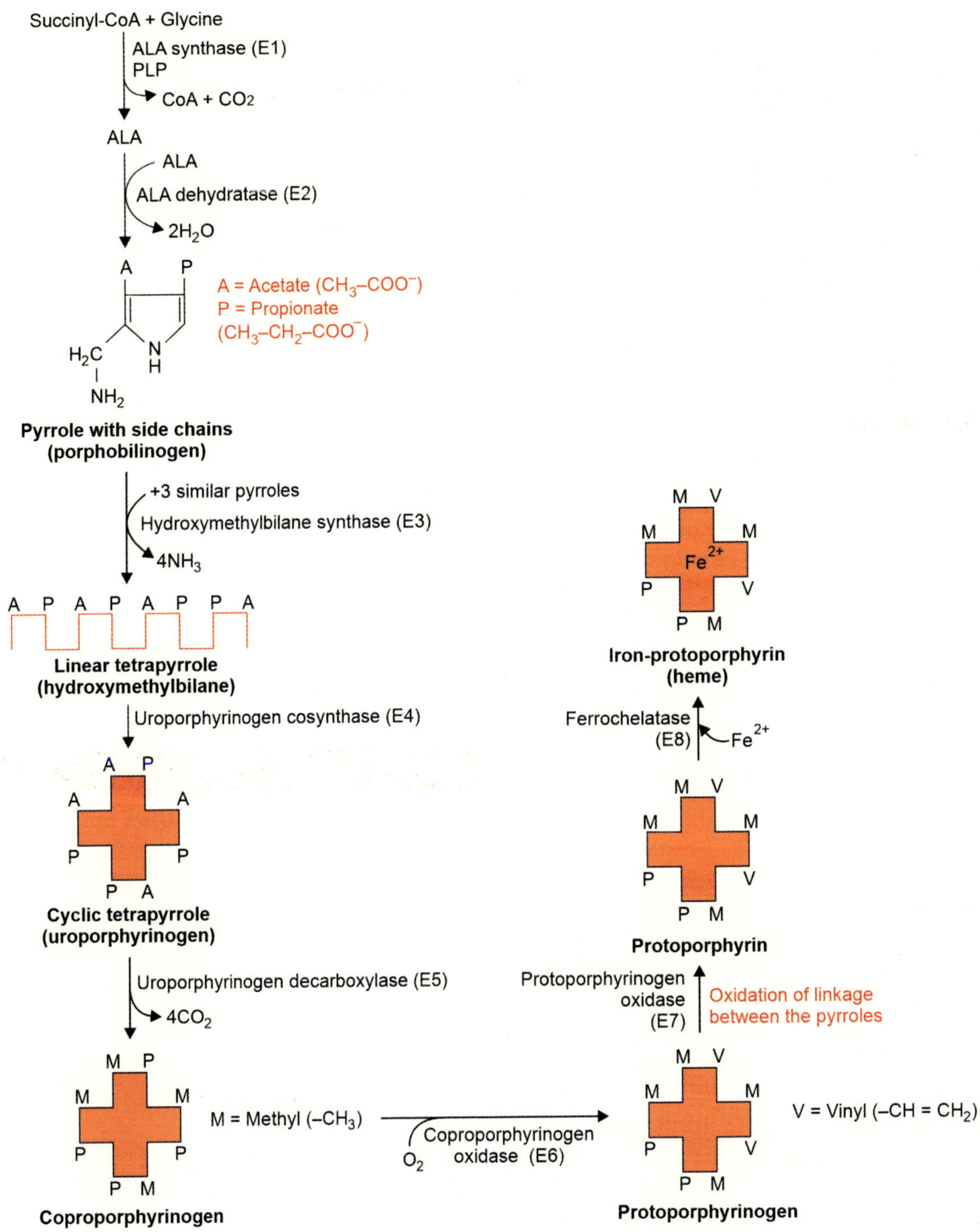

Fig. 29.3: Heme biosynthesis

pyridoxal-phosphate (PLP) as a coenzyme. This is the rate-limiting step in heme synthesis.

2. In the next step, **two molecules of ALA condense** asymmetrically, and **form porphobilinogen**. This reaction is catalyzed **by aminolevulinic acid dehydratase** (ALA-dehydratase or **E2**). It is a zinc-containing enzyme, present in cytosol.

   ALA-dehydratase is sensitive to heavy metals, particularly **lead**. Hence, **ALA levels are increased in lead poisoning**.

3. **Porphobilinogen undergoes deamination by porphobilinogen deaminase** (hydroxymethylbilane synthase, also called uroporphyrinogen I synthase or **E3**) and **leads to the formation of** a linear tetrapyrrole called **hydroxymethylbilane**.

4. With the ring closure, catalyzed **by uroporphyrinogen-I co-synthase (E4), hydroxymethylbilane is converted to uroporphyrinogen-I**.

   Alternatively, **uroporphyrinogen-III co-synthase converts hydroxymethylbilane to uroporphyrinogen-III**.

Note: Only types I and III are found in nature. **Porphyrins with symmetric arrangement of the substituent groups on its four rings are classified as type I** porphyrins while **those with asymmetric substitutions are classified as type III porphyrins** (Fig. 29.4).

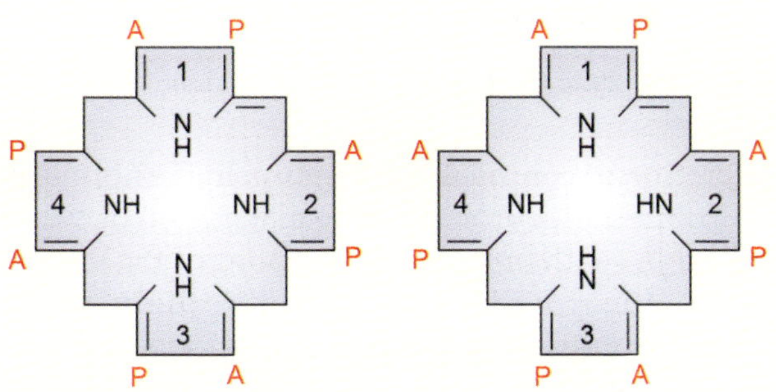

Fig. 29.4: Type I and type III porphyrinogen

Under normal conditions uroporphyrinogen formed is almost, exclusively the type III isomer.

Heme is also a type III porphyrin.

5. **Uroporphyrinogen-I**, or type III is **converted to** the respective **coproporphyrinogen by uroporphyrinogen decarboxylase** (E5).

   This enzyme is inhibited by iron salts.

6. **Coproporphyrinogen-III** enters mitochondria, where it **is converted to protoporphyrinogen-IX**. This reaction is catalyzed **by coproporphyrinogen oxidase** (E6).

   The enzyme E6 requires molecular oxygen and does not act on coproporphyrinogen I.

   These porphyrins are identified as belonging to series IX, since they were designated ninth in a series of the postulated isomers.

7. **Protoporphyrinogen oxidase** (E7) **acts on protoporphyrinogen-IX**, which is converted to protoporphyrin-IX, in the mitochondria.

   Protoporphyrin-IX is water insoluble and its excessive amounts are excreted, by the biliary system, into the intestinal tract.

8. In the final step of heme synthesis, **ferrous iron (Fe^{2+}) is inserted into protoporphyrin-IX by ferrochelatase** (E8).

   E8 requires reducing substances and is sensitive to heavy metals, especially, lead. It is also sensitive to iron deprivation.

   Accordingly, heme is an iron centered cyclic tetrapyrrole.

Porphyrias

Porphyrias are a group of disorders due to abnormalities in the pathway of heme biosynthesis. These can be genetic or acquired. Based on the site of overproduction, porphyrias are either hepatic or erythropoietic, or sometimes mixed (Table 29.1).

Table 29.1: Types of porphyrias (deficient enzyme is given in parentheses)

Hepatic porphyrias	*Erythropoietic porphyrias*
• ALA dehydratase deficiency (E2)	• X-linked sideroblastic anemia (E1)
• Acute intermittent porphyria (E3)	• Congenital erythropoietic porphyria (E4)
• Porphyria cutanea tarda (E5)	• Erythropoietic protoporphyria (E8)
• Hereditary coproporphyria (E6)	
• Variegate porphyria (E7)	

HEME DEGRADATION

As we know, red blood cells (RBCs) have a limited lifespan of, approximately, 100–120 days. The senescent cells are recognized by their membrane changes, removed and engulfed by the reticuloendothelial system at the extravascular sites.

- Degradation of RBC occurs, mainly, in the spleen, bone marrow, liver and lymph glands.
- After an aged RBC is recognized by a macrophage, it is rapidly engulfed to form a phagosome. This, in turn, fuses with a primary lysosome and forms a secondary lysosome.
- In the lysosomes cathepsins result in complete degradation of cellular proteins, including globin of hemoglobin to the constituent amino acids, which are utilized for general metabolic needs.

- Heme is released and converted to bile pigments in the endoplasmic reticulum of the cell.
- Degradation of heme leads to the synthesis of bilirubin (Fig. 29.5).

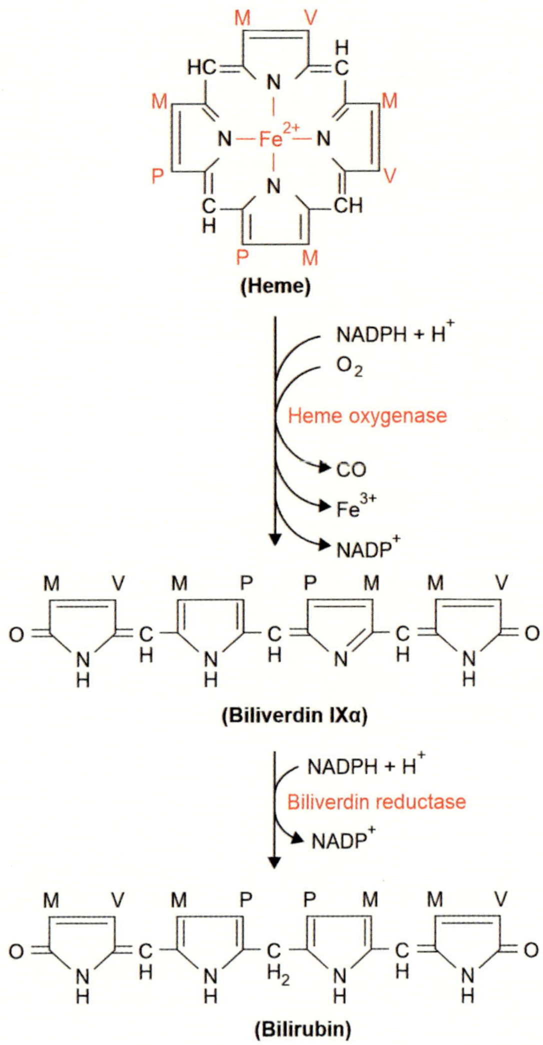

Fig. 29.5: Formation of bilirubin from heme

Hemolytic Anemia

Decreased lifespan of circulating erythrocytes results in a condition referred to as hemolytic anemia.

Symptoms of hemolytic anemia include abnormal paleness, or lack of color of the skin, yellowish skin, eyes and mouth (jaundice); dark-colored urine; fever, weakness, dizziness, confusion, enlarged spleen and liver; increased heart rate (tachycardia) and heart murmur.

There are two main types of hemolytic anemia:

- **Inherited:** In inherited type of the disease, parents pass on the genes, for the condition, onto their children. Two common causes are sickle cell anemia and thalassemia. These conditions produce red blood cells that do not live as long as normal red blood cells.
- **Acquired:** Acquired hemolytic anemias may develop as a result of the immunological reactions consequent on administration of certain drugs.

METABOLISM OF BILIRUBIN

At physiological pH, bilirubin is poorly soluble in aqueous solution. In serum some of the bilirubin is unconjugated while a large concentration of it is conjugated.

- **Unconjugated bilirubin:** Normally, bilirubin is bound to albumin and is transported to the liver. This is referred to as unconjugated bilirubin.
- **Conjugation of bilirubin in the liver:** Hepatocytes trap bilirubin by means of a specific binding protein called protein-Y, or ligandin (a family of glutathione-S-transferases).

  In the hepatocytes, propionyl side chains of bilirubin are conjugated with UDP-glucuronate, which is derived from the oxidation of UDP-glucose. This reaction is catalyzed by UDP-glucuronyl-transferase and results in the formation of conjugated bilirubin (Fig. 29.6).

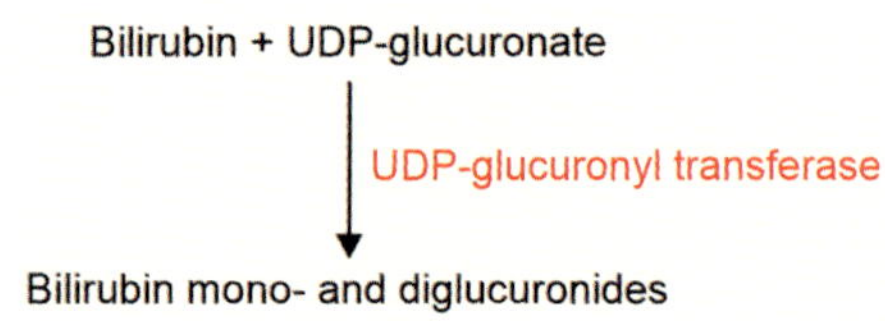

Fig. 29.6: Conjugation of bilirubin in the liver

- **Secretion of conjugated bilirubin:** In the normal bile, bilirubin-diglucuronide is the major form of excreted bilirubin (with only a small amount of the bilirubin-monoglucuronides). As bilirubin diglucuronide is much more water soluble than free bilirubin, transferase, thus, facilitates excretion of bilirubin via bile duct into the intestine.
- **Synthesis of urobilinogens:** As bilirubin-diglucuronide is poorly absorbed by the intestinal mucosa, glucuronide residues are released in the terminal ileum and large intestine by intestinal β-glucuronidases as well as by the enzymes produced by anaerobic bacteria. The released bilirubin is reduced to colorless linear tetrapyrroles called stercobilinogen, mesobilinogen and urobilinogen. These compounds are collectively referred to as urobilinogens. A large portion of the urobilinogens is excreted in the feces.
- **Enterohepatic circulation of urobilinogen:** Some of the urobilinogens (up to 2%) are passively reabsorbed from the intestine and return to liver, via portal venous blood. A majority of these (re-circulating) pigments are taken up the liver and re-excreted in the bile, thereby, completing the enterohepatic circulation of urobilinogen.

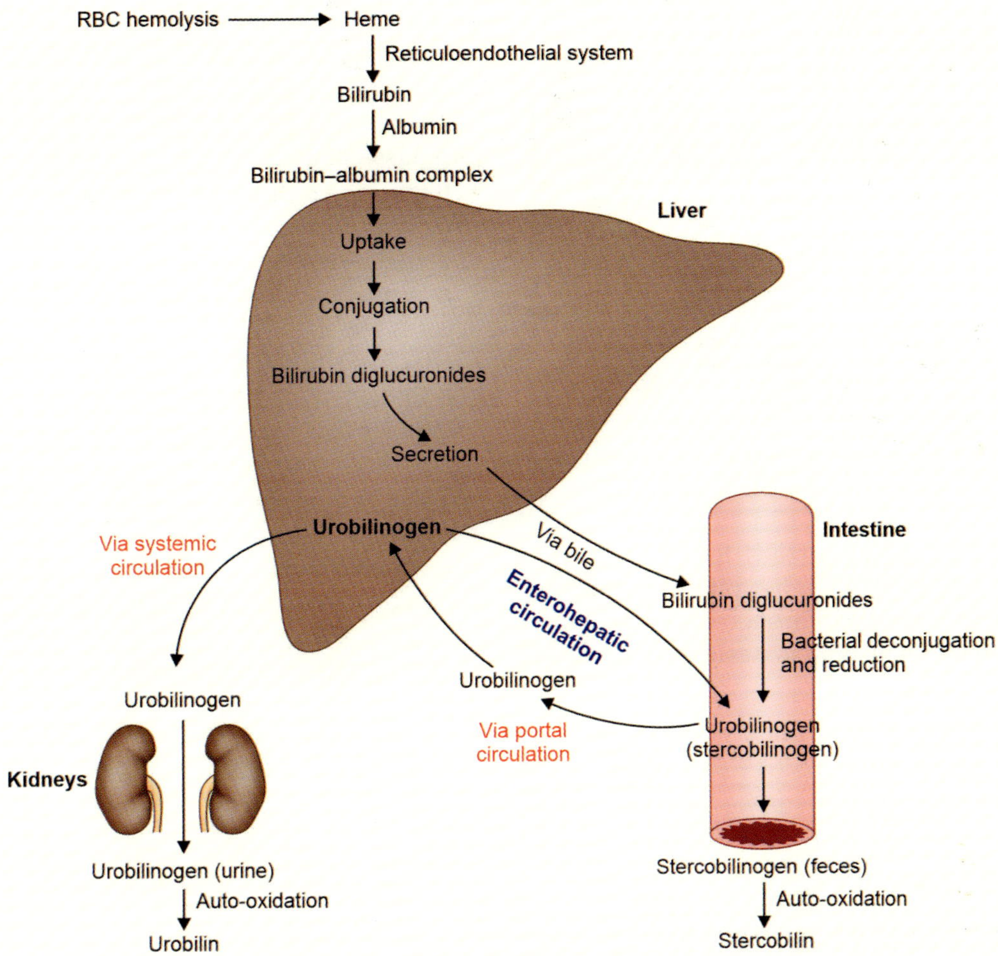

Fig. 29.7: Bilirubin metabolism

- **Formation of urobilin:** Most of the reabsorbed urobilinogen is taken up by the liver and is re-excreted in bile. A small portion of urobilinogens (2–5%), however, escapes hepatic extraction, reaches peripheral circulation and is excreted in urine.

Fecal and urinary urobilinogens are auto-oxidized to form orange/yellow-colored compounds, called urobilins or stercobilins (Fig. 29.7).

Hemoglobinopathies

Hemoglobinopathies refers to a group of **pathological conditions** (such as **methemoglobinemia, sickle cell anemia,** etc.) that may be a **result of structurally and/ or functionally abnormal hemoglobin**. The pathological relevance may be due to genetic or acquired defect, in heme (referred to as hemopathy) or globin structure (called globinopathy).

Methemoglobinemia: Methemoglobin (Met-Hb) is a nonfunctional hemoglobin with Fe^{3+} instead of Fe^{2+}. Normally, Met-Hb levels are <1%. Spontaneously formed Met-Hb is reduced (regenerating normal hemoglobin) by protective enzyme systems, e.g. NADH-methemoglobin reductase (cytochrome b5 reductase, major pathway) and NADPH-methemoglobin reductase (minor pathway).

Sickle cell disease: The most common of all hemoglobinopathies is sickle cell disease, which is characterized by the presence of sickle cell hemoglobin (hemoglobin S or HbS). HbS is a variant form of the normal adult hemoglobin (HbA_1), in which a substitution occurs in the sixth position of the β-globin chain. Whereas in HbA_1, this position is occupied by a glutamic acid residue, in HbS it is substituted by valine (β_6 Glu → Val). The molecular basis for this is a point mutation, i.e. a change in a single nucleotide within the codon from GAA or GAG (which codes for glutamic acid) to GUA or GUG (which codes for valine).

Due to the presence of valine, in place of glutamic acid, **sickle cell hemoglobin has a lower negative charge** than normal hemoglobin. As a result, HbS **gets polymerized and precipitate within the RBCs**, particularly, in the deoxygenated state. This, in turn, **makes the red blood cells assume a sickle-shape**, instead of the normal biconcave shape (Fig. 29.8).

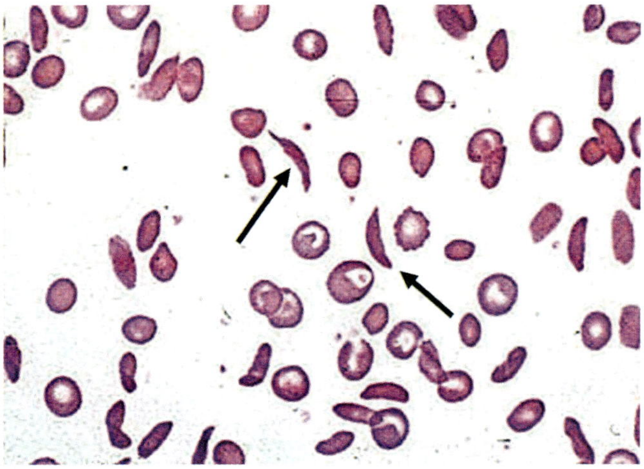

Fig. 29.8: Sickled red blood cells (arrows) in a peripheral blood smear

The **sickle-shaped** (distorted) **RBCs lose their deformability, resulting in higher rate of hemolysis,** particularly, while negotiating through microcirculation. This type of hemolytic anemia is **designated as sickle cell anemia**.

Thalassemias: Thalassemias are a family of related genetic disorders **due to defective synthesis of the globin chain(s)**. Thalassemias arise **due to the deletion of one or more globin-like genes** in either the globin gene clusters or due to a defect in transcription and/or processing of mRNA of the globin gene.

These may be grouped as **α-thalassemia** and **β-thalassemias**.

- If there is a reduced synthesis or total lack of synthesis of α-globin mRNA, the disease is classified as α-thalassemia. The α-thalassemia patients may be missing one to four α-globin genes and have different subtypes.
- If β-globin mRNA level is affected, it is called β-thalassemia. β-thalassemias also exhibit different degrees of severity and can be caused by a variety of defects or deletions.

Thalassemias are also grouped as thalassemia major and thalassemia minor.

- When the child inherits the defective gene from one parent, there are usually minor symptoms, and it is called thalassemia minor or trait (whether α or β).
- On the other hand, **if inheritance of the defective genes is from both the parents** and results in a symptomatic disease requiring treatment, it is called **thalassemia major** (α or β).

Some Important Questions

1. **Describe the process of heme synthesis.**
2. **What is porphyria? Describe various types of porphyrias.**
3. **Describe the process of heme degradation.**
4. **Write notes on:**
   i. Hemoglobin S
   ii. Sickle-cell anemia
   iii. Hemoglobinopathies
   iv. Thalassemias

Chapter

30

Plasma Proteins

Plasma contains over 300 proteins and that the **total plasma protein concentration varies from 6.3–8.0 g/dL**.

CLASSIFICATION OF PLASMA PROTEINS

As mentioned above, plasma contains a large number of proteins (more than 300 in number). Some of these include, **albumin, globulins**, fibrinogen, apolipoproteins (present in lipoproteins), protein hormones (such as insulin, prolactin, etc.), enzymes and coagulation proteins, etc.

Albumin and globulins are the **major plasma proteins**, which are **synthesized in the liver** (except γ-globulins). Serum concentrations of various proteins are given in Table 30.1.

Table 30.1: Serum concentrations of various proteins

Serum protein	*Concentration (g/dL)*
Albumin	3.7–5.3
Globulins (total)	1.8–3.7
α_1 plus α_2-Globulins	0.4–1.4
β-Globulin	0.5–1.3
γ-Globulin	0.6–1.5

FUNCTIONS

Albumin: Albumin performs following functions:

- **Maintenance of plasma colloidal osmotic pressure:** Albumin is important in the maintenance of osmotic pressure. Hence, it plays an important **role in the regulation of blood volume**.
- **Transport of substances:** Several substances, such as **long chain fatty acids, unconjugated bilirubin, steroids, Cu^{2+} and various drugs like salicylates, barbiturates, penicillin, sulfonamides and warfarin**, etc. bind to albumin and are transported from liver to different parts of the body.
- **Act as an antioxidant: Due to the presence of** the sulfhydryl **(–SH) groups**, albumin acts as plasma antioxidant.

Globulins: Various globulins also perform different functions, which include:

- **Transport of substances:** α **and β-globulins** plays an important role in the **transport** of **various molecules, such as hormones, copper, iron, etc.** (Table 30.2).
- **Defence proteins:** γ-Globulins constitute combat antigenic challenge, and thus, act as defence proteins.

DISORDERS

Hypoalbuminemia: Hypoalbuminemia refers to low plasma albumin concentration. It may be due to a number of reasons, such as:

- **Protein malnutrition**, e.g. **kwashiorkor and marasmus**.
- **Malabsorption**, e.g. **inflammatory bowel disease** or **condition following bowel resection**.

Table 30.2: Transport proteins and their ligands

Protein	*Ligand*
Albumin	Cu^{2+}, Fe^{3+}, bilirubin, free fatty acids, steroids, heme
Ceruloplasmin	Copper
Transferrin, ferritin, hemosiderin	Iron
Haptoglobin, hemopexin	Free hemoglobin
Thyroid binding globulin	Thyroid hormones
Cortisol binding globulin	Cortisol
Sex hormone binding globulin	Androgens, estrogens

- **Impaired synthesis** in chronic liver disease, e.g. **cirrhosis**.
- **Excessive losses**, such as in urine **(nephrotic syndrome)**, stool (protein-losing enteropathy), or through skin **(severe burns)**.
- **Leakage and trapping in extravascular sites**, also known as **third space fluid losses**, e.g. **ascites** (accumulation in peritoneal cavity) and **pleural effusion** (accumulation in pleural cavity).
- **Increased catabolism**, such as **after major surgery or trauma, sepsis, malignancy, or following repeated radiation therapy**.
- **Overhydration (artifact causes)**, e.g. pregnancy or dilution of sample due to taking a blood sample from a site close to an intravenous infusion.

Hyperglobulinemia: Hyperglobulinemia refers to an increase in globulin concentration. A liver disease, chronic infection or an autoimmune disease, such as rheumatoid arthritis, give rise to sustained stimulation of B- lymphocytes and, hence, an increased production of γ-globulins. It occurs most commonly in conditions, such as:

- **Advanced liver disease**, e.g. **cirrhosis**.
- **Chronic diseases**, which may be **infectious** (like **tuberculosis** and **viral hepatitis**) or **non-infectious** (such as **rheumatoid arthritis**).
- **Multiple myeloma**

SEPARATION OF PLASMA PROTEINS

Separation of albumin and globulins by precipitation with salt.

Proteins are the large molecular weight substances and that albumin can be easily separated from globulins from a protein solution, such as from plasma, **by the addition of a salt solution**. This process is **known as salting out**. Highly soluble salts, **like sodium chloride** (NaCl) **or ammonium sulfate** [$(NH_4)2SO_4$], **can be used** for this purpose.

For the separation of globulins from plasma or egg white, **add equal volume of saturated solution of ammonium sulfate** to the egg white solution. **Mix, and wait for 10–15 minutes. Filter the precipitate**. Residue on the filter paper contains globulins.

For the precipitation of albumin, add some ammonium sulfate powder to the filtrate, to saturate it completely. Now, albumin is precipitated.

This shows that albumin is more soluble in water than globulin, since, at half saturation only globulins precipitate, whereas at full saturation albumin precipitates. Precipitation of protein by a salt solution is, apparently, due to neutralization of the charges as well as dehydration of the protein molecule. It is known that protein, which has been precipitated by a salt solution, remains native and, usually, gets redissolved, when put in the solvent, again.

Estimation of Serum Albumin

Dyes such as **bromocresol green** (BCG), bind very specifically to albumin. After the addition of alkali, color of BCG is changed from green to blue, intensity of which is proportional to the amount of albumin present in serum. **Serum albumin thus, can be estimated by dye-binding method, using bromocresol green**.

Albumin/globulin Ratio

Albumin: Globulin ratio **(A/G ratio)** refers to the **ratio of serum concentration of albumin to the serum concentration of globulins**. A : G ratio **can be calculated by estimating albumin** and then **subtracting its value from the value of the total serum proteins**. Normal serum A/G ratio is 1.2–2.0:1.

A/G ratio is altered in a number of conditions.

Separation of Plasma Proteins by Electrophoresis

Electrophoresis is a technique for the **separation of the charged particles by means of electric current**. A **charged particle**, when placed in an electric field, **migrates either towards the anode or the cathode, depending upon the net charge carried by the particles**. Different molecules migrate at different speeds depending upon their charge, particle size and shape. Their movement occurs in a liquid medium (a buffer), supported on an inert material, like filter paper, cellulose acetate strip, agar gel, starch gel or polyacrylamide gel.

In paper electrophoresis, a **strip of filter paper** is **dipped in a buffered solution** (barbitone buffer, pH 8.6) and is laid on a platform. Two ends of the strip are dipped in the buffer. Entire apparatus is covered with a sheet to minimize evaporation. Two electrodes are also dipped in two compartments containing buffer. **Current is supplied through a power supply** which either supplies constant current and/or voltage. Current is **carried by the charged particles** and **depending upon the charge, protein migrates towards either anode or cathode**, at different rates. At the end, their **positions are revealed by** some dye, such as **bromophenol blue**, which stains proteins. Different proteins form separate bands on the paper strip.

In the **normal serum five bands** are observed. Starting from anode, these bands are designated as **albumin, α_1-globulin, α_2-globulin, β-globulin and γ-globulin**. Pattern of serum protein on electrophoresis may be used in the diagnosis of a disease (Fig. 30.1).

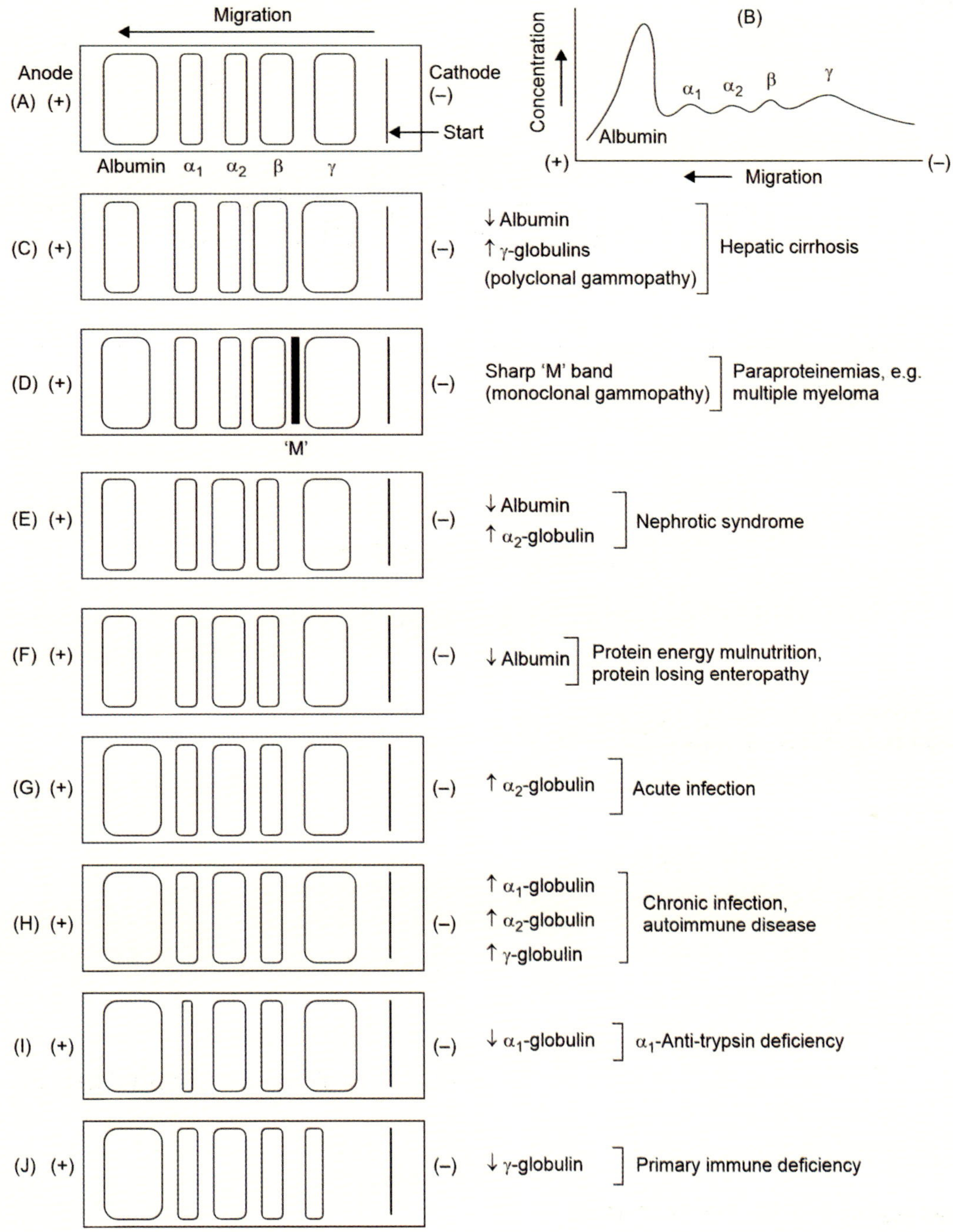

Fig. 30.1: Plasma proteins pattern on electrophoresis in some of the diseases. (A: Electrophoresis bands in normal serum; B: Bands on densitometer; C: Pattern in hepatic cirrhosis; D = Multiple myeloma; E: Nephrotic syndrome; F: Protein energy malnutrition (PEM); G: Acute infection; H: Autoimmune disease; I: α_1-Anti-trypsin deficiency; J: Primary immune deficiency

Some Important Questions

1. What are plasma proteins? Describe the functions of albumin.

2. Write notes on:

i. A/G ratio
ii. Functions of plasma albumin
iii. Paper electrophoresis

Chapter 31

Immunoglobulins

Immunoglobulins are a **diverse group of glycoproteins synthesized by the mature B lymphocytes**, called plasma cells. They are **present either in the free form in plasma** (constituting ≈20% of total plasma proteins, mainly the γ-globulins) and other biological fluids, or **bound to the surface of B cells**, where they **act as receptors for antigens**. Since, these are the globulins which bind to specific antigens, these are **also referred to as antibodies**.

STRUCTURE OF IMMUNOGLOBULIN

Salient features of the structure of an immunoglobulin molecule are summarized in Table 31.1.

Table 31.1: Salient features of the structure of an immunoglobulin molecule

1. An immunoglobulin has **four peptide chains**, which include **two H chains** and **two L chains**.
2. Each chain has **two regions** referred to as the **variable region** and the **constant region**.
3. Each variable region has **hypervariable sequences**.
4. An immunoglobulin has a **Y-shape** structure with **two arms** (called Fab fractions) and **a stem** (Fc fragment).
5. **Fab segments** are linked to **Fc segment** with **hinge region**.

IMMUNOGLOBULINS HAVE FOUR PEPTIDE CHAINS

An immunoglobulin molecule has four peptide chains, which are **bound to each other by the disulfide** (–S–S–) **linkages** (Fig. 31.1).

Out of these four peptide chains (subunits), each immunoglobulin is comprised of **two small peptide chains**, called **L-chains (light chains)**, and **two large peptide chains**, referred to as **H-chains (heavy chains)**.

Light Chains

There are **two types** of the L-chains found in an immunoglobulin, which are designated as the **kappa chain** (κ-chain) and the lambda chain (λ-chain).

- Each immunoglobulin molecule has **two identical L-chains**, i.e. it may have **either two λ-chains** (as λ2) **or two λ-chains** (as λ2), but **never one κ-chain and one λ-chain** (i.e. as κλ).
- Each **L-chain has**, nearly, **220 amino acids**.

Heavy Chains

There are **five types** of the H-chains found in immunoglobulin molecules. These are designated as **gamma** (γ), **alpha** (α), **mu** (μ), **delta** (δ) and **epsilon** (ε) chains.

- Each of these H-chain is **specific to a class of immunoglobulin** (Ig). Accordingly, depending upon the presence of the H-chain, **immunoglobulins** are classified into **five groups**, and are designated as **IgG, IgA, IgM, IgD and IgE**.
- Each **H-chain has**, nearly, **440–450 amino acids**.

These **L-chains and H-chains are synthesized separately**, which are, **subsequently, assembled to form a mature immunoglobulin** molecule, forming a tetramer, within the plasma cells. During assembly, each H-chain is associated with the L-chain as well as to each other by the –S–S– linkages. An L-chain is joined to an H-chain in such a way that they run parallel to each other.

Variable Regions and Constant Regions

In the structure of the antibody molecule, all the **four chains are present in the folded form in several** discrete regions, called **domains. Each domain has**, nearly, **110 amino acids**.

An **L-chain**, normally, **has two domains**, while depending upon the class of the immunoglobulin, each of the **H-chain has four (or five) domains. Each** of these **domains is referred to as the variable region and the constant regions**.

- **Variable regions:** Amino acid sequences in the N-terminal half of the L-chain and one-quarter of the H-chains are highly variable between different immunoglobulin molecules. Therefore, these N-terminal regions are called the variable regions (V-regions).
  - These variable regions are **heterogeneous** to the extent that **no two V-regions, from different humans, have identical amino acid sequences**.
  - V-region **determines antigenic specificity** of the antibody.
  - These regions, in the **L-chains** and the **H-chains**, are designated as V_L and V_H, respectively.

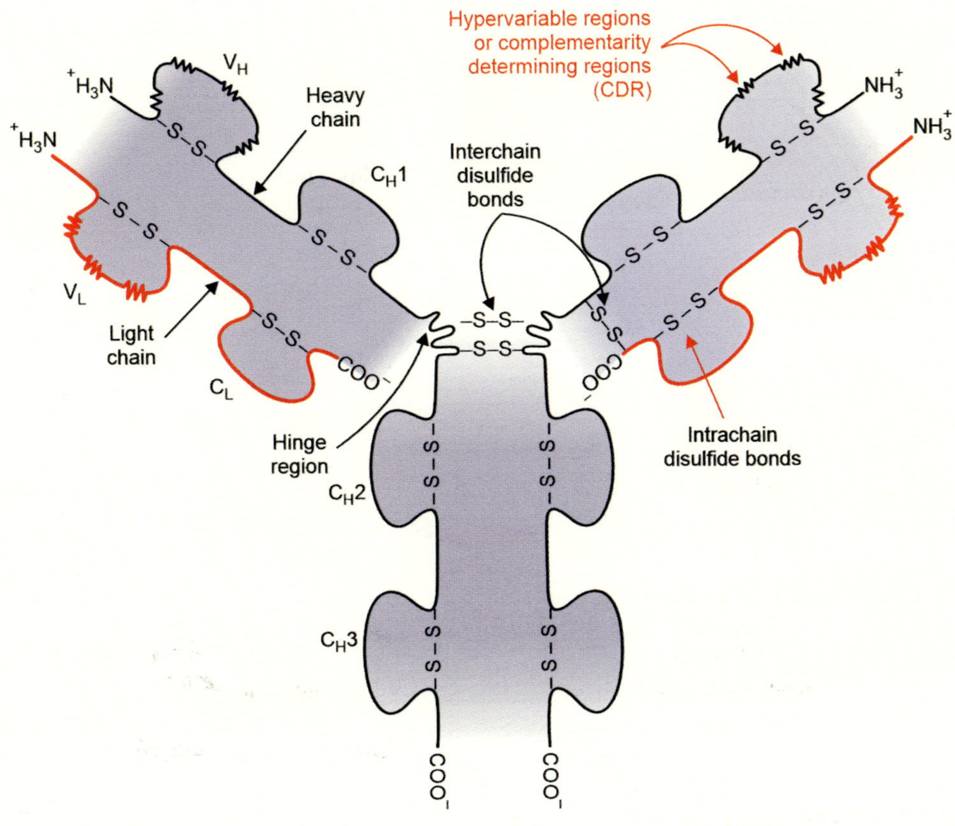

Fig. 31.1: Structure of an immunoglobulin

- **Hypervariable regions: Antigenic specificity of an immunoglobulin** molecule **is responsible for the recognition and binding** of an antigen with the antibody. **This ability** of the antibody to recognize antigen **resides in several short sequences** that are **located in small loops** (short segments) **within the V-regions**. These sequences are **referred to as hypervariable regions, or hypervariable sequences.**
  - Nearly, **only 5–10 amino acids in each hypervariable sequence contribute to the site**, where an **antigen binds.**
  - This segment is **referred to as antigen binding site (ab site).**
  - It is **complementary to the topology of the antigen structure** and, hence, it is **called complementarity-determining region** (CDR or complementarity determinant).
  - Three hypervariable sequences are, commonly, found in the VL-regions, while each of the VH-region, depending upon the type of antibody, has three or four hypervariable sequences.
- **Constant regions: Remainder of the immunoglobulin molecule,** i.e. the **C-terminal half of the L-chain and the C-terminal three-quarter of the H-chain,** are **homologous in sequence** with the other L-chain or the H-chains of the same class of immunoglobulin. These regions are called the constant regions (C regions).
  - The constant regions in the **L-chains and the H-chains** are designated as **C_L and C_H**, respectively.
  - The **constant region in the H-chains is further subdivided into three homologous sequences** of about 110 amino acids each, which are designated as **C_H1, C_H2 and C_H3**, respectively.
  - Significance of the C_H region
    - The C_H region **determines class of an immunoglobulin.**
    - It also **provides site for binding of a complement protein.**
    - It is also the **site for the antibodies to cross the placental membrane.**
    - Depending upon the class of an immunoglobulin, **variable amounts of carbohydrates** (2–15%) **are attached to C_H2 region.**
    - Amino acid sequences in the C_H region also **promote polymerization of the basic molecular structure** (L_2H_2), such **as in IgA and IgM.**
    - In a polymer, different molecules are **covalently linked with** each other with a peptide, referred to as the **joining chain** (J-chain; Fig. 31.2).

Fab and Fc Segments

An antibody is a **Y-shape structure**, i.e. it **has two arms,** referred to as the **antigen binding fragments (Fab fragments),** and a stem, called **crystallizable fragment (Fc fragment).**

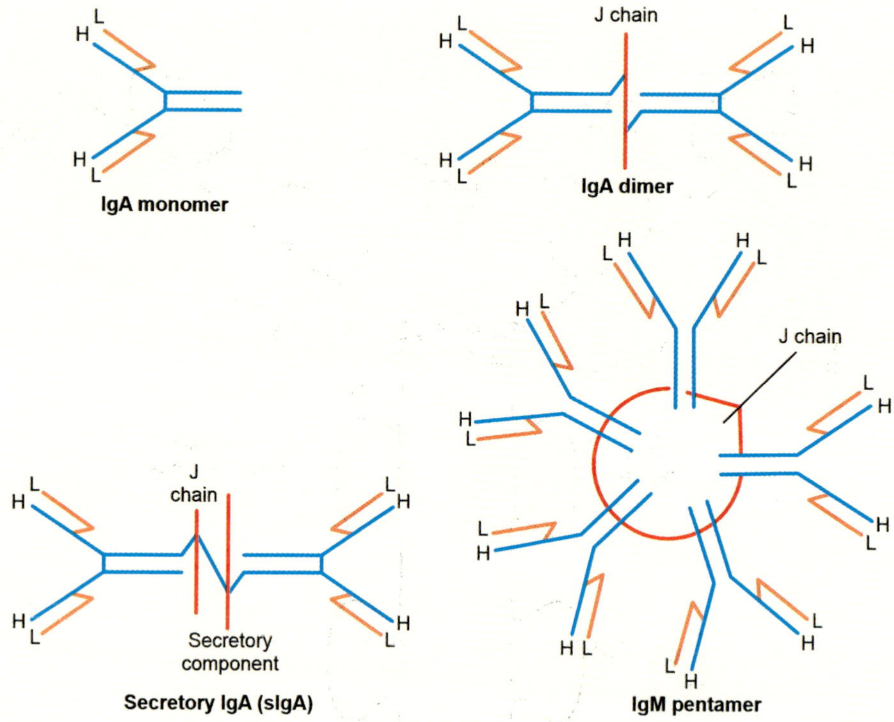

Fig. 31.2: Polymerization of immunoglobulin molecules

When **hydrolyzed by the enzyme papain**, an **immunoglobulin molecule**, such as IgG, **is cleaved into three fragments** of nearly 50 kD each.

- **Two identical fragments are obtained from the two arms**, which are the sites, **where antigen can bind**. Hence, these two fragments are **called antigen binding fragments (Fab)**. Accordingly, **an immunoglobulin can bind two molecules of an antigen**, simultaneously. Therefore, an antibody is **termed as divalent**.
- The **fragment which is obtained from the stem is called crystallizable fragment or Fc.**

On the other hand, when pepsin (a proteolytic enzyme) acts on an immunoglobulin molecule, it hydrolyzes the Fc fragment to its constituent amino acids, thereby leaving the two Fab fragments intact (Fig. 31.3).

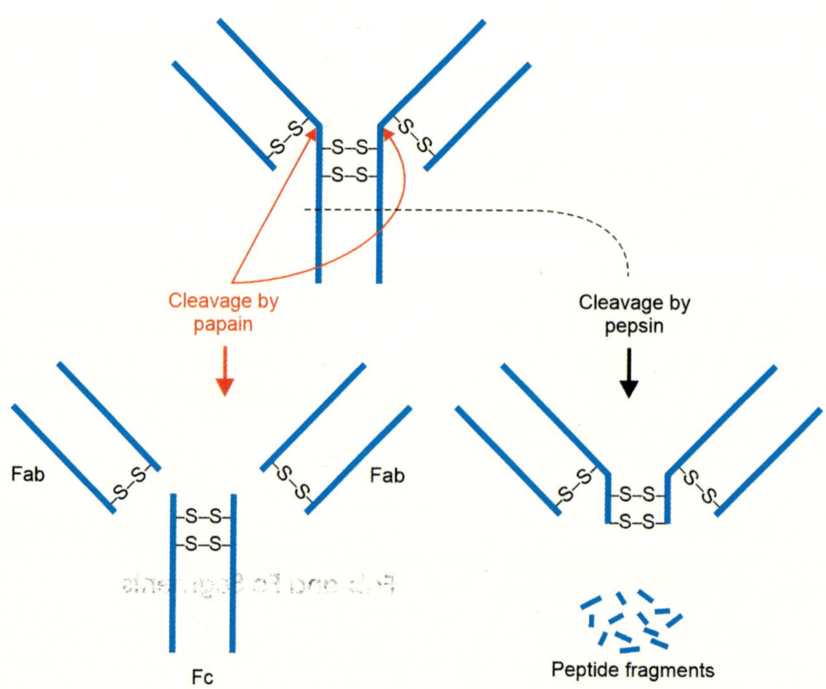

Fig. 31.3: Hydrolysis of an immunoglobulin molecule by papain and by pepsin

Hinge Region

The **two Fab segments are linked to the Fc segment with a flexible** region, called **hinge region**, which **confers flexibility to the antibody molecule** and allows the two Fab fragments to move independently (Fig. 31.4).

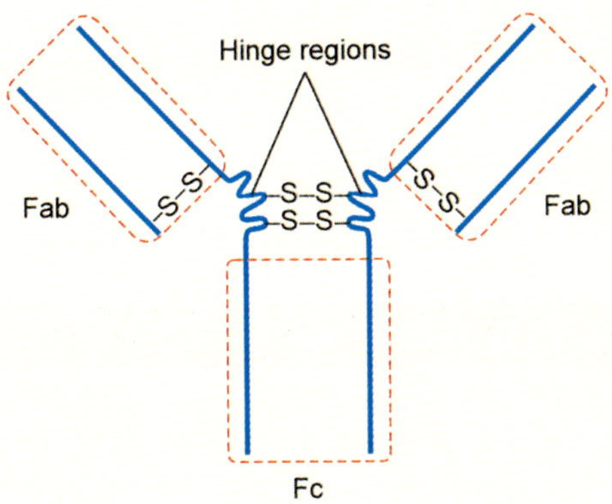

Fig. 31.4: Antigen binding (Fab) and crystallizable (Fc) fragments of immunoglobulin

CLASSIFICATION OF IMMUNOGLOBULINS

As mentioned above, there are five classes of immunoglobulins called **IgG, IgA, IgM, IgD and IgE**. Each one of it differs from the other with respect to the type of its H chain (Table 31.2).

Immunoglobulin G (IgG)

Immunoglobulin G (IgG) is a **major immunoglobulin produced by plasma cells**. It accounts for 70–75% of the total immunoglobulins found in serum.

- IgG has **four subclasses**, which are referred to as **IgG$_1$, IgG$_2$, IgG$_3$ and IgG$_4$**. These subclasses differ, primarily, in the hinge region.
- IgG is the **most important** class **in secondary immune response** and is distributed evenly between the intravascular and the extravascular pools.
- It is **produced in response to most bacteria and viruses**, binds to macrophages and neutrophils, and promotes phagocytosis.
- The major effector mechanism is the **activation of the classical pathway of a complement.**

Immunoglobulin A (IgA)

Immunoglobulin A (IgA) accounts for about **15–20% of the total** serum immunoglobulins.

- IgA has **two subclasses** designated as **IgA$_1$ and IgA$_2$**.
- In human serum IgA$_1$ is predominant. It accounts for about **75–90% of the total IgA** in many secretions, such as in nasal secretion, tears, saliva, and milk.
- **Secretory IgA:** Secretory IgA (sIgA) is the **predominant immunoglobulin in seromucus secretions**, such as saliva, colostrum, milk, and tracheobronchial and genitourinary secretions. It exists, mainly, **in dimeric form, in association with** another protein that is known as the **secretory component.**

Immunoglobulin M (IgM)

Immunoglobulin M (IgM) accounts for, nearly, **5–10% of the total** circulating immunoglobulins.

- IgM is **found as a pentamer**, consisting of five Y-shaped monomeric molecules, which are arranged around the J chain.
- It is the **first immunoglobulin**, which is **synthesized by the cells on introduction of an antigen into the host.**
- Thus, IgM is **called the first line of defense.**
- IgM is a potent **activator of the classical pathway of a complement.**

Immunoglobulin D (IgD)

Immunoglobulin D (IgD) accounts for less than 1% of the total serum immunoglobulins.

- IgD is the **major component of the surface membrane of many B cells.**
- It plays a role in **antigen-triggered lymphocyte differentiation.**

Immunoglobulin E (IgE)

Immunoglobulin E (IgE) is, normally, **present in blood in minute concentration only.**

Table 31.2: Types of immunoglobulins (Ig)

Ig class	*Approximate molecular weight (kD)*	*H chain*	*Carbohydrate content (%)*	*Serum concentration (mg/dL)*	*Physiological functions*
IgG	146	γ	2–4	800–1500	• Placental transfer • Provides immunity to neonates
IgA	160–380	α	5–9	150–250	• Protects outer surfaces • sIgA is present in mucus secretions
IgM	970	μ	8–12	70–150	• First line of defense and is synthesized in neonates
IgD	160	δ	8–12	3–5	• Primary function unknown, acts as B cell receptor
IgE	190	ε	10–15	0.01–0.05	• Reaginic antibodies, implicated in allergic reactions • Release of histamine and other vasoactive amines

- IgE is **found on the surface membrane of the basophils** and the **mast cells.**
- It is commonly **associated with the allergic diseases**, such as hay fever and asthma.
- **After an antigen links IgE, mast cells** are stimulated to release histamine and other vasoactive amines, which, in turn, are **responsible for the vascular permeability** and smooth muscle contraction.
- IgE also **sensitizes cells on the mucosal surfaces**, such as conjunctival, nasal, and bronchial mucosa, and, thus, **protects the host against parasites**.

FUNCTIONS OF IMMUNOGLOBULINS

Each immunoglobulin class has different physiological functions (Table 31.2).

- **IgG** can **cross placenta** and **confer high degree of passive immunity to the newborn**.
- **sIgA is predominant in seromucous secretions**, such as saliva, colostrum, milk, and tracheobronchial and genitourinary secretions and, thus, **protects the outer surfaces**. Thus, it provides initial defense against invading viral and bacterial pathogens, prior to their entry into the internal spaces.
- **IgM** is the only immunoglobulin that a **neonate, normally, synthesizes**. It is also the **predominant antibody in primary immune response**.
- **IgD** is the **major component of the surface membrane of many B cells** and plays a role in antigen triggered lymphocyte differentiation.
- **IgE is commonly associated with the allergic diseases**, such as hay fever and asthma. It **stimulates the mast cells to release histamine** and other vasoactive amines, which, in turn, are responsible for **vascular permeability and smooth muscle contraction**.

MECHANISM OF ACTION

Immunoglobulins destroy pathogens in the following three ways:

1. They **bind to the specific molecules on the surface of the pathogen**, thereby, neutralizing the pathogen. This, in turn, prevents entry of the pathogen to the cell.
2. Thereafter, the antibody-bound pathogens are subjected to **phagocytosis by the macrophages** and other cells, **by** the process called **opsonization**.
3. The binding of antibodies to the pathogens also **activates the complement system**. During this process, the complement proteins bind to the antibody-bound pathogens and recruit the phagocytic cells.

Antigen

Any **molecule that triggers an immune response** is called an immunogen. It may be an **antigen, hapten or allergen** that can **bind to its corresponding antibody**. An antigen **may be a protein, carbohydrate or nucleic acid** and can be specifically recognized by the adaptive elements of the immune system, i.e. by the B-cells or the T-cells, or both.

- Antigen molecules are **recognized by the receptors** present on the lymphocytes.
- B-lymphocytes, usually, recognize intact antigen molecules, while T-lymphocytes recognize antigen fragments on the surface of the cells.
- Each **antibody binds to** a restricted part of the antigen, called **an antigenic determinant (epitope)**.

MONOCLONAL ANTIBODIES

Monoclonal antibodies (mAbs) refer to **proteins which are made in the laboratory but act like antibodies.** These are the **clones** (exact copies) **of one antibody and bind to only one antigen**.

Monoclonal Antibodies as Therapeutic Agents

Monoclonal antibodies target specific epitopes implicated in disease processes and, hence, **are employed as drugs.** By convention, the suffix **mAb** (for monoclonal antibody) is tagged with the drug. They are useful in the treatment of diverse clinical conditions:

- **Autoimmune diseases:** Infliximab for Crohn's disease and rheumatoid arthritis.
- **Age-related macular degeneration:** Ranibizumab.
- **Postmenopausal osteoporosis:** Denosumab.
- **Allergic bronchial asthma:** Omalizumab.
- **Renal transplant rejection:** Muromomab.
- **Cancer:** Trastuzumab (breast cancer), rituximab (lymphoma, leukemia).

AUTOIMMUNE DISEASES

Immune system of the body is geared to detect an antigen that is foreign to the body, or say that **it distinguishes the self, from the nonself** antigenic determinants, so as to avoid autoreactivity. However, **due to various reasons** such as loss of self-tolerance, genetic mutation, interaction with drugs or certain types of infections, the **immunological machinery of an individual sometimes starts forming antibodies against one's own tissues** or cells. Such a disorder is referred to as an autoimmune disease.

Autoimmune diseases range from **single organ** (or cell) type disorder, which involves specific immune reaction directed against only a particular organ or cell type (such as Graves' disease or insulin dependent diabetes mellitus) to multisystem disease, which are characterized by lesions in many organs and are associated with multiple autoantibodies (e.g. rheumatoid arthritis).

Some of the autoimmune diseases are listed in Table 31.3.

Table 31.3: Some autoimmune diseases

Autoimmune disease	*Target tissue*	*Effects*
Graves' disease	Thyroid gland	↑ Thyroid hormone secretion
Insulin-dependent diabetes mellitus	Pancreatic β-cells	↓ Insulin secretion
Addison's disease	Adrenal cortex	↑ Na^+ excretion, K^+ retention
Myasthenia gravis	Acetylcholine receptor at neuromuscular junctional synapse	Progressive muscle weakness
Rheumatoid arthritis	Joint connective tissue	Inflammation of joints (arthritis)
Systemic lupus erythematosus	Tissue components, e.g. DNA, phospholipids, etc.	Joint and muscle pain, anemia, neurological disturbances
Pernicious anemia	Gastric parietal cells or intrinsic factor	Megaloblastic anemia

Some Important Questions

1. **What are immunoglobulins? Describe the structure of an immunoglobulin.**
2. **Classify immunoglobulins. Describe the functions of each class of immunoglobulin.**
3. **Write notes on:**
   i. Autoimmune diseases
   ii. Hypervariable sequences
   iii. Antigen
   iv. Hinge region

Unit IX

Medical Biochemistry

Chapter
32

Regulation of Blood Glucose

Several hormones regulate blood glucose concentration, as a result of which blood glucose level is maintained within the **normal range of 60–90 mg per 100 mL in the fasting** (post-absorptive) state.

HORMONAL REGULATION

Hormones which regulate blood glucose concentration are divided into two groups, i.e. (i) those which **lower blood glucose** level, and (ii) those which **increase blood glucose** level (Fig. 32.1).

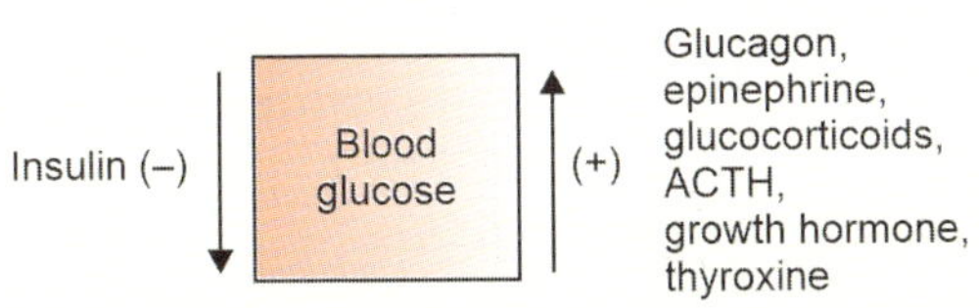

Fig. 32.1: Regulation of blood glucose by hormones

i. Hormones which Lower Blood Glucose Level

Insulin is the only hormone which lowers blood glucose level, i.e. **has hypoglycemic action.**

- Insulin is **released** into the blood stream **under the direct influence of hyperglycemia.**
- Insulin is a **polypeptide containing 2 chains.**
- It is **produced by the β-cells of the islets of Langerhans** of the pancreas.
- Insulin **lowers blood glucose concentration** by various mechanisms:
  - Insulin **promotes uptake of glucose by the extrahepatic tissues.**
  - It also **promotes glycolysis and glycogenesis,** both **in the liver and** the **muscle.**
  - Insulin also **suppresses glycogenolysis in the liver** and the **kidney.**
  - It also **suppresses gluconeogenesis.**
  - Insulin also **promotes transport of amino acids** across the cell membrane and, thus, **stimulates protein synthesis.**
  - It also **inhibits ketogenesis** and **promotes lipogenesis.**

ii. Hormones which Increase Blood Glucose Level

Several hormones are known to increase blood glucose level and are referred to as **hyperglycemic hormones** or **diabetogenic hormones.** These include **glucagon, epinephrine, glucocorticoids, growth hormone and thyroxine.**

- **Glucagon:** Glucagon is **produced by the α-cells of the islets of Langerhans** of the pancreas.
  - Glucagon **synthesis is stimulated under the influence of hypoglycemia.**
  - It **acts only in the liver,** where it **promotes glycogenolysis.**
  - Glucagon also **promotes gluconeogenesis from amino acids and lactate.**
- **Epinephrine:** Epinephrine, also called **adrenaline,** is a derivative of tyrosine. It is **secreted by the adrenal medulla.**
  - Epinephrine is a hormone in the **first line of defense against hypoglycemia.**
  - It **promotes glycogenolysis,** both **in the liver and muscle.**
  - Epinephrine also **promotes gluconeogenesis in the liver.**
  - It also **inhibits the release of insulin from the pancreas,** which, in turn, reduces the **transport and utilization of glucose** in different tissues.
  - At the same time, epinephrine also **stimulates secretion of glucagon.**
- **Glucocorticoids:** Glucocorticoids are **steroids, secreted by the adrenal cortex.**
  - Glucocorticoids are **antagonist to insulin.**
  - **Cortisol is a major glucocorticoid** present in blood.
  - Cortisol **stimulates protein catabolism in muscle** and **promotes gluconeogenesis in the liver.**
  - It also **stimulates lipolysis and inhibits glucose oxidation** by the liver.
  - Cortisol also **facilitates action of other hyperglycemic hormones** (permissive effects) such as glucagon, epinephrine, and growth hormone, **which**

further inhibit uptake and utilization of glucose by the peripheral tissues.

- **Growth hormone:** Growth hormone is **secreted by the anterior pituitary**.
  - **Secretion** of growth hormone is **stimulated under the influence of hypoglycemia**.
  - Prolonged administration of the growth hormone also **stimulates the secretion of insulin**. As a result of which, **β-cells are exhausted**, thereby **producing a diabetes-like situation**.
  - Growth hormone also **decreases glucose uptake and utilization by muscles**.
  - It also **promotes lipolysis in the adipose tissue**.
- **Thyroxine:** Thyroxine is **secreted by the thyroid gland**.
  - Thyroxine **stimulates intestinal absorption of glucose**.
  - It also **promotes glycogenolysis** as well as **gluconeogenesis in the liver**.

DIABETES MELLITUS

Diabetes mellitus (DM) is a major disorder of carbohydrate metabolism. It is **characterized by persistent hyperglycemia** with or without **glycosuria** (glucosuria). It is the commonest endocrine disease, which is caused by the **deficiency in secretion** and/or **action of insulin**. It may be a **result of the genetic and/or environmental factors**. Thus, it is a multifactorial disease Metabolic derangement is due to elevated glucagon/insulin ratio. In addition, there may be weight loss in IDDM.

There are **two** major clinical **types** of diabetes mellitus. These are referred to as insulin dependent diabetes mellitus (IDDM) and noninsulin dependent diabetes mellitus (NIDDM).

Insulin dependent diabetes mellitus: Insulin dependent diabetes mellitus (IDDM) or **type I diabetes** is also called **juvenile-onset diabetes** because it usually appears in the childhood or in younger age group (commonly less than 40 years of age). There is **absolute deficiency of insulin**, due to a gradual depletion of β-cells of the pancreas, which may get destroyed by an autoimmune process.

IDDM is characterized by **hyperglycemia, hyperlipoproteinemia** (raised chylomicron and VLDL) and severe ketoacidosis. This, in turn, suggests that besides defects in carbohydrate metabolism there are abnormalities in fat and protein metabolism also in such patients.

- **Hyperglycemia** in IDDM is a result of **inability of the insulin-dependent tissues to take up glucose** as well as due to **accelerated hepatic gluconeogenesis from amino acids** (derived from muscle protein).
- **Increased lipolysis** (in the adipose tissue) and accelerated **fatty acid oxidation** (in the liver) result in **ketoacidosis**.
- Insulin deficiency also **reduces lipoprotein lipase** activity, thereby, resulting in **hyperchylomicronemia**.
- Patients with IDDM can usually be recognized by abrupt appearance of **polyuria** (frequent urination), **polydipsia** (excessive thirst) and **polyphagia** (excessive hunger), often triggered by the stress or some other illness. These symptoms are usually accompanied with **fatigue, weight loss and weakness**.
  - Its **diagnosis is confirmed by high fasting blood glucose**, commonly accompanied with **ketoacidosis**.
  - **Insulin injection**, though does not cure the disease but promotes glucose uptake by the tissues and **inhibits gluconeogenesis, lipolysis and proteolysis**.
  - **Life span of the patient is reduced** as a result of the degenerative complications, such as **kidney malfunction, nerve impairment** and **cardiovascular disease**.
  - Hyperglycemia also leads to **blindness** through **retinal degeneration** and **glycosylation of the lens proteins**, which, in turn, causes **cataract**.
- **Noninsulin dependent diabetes mellitus: Majority of the diabetic patients** (over 80%) suffer from noninsulin dependent diabetes mellitus **(NIDDM)** or **type II diabetes**. It is also called **maturity-onset diabetes**, since it, usually, occurs in the middle age group (usually more than 40 years of age), in those who are, generally, obese.
  - **Occurrence of NIDDM is**, almost completely, **determined by genetic factors**.
  - It **develops gradually**, without obvious symptoms.
  - **Metabolic alterations are milder** than IDDM.
  - NIDDM is characterized by **hyperglycemia**, often **with hypertriglyceridemia**.
  - Hyperglycemia is, mainly, a result of **the poor peripheral utilization of glucose**, especially in muscle.
  - **Blood glucose concentration is much higher** than normal, particularly, after a meal.
  - **These patients are insulin resistance**, which **due to increased expression of the tumor necrosis factor-α** in the adipocytes of obese individuals.
  - **Ketoacidosis does not develop**, because adipocytes remain sensitive to the effect of insulin.
  - Rapid *de novo* **synthesis of fatty acids and VLDL leads to hypertriglyceridemia** without hyperchylomicronemia.
  - **Weight reduction and dietary modifications** often correct hyperglycemia of type II diabetes.
  - Hypoglycemic agents, such as sulphonylureas, may be required to achieve a satisfactory fall in blood glucose level.
  - **Long-term complications** of the disease include **acute myocardial infarction** (diabetic patients often present with painless acute myocardial infarction, i.e. silent MI), due to accelerated atherosclerosis and coronary heart disease, **nephropathy, retinopathy, neuropathy, infections and delayed wound healing**.

Salient features of diabetes mellitus are shown in Table 32.1.

Table 32.1: Salient features of the two types (IDDM and NIDDM) of diabetes mellitus

	IDDM	*NIDDM*
Type of diabetes	Juvenile onset (Type I)	Maturity-onset (Type II)
Prevalence	About 20%	About 80%
Age of onset	<40 years	>40 years
Body habitus	Normal to wasted (weight loss)	Obese
Plasma insulin	Low (due to β-cell destruction)	Normal to high (insulin resistance)
Plasma glucagon	High (suppressible)	High (resistant)
Acute complications	Ketoacidosis	Hyperosmolar coma (ketoacidosis is rare)
Insulin therapy	Responsive	Resistant
Oral hypoglycemic agents	Unresponsive	Responsive

Insulin and Maturity Onset Diabetes

Insulin level in circulation is normal or high, in most of the cases of maturity onset diabetes. In spite of normal or high level of insulin, **glucose levels are poorly controlled** because of the **lack of normal response to insulin**. It is due to the reason that these patients are **insulin resistant**.

Diabetes and Related Disorders

Metabolic Syndrome

Obesity and **insulin resistance**, resulting in either glucose intolerance or diabetes, may coexist with **dyslipidemia** and **increased arterial blood pressure**. Such combination is referred to as metabolic syndrome and **is associated with an increased risk of cardiovascular disease**.

Diabetic Ketoacidosis

Diabetic ketoacidosis is a **common feature**, which is observed **in patients with insulin dependent diabetes mellitus**. This is **due to severe deficiency of insulin** with **excess of glucagon** and other hyperglycemic hormones, such as **epinephrine, cortisol and growth hormone**. As a result of it, **plasma free fatty acids concentration is increased**. This, in turn, leads to **increased production of ketone bodies** by the liver. There is also marked **hyperglycemia, ketonemia, ketonuria**, and **water and electrolyte imbalance**. Various features of the disease can be corrected by insulin administration.

EVALUATION OF GLYCEMIC STATUS

As mentioned above, normal value for blood glucose remains in the range of 60–100 mg/100 mL. When this value exceeds it is called **hyperglycemia**. Persistent hyperglycemia may be a result of **diabetes mellitus**. It can be assessed by estimating glycemic status of the individual.

Glycemic status of the person can be assessed by several means, such as by **estimating blood glucose level, glucose tolerance test** (GTT) and **glycated hemoglobin** (Hb1Ac) level.

Glucose Tolerance Test

For performing a glucose tolerance test **(GTT)** glucose is given to the subject and blood samples are withdrawn at certain time intervals to determine how quickly glucose is cleared from blood. The test is usually, done to assess diabetes, insulin resistance, impaired beta-cell functions, and sometimes, reactive hypoglycemia and acromegaly, or some other rare disorder of carbohydrate metabolism.

Oral glucose tolerance test: Normally, **oral glucose tolerance test** (OGTT) is performed by giving a load of glucose, orally. It is helpful in confirming the diagnosis of diabetes in those patients whose fasting blood glucose concentration is in the upper normal limit, with transient or sustained glycosuria, but without the symptoms of diabetes, or with family history of the disease.

For performing OGTT fasting venous blood sample (after 12–16 hours of fast) is withdrawn and thereafter, 75 g of glucose (about 1 g/kg body weight) is given in nearly 200–300 mL of water. After oral administration of glucose, blood samples are again withdrawn after every 30 minutes, till 2 to 2½ hours. Urine specimen may also be collected, simultaneously. Each blood sample is analyzed and sometimes insulin levels are also assessed. The intervals and number of samples may vary according to the purpose of the test. For evaluation, glucose tolerance curve is plotted (Fig. 32.2).

Fasting blood glucose concentration, maximum blood glucose value after a glucose load, and the rate at which it returns towards the fasting value, gives an idea about the disease.

Normal GTT: For a normal individual, fasting blood glucose value should be within the normal limit. This value is increased by about 50%, within 60 minutes, and returns toward the fasting value, after, nearly, 2 hours. Glycosuria is, generally, not observed at any time.

Any deviation from the above is referred to as an **abnormal glucose tolerance curve**.

- **Mini GTT:** International Committee of Diabetologists has recommended the estimation of blood glucose

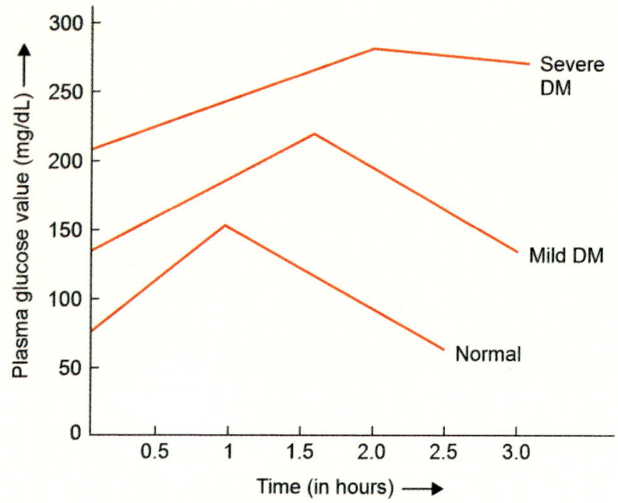

Fig. 32.2: Glucose tolerance curves

in the **overnight fasting and postprandial samples** (2 hours after 75 g of a glucose load) to confirm the diagnosis of diabetes mellitus. It is referred to as **mini GTT** and is sufficient to diagnose or exclude all forms of diabetes mellitus.

- Accordingly, an individual is said to be **normal**, if fasting blood glucose value is less than 100 mg/100 mL while the 2-hour's value is below 140 mg/100 mL.
- A fasting value of 126 mg/100 mL or higher, and the 2 hours' value of more than 200 mg/100 mL is diagnostic of **diabetes mellitus**.
- Fasting value between 100 and 125 mg/100 mL and/or the 2 hours' value between 140 and 200 mg/100 mL is referred to as **impaired glucose tolerance**.

- **Glycated-hemoglobin:** Glycated-hemoglobin (HbA1c) **reflects** the **average blood sugar concentration for a time period of 8–10 weeks** and remains unaffected by the short-term fluctuations in blood sugar. Compared with the repeated daily blood sugar test, HbA1c **helps in evaluating the adequacy of diabetic control**.
  - An **elevated HbA1c** level may signal the **need** for a **change in insulin regimen** or **meal plan**. However, target HbA1c goal may vary depending on age and various other factors. HbA1c can be measured by ion exchange method or HPLC.
  - **Reference range** for Hb1Ac **is 4.0–6.0%**.
  - **Higher levels** are directly **linked to** the microvascular complications, like **retinopathy and nephropathy**.
  - High HbA1c are **also** seen **in iron deficiency anemia**, probably because of high proportion of old erythrocytes.
  - **Decreased levels** may be seen **in hemolytic disease** or in other conditions with shortened red cell survival.

Some Important Questions

1. Define diabetes mellitus. Differentiate between type I and type II diabetes.

2. Write notes on:

i. Hormonal regulation of blood glucose
ii. Glycated hemoglobin
iii. Oral glucose tolerance test
iv. Mini glucose tolerance test
v. Diabetic ketoacidosis

Chapter

33

Lipoproteins

Lipoproteins or proteolipids are the lipid-protein complexes. Since, lipids are **not soluble in** the aqueous **plasma**, hence, they are **transported in** the body in **association with proteins in the form of lipoproteins.** These are **globular micelle-like particles**, consisting of **nonpolar core of triacylglycerols and cholesterol esters,** which are **surrounded by the amphiphilic coating** that consists **of proteins, cholesterol and phospholipids**.

CLASSIFICATION OF LIPOPROTEINS

Lipoproteins are **classified into** four groups.

- **Chylomicrons**
- **Very Low-Density Lipoproteins**
- **Low-Density Lipoproteins**
- **High-Density Lipoproteins**

Various lipoproteins can be separated according to their density by ultracentrifugation. They can also be separated according to their protein content by electrophoresis (Table 33.1).

FORMATION, FUNCTIONS AND TURNOVER OF LIPOPROTEINS

Chylomicrons

Chylomicrons are triglyceride-rich particles that are assembled in the intestinal mucosal cells. **They carry dietary triacylglycerols, cholesterol and cholesteryl esters to peripheral** (extrahepatic) **tissues**.

- **Intestinal mucosal cells** release **nascent chylomicrons**. These particles, contain **apo B-48**, which is synthesized in the intestine.
- Thereafter, these **nascent chylomicrons receive apo E** and **apo C from** the circulating HDL and **are converted to chylomicrons**.
- **Apo C-II**, in turn, **activates lipoprotein lipase** and **hydrolyzes triacylglycerols** (present in chylomicrons) to monoacylglycerols, free fatty acids and glycerol.
- As a result of **hydrolysis of triacylglycerols**, chylomicrons decrease in size and increase in density.
- Thereafter, **apo C is returned to HDL** and the leftover particles are called **chylomicron remnants**.
- Chylomicron remnants bind to apo E receptors on hepatocytes.
- They are then **internalized** and **their lipids**, including cholesteryl esters, are either **utilized or stored**, intracellularly.
- A small amount of the released **free fatty acids enters the circulation** and contributes to plasma free fatty acid pool.

Table 33.1: Properties and functions of lipoproteins

Lipoprotein class	*Density on ultracentrifugation*	*Diameter (nm)*	*Protein/ lipid (%)*	*Major apoproteins*	*Major lipids*	*Source*	*Functions*
Chylomicrons	<0.95	100–1000	2/98	B-48, A	TG	Small intestine	Transport dietary TG from intestine to extra-hepatic tissues
Very low-density lipoproteins (VLDL)	0.95–1.006	30–80	10/90	B-100	TG	Liver	Transport hepatic TG to extrahepatic tissues
Low-density lipoproteins (LDL)	1.006–1.063	18–28	25/75	B-100	CHOL	Circulating VLDL and IDL	Transport CHOL to various tissues
High-density lipoproteins (HDL)	1.063–1.21	10–20	33/67	A, C	CHOL, PL	Liver	Reverse CHOL transport from peripheral tissue to liver

TG: Triacylglycerol; CHOL: Cholesterol; PL: Phospholipids; FFA: Free fatty acids

Very Low-Density Lipoproteins

Very low-density lipoproteins **(VLDL)**, also called **pre β-lipoproteins**, are **composed of triacylglycerols**, like chylomicrons, but their function is to **transport lipid from liver to the peripheral tissues**.

- VLDL is released from the **liver** as **nascent VLDL**, similar to the release of nascent chylomicrons from the intestinal mucosa. Nascent VLDL particles contain **apo B-100 and apo A-1**.
- Subsequently, they **acquire apo C-II and apo E from** the circulating HDL and **converted** to **VLDL**.
- During circulation, **lipoprotein lipase hydrolyses triacylglycerols** and releases **free fatty acids**, which are **taken-up by the peripheral tissues**.
- **Apo C and apo E are transferred to HDL**.
- In addition, **cholesteryl esters**, which are synthesized in the plasma as a result of the action of lecithin cholesterol acyltransferase (LCAT), are **transferred from HDL to VLDL** and IDL, via cholesteryl ester transfer protein (CETP).
- As a result of it, their particle size is reduced and density is increased. VLDL particles are, hence, converted to **VLDL remnants**, which are also designated as intermediate density lipoproteins (IDL).
- IDL particles are removed by the liver or converted to the LDL.

Low-Density Lipoproteins

Low-density lipoproteins (LDL) **contain high concentration of cholesterol**. They retain apo B-100 and lose other apoproteins to HDL. **Primary function** of LDL **is to transport cholesterol from liver to the extrahepatic tissues**.

- LDL **binds to its receptors**, which are present in the cell membrane. The LDL receptors are negatively charged glycoproteins that are clustered in the pit on the cell membrane and **recognize apo B-100**, which, in turn, acts as a ligand between the IDL and its receptor. The intracellular side of the pits is coated with a protein, called clathrin, which stabilizes shape of the pit. Ability of the tissues to take up LDL depends upon the rate of transcapillary transport as well as the number of receptors. The number of these receptors is regulated by cholesterol content of the cell.
- After binding, **LDL particles are internalized by endocytosis**, in the form of vesicles. These vesicles rapidly **loose clathrin coat, fuse with the other vesicles and form endosomes** (large vesicles). This, in turn, results in **separation of LDL particles from their receptors**.
- **Receptors are recycled**, whereas **endosome contents are degraded**, resulting in release of cholesterol, free fatty acids, phospholipids and amino acids.
- **Free cholesterol is used for membrane biosynthesis or converted to steroid hormones**. Excess of the cholesterol, however, is re-esterified by acylcholesterol acyltransferase (ACAT) and is stored.
- In man, 70–80% of LDL is removed by LDL receptors while rest of it is removed by the nonspecific endocytosis via the scavenger pathway. The latter is also a receptor-mediated process involving phagocytic cells in the reticuloendothelial system.

High-Density Lipoproteins

High density lipoprotein (HDL) particles are **synthesized in the liver** and are **released into the blood stream by exocytosis**.

- Secretory HDL particles are called **nascent HDL** and are discoid in shape. Nascent HDL is composed of **apo A, apo E, phospholipids and free cholesterol**.
- There also occurs transfer of **apo C** from the chylomicrons and VLDL to nascent HDL, which is converted to **mature HDL**, also called HDL_3.
- From HDL_3, **cholesteryl esters** (produced by the action of LCAT) **are shifted to VLDL and IDL**.
- At the same time, HDL_3 **acquires triacylglycerols** and is converted to LDL.

Metabolism of various lipoproteins is outlined in Fig. 33.1.

HYPERLIPOPROTEINEMIAS

Hyper-lipoproteinemias **(hyperlipidemias)** refers to the **increased levels of lipoproteins in the blood**. It may be a **result of either increased rate of synthesis of lipoproteins or their reduced clearance from the blood**. As we know, lipoproteins are the complex particles consisting of lipids (triglycerides and cholesterol) and proteins (apoproteins), accordingly, **hyper-lipoproteinemias can be detected by measuring various parameters of the lipid profile** (Table 33.2).

There are **several types of hyper-lipoproteinemias**, depending upon the type of the lipid affected.

Type I hyperlipoproteinemia: This condition is also called **hyper-chylomicronemia** or **familial fat-induced hyperlipemia**. This is **due to the accumulation of chylomicrons**. These patients have **very high levels of triacylglycerols** (over 1000 mg/dl) **with a proportionally smaller increase in cholesterol** in their plasma. Type I hyperlipoproteinemia may be due to three different types of genetic abnormalities:

- **Familial lipoprotein lipase deficiency:** It is, usually, **present in infancy or childhood**. There are **recurrent episodes of abdominal pain**, due to attacks of acute pancreatitis, which are triggered by very high plasma levels of triacylglycerols. **Patients may also have** skin lesions called **eruptive xanthomata** which appear **on buttocks, back, knees and elbows**. These lesions **contain a lot of triacylglycerols**, due to the deposition of chylomicrons. Its **diagnosis can be confirmed by**

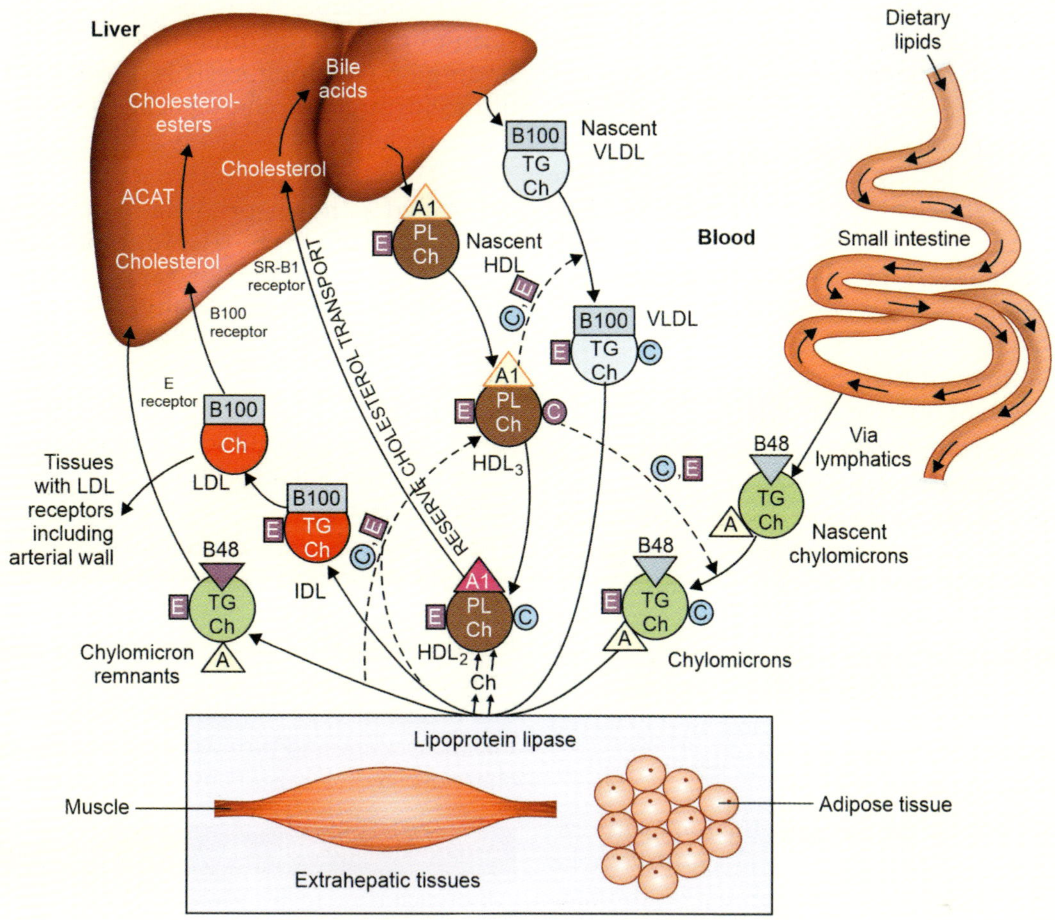

Fig. 33.1: Outline of lipoproteins metabolism

Table 33.2: Classification of hyperlipoproteinemias	
Type	↑ *Lipoproteins*
Primary	
I. Exogenous hypertriglyceridemia	Chylomicrons
IIa. Hypercholesterolemia	LDL
IIb. Combined hyperlipidemia	LDL + VLDL
III. Remnant hyperlipidemia	Remnant VLDL
IV. Endogenous hyperlipidemia	VLDL
V. Mixed hyperlipidemia	VLDL + Chylomicrons
Secondary	
Type IV pattern: Diabetes mellitus, alcoholism, von Gierke's disease, lipodystrophies, acromegaly, oral contraceptives, uremia, hypothyroidism, high carbohydrate diet	VLDL

measuring lipoprotein lipase activity in the plasma after a bolus injection of heparin.

- **Familial Apo C2 deficiency:** It is a rare condition which is inherited as an **autosomal recessive disorder**. It is due to the deficiency of Apo C2 which is essential for the activation of lipoprotein lipase. Hence, there is impaired removal of, both, **chylomicrons and VLDL from the plasma**. This, in turn, results in the lipoprotein pattern which may be of type I or type V. It is an **autosomal dominant** condition of the type I hyperlipoproteinemia. The patient has low post-heparin plasma lipolytic activity **but high levels of lipoprotein lipase in the adipose tissue**. Plasma of the affected individuals contains a nondialyzable, heat stable inhibitor of lipoprotein lipase. Occasionally, subjects with type I phenotype may also show a type V pattern, due to the **accumulation of VLDL in their plasma**. This is common, if they ingest a high carbohydrate diet.

Type II hyper-lipoproteinemia: It may be further sub-classified as:

- **Type IIa hyperlipoproteinemia:** It is also called **familial hypercholesterolemia** or **familial hyper-beta-lipoproteinemia**. There is **high cholesterol** in fasting plasma **without increase in triacylglycerols. Electrophoretic pattern** also **shows an increase in β-lipoproteins**.

It may be a primary disorder due to some genetic abnormality or a secondary lipoprotein disorder.

- **Primary type IIa hyper-lipoproteinemia,** also called as **familial type IIa hyperlipoproteinemia,** may be **seen in heterozygotes or homozygotes.**
  - Heterozygous familial type IIa hyperlipoproteinemia is an **autosomal dominant** inherited disease, usually, from many different **genetic mutations affecting the gene for LDL, for Apo B and Apo E receptors**. These patients **have very high levels of plasma cholesterol and LDL**. Some of these patients may also show moderate elevation of triacylglycerols.

    Mutations for LDL receptor gene can cause **four different types of disorders:**

    a. The **most common type** is **mutant allele,** where **no receptors are synthesized.**

    b. **Second type** of disorder is the one where **receptors are synthesized,** but are **transported slowly from the endoplasmic reticulum to the Golgi apparatus.**

    c. **Receptors** are processed and reach the cell surface but **fail to bind LDL.**

    d. **Receptors** reach the surface and bind LDL, but **fail to cluster in the coated-pits,** and cannot be internalized.
  - **Homozygous familial type IIa hyper-liporoteinemia** is, generally, seen in **children** who present **with planar or tuberous xanthomata since birth. Yellowish plaques or lumps occur on buttocks, knees, elbows and hands. Cardiovascular disease may develop before the age of 10 years.**
- **Secondary type IIa hyper-lipoproteinemia** results in **hypercholesterolemia,** which can be caused by several common disorders unrelated to familial conditions, such as **Cushing's syndrome, hypothyroidism, anorexia nervosa, nephrotic syndrome, primary liver cell carcinoma or diabetes mellitus.**

• **Type IIb hyper-lipoproteinemia:** It is also called **familial combined hyper-lipidemia** or **multiple lipoprotein type hyper-lipidemia.** There is an **increase in total plasma cholesterol and triacylglycerols.** On electrophoresis, there is an increase in the **intensity of both β- and pre-β-bands, due to increased production of VLDL and LDL.** Composition of the individual lipoproteins is normal. Obesity, high serum uric acid levels and glucose intolerance are common in patients with this pattern.

Type III hyperlipoproteinemia: It is also called **dysbetalipoproteinemia** or **remnant hyperlipoproteinemia,** or **broad, floating beta disease** or **familial type III hyperlipoproteinemia.** There is a **moderate hypercholesterolemia** while hyper-triacylglyceridemia is relatively uncommon. This is **associated with the presence of chylomicron remnants and IDL in plasma.** The disease rarely manifests itself before early adult life in males or before the menopause in females. Fasting serum or plasma is often turbid. The characteristic finding on electrophoresis is a **broad β-band** but on ultracentrifugation these particles are isolated in the VLDL region.

Type IV hyper-lipoproteinemia: This condition is also called as **hyper-pre-beta-hyper-lipoproteinemia** or **endogenous hyper-lipidemia** or **diet-induced hypertriglyceridemia** or **familial type IV hyper-lipoproteinemia.** These patients have a marked **elevation of plasma triacylglycerols in VLDL.** In some families, there is excessive **VLDL secretion** while in others the **removal rate of VLDL from plasma is reduced.** Fasting serum or plasma is turbid. On electrophoresis, there is a **marked pre-β-band** with **normal** β- and a **normal or reduced** α**-band.**

Type V hyper-lipoproteinemia: It is also called mixed hyper-lipidemia, since large amounts of, both, chylomicrons and VLDL are seen in the fasting plasma. It is occasionally seen in patients whose characteristic pattern is like type I (due to lipoprotein lipase deficiency) but rarely of type IV. Whole blood may be lipemic. Plasma is white and turbid. The electrophoretic pattern is characterized by raised chylomicrons and VLDL levels.

ATHEROSCLEROSIS

Atherosclerosis (arteriosclerosis) is a disease of arterial wall. It is characterized by the accumulation of cholesterol and its esters of lipoproteins containing Apo B-100 in cells which are derived from monocyte macrophage that line smooth muscle cells. This, in turn, results in the formation of atherosclerotic plaque, which narrows the blood vessels and serves as the site of thrombus formation (Fig. 33.2).

- **Important contributory factors,** favorable in the development of atherosclerosis, include **high calorie diet** or **diet rich in saturated fat and cholesterol, hypercholesterolemia, sedentary lifestyle, stress and strain, obesity, hypertension and smoking.**
- **Risk of developing the disease** is **directly related to the concentration of the LDL-cholesterol (bad cholesterol) in plasma.** It is also **inversely related to the plasma concentration of HDL-cholesterol (good cholesterol).**
- Besides, diseases with prolonged elevated level of LDL, VLDL, IDL or chylomicron remnants in blood, like **diabetes mellitus, hypothyroidism, lipid nephrosis,** etc. **are associated with severe atherosclerosis.**
- **Lipoprotein(a)** or Lp(a) is also an independent risk factor. It contains apo(a) which is similar to plasminogen in structure. It competes with plasminogen for conversion to plasmin which degrades fibrin in the blood clots. This apo(a) is different from Apo A of HDL.
- **Indians are genetically predisposed and are at an increased risk of developing atherosclerosis** at an

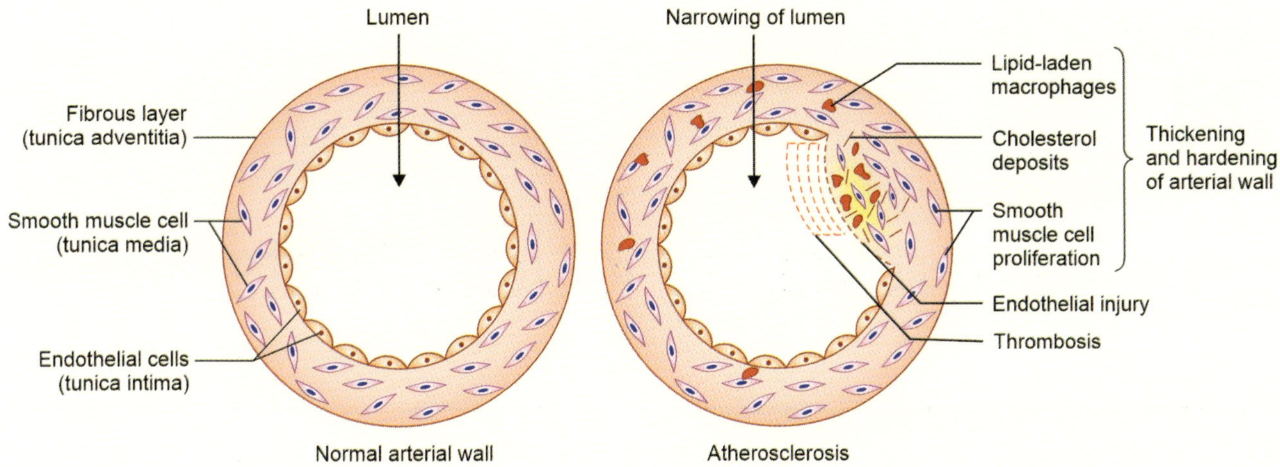

Fig. 33.2: Atherosclerosis

early age, hence, sometimes known as premature atherosclerosis. About 40% Indians have higher levels of Lp(a).

Dietary Recommendations

- **Reduce the total amount of fat.** Not more than 30% of total energy intake should come from fat.
- **Reduce the use of animal fat.** Not more than one-third of the total fat (less than 10% calories/day) should come from saturated fat, with the remainder from unsaturated fat.
- **Reduce the intake of cholesterol.** Dietary cholesterol should be less than 300 mg/day.
- **Trans-fatty acid intake should limit to less than 1%** calories/day.
- **Increase omega-3 fatty acid intake** from dietary or supplementary fish oil.
- **Eat five or more servings of fruits** and vegetables/day.
- **Reduce salt intake.**

Other Lifestyle Interventions

- **Promotion of physical activity**, e.g. adults should perform at least 30 minutes of moderate activity (brisk walking), at least 5 days per week.
- **Maintaining ideal body weight** emphasizes activity.
- **Limit sedentary activities**
- **Give up smoking.**

LIPID PROFILE

Serum lipids and lipoprotein fractions are, generally, measured after 12 hours of fasting, to allow complete clearing of chylomicrons. Serum may appear hazy when serum triglycerides exceed 200 mg/dL. Chylomicrons can be easily detected because they form a white supernatant after refrigeration.

The following **parameters are included under a serum lipid profile** or lipidogram:

- **Total cholesterol** (which is a sum of cholesterol distributed in LDL, VLDL and HDL): 150–220 mg/dL (desirable **140–200 mg/dL**)
- **LDL-cholesterol: 60–160 mg/dL**
- **VLDL-cholesterol: <32 mg/dL**
- **HDL-cholesterol: 30–60 mg/dL**
- **Triglycerides: 50–160 mg/dL**

Friedwald's formula

According to **Friedwald's formula, VLDL-cholesterol is** calculated by **triglycerides/5** (provided triglycerides are <400 mg/dL).

Thereafter, **LDL-cholesterol can be calculated**, as follows:

LDL-cholesterol = Total cholesterol – [HDL cholesterol + Triglycerides/5]

- **Cardiac risk ratio:** It is the **ratio of total cholesterol to HDL-cholesterol**. A **ratio >5 indicates an increased cardiovascular risk**.
- **Special investigations:** In several cases, some special investigations may also be performed. These include plasma **troponin, myoglobin, homocysteine, lipoprotein(a)** and **C-reactive protein**, etc.

Some Important Questions

1. **Define lipoproteins. Describe their formation, functions and turnover.**
2. **Write notes on:**
   i. Atherosclerosis
   ii. Lipoproteins
   iii. Lipid profile
   iv. Hyper-lipoproteinemias

Chapter 34

Thyroid Function Tests

Thyroid gland is **located in the neck**. Its **main function is the synthesis of thyroid hormones** referred to as thyroxine **(T_4)** and triiodothyronine **(T_3)**.

- In order to synthesize T_4 and T_3, thyroid gland **requires iodine**.
- Iodine is taken up from the bloodstream into the thyroid gland, where it undergoes different chemical reactions, and produce T_4 and T_3.
- **T_4 has four atoms of iodine** while **T_3 has three atoms of iodine**.
- In the cells and tissues of the body **most of the T_4 is converted to T_3**.
- **T_3 is biologically more active** than T_4.

HYPERTHYROIDISM

Hyperthyroidism, often called **overactive thyroid**, is a condition in which the **thyroid gland produces and secretes excessive amounts** of the **thyroid hormones** (T_4 and/or T_3).

Hyperthyroidism may be **caused by various conditions**, such as **Graves' disease** (an autoimmune disorder). Other causes include **excessive intake of iodine** (needed to make T_4 and T_3), **inflammation of the thyroid gland** (thyroiditis which causes T_4 and T_3 to leak out of the gland), **tumor of the thyroid or pituitary gland**, or **taking large amount of thyroxine** (as medication).

Graves' disease: Graves' disease is the most common form or cause of hyperthyroidism. In this condition **antibodies stimulate thyroid gland to secrete too much of the thyroid hormones** (T_4 and T_3). Clinically, **eyes look enlarged**, because eye muscles swell and push the eye forward, called **exophthalmos**. Some patients also have **swelling of the front of the neck** from an enlarged thyroid gland. It occurs more often in women and tends to run in families. Other symptoms include **weakness, irregular heartbeat, difficulty in sleeping, itching, hair loss, nausea and vomiting,** besides breast development in men.

Thyrotoxicosis: Thyrotoxicosis is a **hypermetabolic clinical syndrome due to elevated serum levels of T_4 and/or T_3**. Thyrotoxicosis can also occur without hyperthyroidism. Some people develop thyrotoxicosis due to **inflammation of the thyroid gland (thyroiditis),** which can lead to the **excessive release of the thyroid hormones,** already stored in the gland (without the accelerated hormone production that characterizes hyperthyroidism). Thyrotoxicosis can also occur after excessive ingestion of exogenous thyroid hormone, in the form of thyroid hormone supplements/medicine. It may be asymptomatic, but if observed, these symptoms are due to an excess of the thyroid hormone.

Major clinical signs of hyperthyroidism include **weight loss** (often accompanied by increase in appetite), **anxiety and intolerance to heat, hair loss** (especially of the outer side of the eyebrows), **muscle aches, weakness, fatigue, hyperactivity, irritability, hyperglycemia, polyuria, polydipsia, delirium, tremor and sweating**.

Biochemical tests that may be performed to evaluate the diagnosis, include estimation of serum cholesterol (which is reduced due to the elevated metabolic rate), T_4, T_3 and TSH (produced by the hypothalamus that stimulates the thyroid gland to produce thyroid hormones).

HYPOTHYROIDISM

Hypothyroidism, often called **underactive thyroid**, is a common endocrine disorder in which thyroid gland does not produce enough thyroid hormone.

- Iodine deficiency is the most common cause of primary hypothyroidism and endemic goiter, worldwide.
- In areas with sufficient dietary iodine, hypothyroidism is most commonly caused by the autoimmune disease such as **Hashimoto's thyroiditis** (chronic autoimmune thyroiditis).

Hashimoto's disease may be associated with goiter. It is characterized by **infiltration of the thyroid gland with T-lymphocytes** and the **autoantibodies** produced against specific thyroid antigens, such as **thyroid peroxidase, thyroglobulin** and the **TSH-receptors. Autoimmune thyroiditis is also associated with** other immune-mediated diseases such as **diabetes mellitus type I, pernicious anemia, myasthenia gravis, rheumatoid arthritis,** etc.

- **Hyperthyroidism,** due to certain types of thyroiditis, **can also,** eventually, **lead to hypothyroidism** (lack of thyroid hormone), as the thyroid gland is damaged.
- **Radioiodine treatment of Graves' disease,** eventually, **can also lead to hypothyroidism.**
- Hypothyroidism can cause a number of **symptoms,** such as **tiredness, poor ability to tolerate cold** and **weight gain.**
- In children, hypothyroidism leads to **delays in growth and intellectual development,** and in severe cases **cretinism.** These children are dwarf and mentally retarded.
- **Diagnosis** of hypothyroidism, when suspected, **can be confirmed** with blood tests **by measuring TSH and thyroxine levels.**

BIOCHEMICAL EVALUATION OF THYROID FUNCTIONS

Biochemical evaluation, to establish if there is any thyroid dysfunction, **can be done by performing several thyroid function tests,** a collective term for blood tests used to check functioning of the thyroid gland (hyperthyroidism or hypothyroidism) or to monitor effectiveness of treatment.

These tests include **measurement of** the thyroid hormones (T_3 and T_4) and **TSH** in serum. Other tests include **radioactive iodine uptake, protein bound iodine, serum cholesterol,** etc.

- **Thyroid hormones:** Thyroid function test panel typically includes thyroid-stimulating hormone (TSH or thyrotropin), thyroxine (T_4) and triiodothyronine (T_3).
  - **Thyroxine:** Thyroxine level is, generally, **elevated in hyperthyroidism** and **decreased in hypothyroidism.** It is also, usually, slightly elevated in pregnancy, secondary to the increased levels of thyroid binding globulin (TBG).
    - Serum T_4 **value in a normal person is in the range of 4.5 to 12.5 mg/dL.**
    - In hyperthyroidism, serum T_4 concentration is increased to >12 mg/dL, whereas in hypothyroidism the value is < 5 mg/dL.
    - **Estimation of free thyroxine (FT_4),** however, provides **more reliable** information than total T_4.
  - **Triiodothyronine:** Similar to T_4, T_3 is also, generally, **elevated in hyperthyroidism and decreased in hypothyroidism.**
    - **Normal value** for serum T_3 varies **between 86 and 187 ng/dL.**
    - Its concentration is **low at birth and rises to near adult level in early childhood** and maintained up to 30 years of age, after which the value again falls.
    - **Estimation of free T_3 (FT_3),** however, provides more reliable information than total T4.
    - Measurement of **reverse T_3** (rT_3, a catabolic product of T_4) may also be helpful in the evaluation of some cases, e.g. in low T_3 syndrome where rT_3 concentration is increased.
- **Thyroid-stimulating hormone:** Thyroid-stimulating hormone **(TSH)** is a **most sensitive test** for the evaluation of thyroid function.
  - TSH is **produced in the pituitary gland.**
  - Production of TSH is **controlled by** thyrotropin releasing hormone **(TRH),** which is produced in the hypothalamus.
  - **Reference value** for serum TSH concentration **is in the range of 0.3–5.0 mIU/L.**
  - TSH levels may be **suppressed by excess free T_3 or free T_4** in the blood.
  - Measurement of TSH is **most useful and sensitive for primary hypothyroidism.**
- **Thyroxine-binding globulin: Reference range** for thyroxine-binding globulin (TBG) is **12–30 mg/L.** Increased TBG results in increased total T_4 and T_3 without an actual increase in the hormonal activity of the thyroid hormones.
- **Thyroid hormone uptake:** Thyroid hormone uptake (T-uptake or T_3-uptake) is **a measure of the unbound thyroxine-binding globulin** in blood, i.e. the TBG which is unsaturated with thyroid hormones. Unsaturated TBG increases with decreased levels of thyroid hormones. It is not directly related to T_3.
- **Stimulation/suppression tests:**
  - **Thyrotropin releasing hormone (TRH) stimulation test:** TRH stimulation test is used to **assess functional state of the TSH secretory mechanism.**
    - **Serum TSH is assayed before,** and **after 20, 30 and 60 minutes of the administration of** a standard dose of **TRH.**
    - **In normal individuals, serum TSH peaks are observed in 30 minutes** and values, generally, range **between 5 and 30 mIU/L.**
    - A **normal response excludes the possibility of thyrotoxicosis.**
    - **In hyperthyroidism, no significant rise in TSH occurs,** because elevated thyroid hormones inhibit TSH production.
    - **In primary hypothyroidism, TSH response to TRH is exaggerated** and is of diagnostic significance.
    - It is often **useful in differentiating between pituitary and hypothalamic lesion** as the cause of secondary hypothyroidism.
  - **Thyroid suppression test:** Normally exogenous thyroid hormone suppresses pituitary TSH secretion, resulting in a decrease in radioactive iodine uptake (RAIU). An **abnormal suppression test is observed**

in hyperthyroidism, irrespective of the underlying cause.

- **Autoimmune profile antibodies against thyroid peroxidase (anti-TPO antibodies): Anti-TPO antibodies** may be **detected in the serum of some hypothyroid patients**. In Graves' disease, long-acting thyroid stimulator (LATS) is detectable in serum.
- **Other tests:** These include RAIU, PBI, BMR, cholesterol, etc.
  - **Radioactive iodine uptake (RAIU):** As iodine plays an important role in the metabolism of the thyroid gland, radioactive iodine uptake (RAIU) is used for thyroid function studies.
    - For this purpose, usually, **10 µci** (microcurie) **of sodium or potassium iodide is administered orally** (^{125}I delivers low radiation dose, hence, it is preferred over ^{131}I).
    - **Radioactivity mixes uniformly with the endogenous iodide in the extracellular fluid.**
    - **Percentage of the iodide entering and leaving the extracellular space per unit time**, which is accumulated by the thyroid in the steady state, **is assessed**.
    - RAIU is, usually, **measured 24 hours after the administration of the isotope**.
    - Normally, **24 hours RAIU uptake is 5–30% of the administered dose**.
    - **Value above the normal range indicate hyperfunctioning** of the gland and are useful in the diagnosis of hyperthyroidism.
    - RAIU is **also used as a part of thyroid suppression test**.
  - **Protein-bound iodine** Serum protein-bound iodine (PBI) is an **indirect measure for assessing thyroid function,** since about 90% of the iodine in serum is bound to thyroxine.
    - PBI value in a **normal subject, ranges from 4 to 8 mg/100 mL**.
    - **In hypothyroidism,** PBI value varies from **0.2 to 2.5 mg/100 mL**, whereas **in hyperthyroidism** PBI value ranges from **9 to 18 mg/100 mL**.
  - **Basal metabolic rate (BMR):** It is a **measurement of oxygen consumption in the basal state**. BMR is **raised in hyperthyroidism** and is **reduced in hypothyroidism**.
  - **Serum cholesterol: Increase** in serum cholesterol is observed **in hypothyroidism**, whereas it is **decreased in hyperthyroidism** or thyrotoxicosis.
  - **Serum calcium: Hyperthyroidism** may result in **increased plasma calcium** along with increased plasma alkaline phosphatase activity.
  - **Glucose tolerance test (GTT):** It is sometimes **abnormal in patients with hyperthyroidism**, who may show a diabetic type of response.

Some Important Questions

1. **What is the biochemical function of the thyroid gland? Explain various biochemical test to evaluate thyroid functions.**
2. **Write notes on:**
   i. Hypothyroidism
   ii. Hyperthyroidism
   iii. Thyroid stimulation test
   iv. Thyroid suppression test

Chapter

35

Liver Function Tests

The **liver is a multifunctional organ** that is involved in a **number of excretory, synthetic and metabolic functions** (Table 35.1).

Table 35.1: Important biochemical functions of the liver
Metabolism of nutrients • Carbohydrates • Proteins • Fats
Synthesis of proteins • Albumin • α- and β-globulins • Clotting factors • Transport proteins
Metabolism and excretion of exogenous substances • Alcohol • Drugs • Toxins
Metabolism and excretion of endogenous substances • Bilirubin • Hormones
Storage of vitamins • Vitamin A • Vitamin B_{12}
Minerals • Iron

FUNCTIONS OF THE LIVER

1. The liver has a major influence on the **flow of nutrients to the rest of the body**. It controls the release of absorbed material into the systemic circulation and **has a central role in carbohydrate, protein and fat metabolism**.
2. The liver is an important site for the **storage of glycogen and for gluconeogenesis**.
3. Most proteins in plasma including **albumin, α and β-globulins, clotting factors and transport proteins are synthesized by the liver**.
4. This is also the **site for urea synthesis**.
5. **Fatty acids and phospholipids are** also taken up from circulation by the liver and are **metabolized** there.
6. **Cholesterol is also synthesized** and **esterified** in the liver.
7. Liver is also a site for the **detoxification of exogenous compounds** (such as alcohol, drugs and toxins) as well as endogenous materials (such as bilirubin and hormones), which are excreted via the kidney or the biliary system.
8. **Bile salts are synthesized** in the liver.
9. Liver stores various substances, such as **vitamins and minerals**, and releases them as and when required.
10. Liver is also one of the biggest reticuloendothelial organs and has important **immune functions.**

LIVER FUNCTION TESTS

Various liver function tests that are **useful in the assessment of a liver disease include** the estimation of **serum protein patterns and the levels of serum enzymes and bilirubin** (Table 35.2).

Table 35.2: Commonly used biochemical tests for the assessment of liver functions
Total proteins **Albumin** **Bilirubin** **Enzymes** • GPT and GOT • Alkaline phosphatase • γ-Glutamyltranspeptidase (γ-GT) • 5′-Nucleotidase • Glutamate dehydrogenase

PLASMA PROTEIN PATTERN

Normal serum concentrations of some of the liver function test parameters, which are done routinely, are shown in Table 35.3.

Table 35.3: Normal serum concentration of some of the liver function test parameters, which are done routinely

Parameters	*Normal values*
Plasma albumin	3.5–5.5 g/dL
SGOT activity	Up to 40 U/L
SGPT activity	Up to 56 U/L
Alkaline phosphatase activity	80–300 U/L
Total bilirubin	<0.8 mg/dL
γ-GT activity	5–35 U/L

As liver is the primary site of the synthesis of plasma proteins, a **disturbance in protein synthesis occurs as a consequence of impaired hepatic function**. Decreased synthesis of protein leads to a decrease in their plasma concentration. **Plasma albumin** concentration **provides** a fairly **good index of the progress of a chronic liver disease**. Pattern of alteration in plasma proteins, however, depends upon the type, severity and duration of the liver injury.

- **In a severe liver disease,** hepatic **synthesis of albumin is decreased.**
- **In chronic hepatocellular damage** also, **serum albumin concentration falls.**
- **Serum protein electrophoresis**, to determine the proportion of different serum proteins, is also helpful in the diagnosis of a liver disease, e.g. α_2- **and** β **globulins are increased in cirrhosis,** due to their increased production and decreased clearance (*see* Fig. 30.1).
- **In cholestasis,** there is a **small increase in serum γ-globulin** with a **more increase in α- and β-globulins**, due, in part, to increased serum lipoproteins.

SERUM ENZYME LEVELS

Serum levels of **several enzymes are elevated in liver diseases,** e.g. **SGPT (ALT), SGOT (AST)**, ALP, γ-GT, etc.

- **SGOT/SGPT: In viral hepatitis and other** forms of a **liver disease**, which may be associated with hepatic necrosis, **serum GPT** (ALT) and **GOT** (AST) **levels are elevated.**
  - **ALT and AST levels are elevated even before the clinical signs and symptoms of the disease appear**. Levels of both the enzymes may reach the values as high **as 100 times the upper normal limit. Peak values occur between day seven and day twelve**. Thereafter, their activities **gradually decrease** and **reach toward normal by the third to fifth weak** of recovery.
  - Five to ten-fold increase in both the enzymes also occur **in patients with primary metastatic carcinoma of the liver.**
  - Although serum levels of both GPT and GOT are elevated in a liver disease, however, GPT levels are, comparatively, more elevated, as it is more liver specific.
- **Alkaline phosphatase:** Serum alkaline phosphatase levels are **important in a hepatobiliary disease** (as well as in bone diseases that are associated with increased osteoblastic activity). As biliary obstruction **results in induction of the enzyme, rise is more marked in extrahepatic obstruction** than in intrahepatic obstruction.
- **γ-Glutamyl-transferase:** γ-Glutamyl-transferase, also referred to as **γ-glutamyl-transpeptidase (γ-GT)**, is **present in high concentration in the serum in intrahepatic or post-hepatic biliary obstruction**.

  Elevated levels of γ-GT are also observed **in the sera of** people who are **heavy drinkers**. This **enzyme** has been shown to be **of significance in the detection of an alcohol-induced liver disease**.
- **Glutamate dehydrogenase:** Glutamate dehydrogenase **(GDH)** is found in the liver, heart, muscle and kidney. It is present only in traces in normal serum but **increased activity is observed in a liver disease with hepatocellular damage**.
- **5′-Nucleotidase:** 5′-Nucleotidase **(5′-NT)** activity is **increased** by two to six folds, **in some of the hepatobiliary diseases**. It may be **due to extrahepatic causes** such as **stone or tumor obstructing the bile duct**, or **in intrahepatic conditions**, e.g. **cholestasis** that may be caused by chlorpromazine, malignant infiltration of the liver or biliary cirrhosis.

SERUM BILIRUBIN

As discussed in Chapter 31, bilirubin is an **orange-yellow pigment**, derived from the **breakdown of red blood cells** in the liver, spleen and bone marrow. **Bilirubin, normally present in the blood is bound to albumin** and is **transported to the liver.** In the hepatocytes, **bilirubin gets conjugated with UDP-glucuronate**. Thus, serum contains two forms of bilirubin, which are referred to as:

1. **Unconjugated bilirubin:** It is lipid-soluble, bound to albumin and is transported from the reticuloendothelial system to the liver.
2. **Conjugated bilirubin:** It is water-soluble and is regurgitated from the liver into the plasma.

Normal value for total bilirubin (sum of the unconjugated and conjugated forms) is 0.1–1.0 mg/ 100 mL of serum or plasma. **Under normal conditions almost all the bilirubin in plasma is unconjugated**.

Disorders of bilirubin metabolism leads to **hyperbilirubinemia,** where serial measurements of bilirubin are helpful in knowing severity of the liver disease. **Bilirubin fractionation is also helpful in** differential diagnosis of jaundice.

JAUNDICE

Jaundice is a physical sign, characterized by the **yellow appearance** of the patient, and is a most characteristic **clinical manifestation of hyperbilirubinemia**.

- Jaundice results from the **deposition of bilirubin** (bile pigment) **in the skin, mucous membrane and sclera** of the patient.
- It is **apparent clinically when serum bilirubin level is more than 2 mg/dL**.
- When serum bilirubin is **below 2 mg/dL**, it is called **latent jaundice (subclinical jaundice)**, since it is not detectable at this stage, clinically.

CLASSIFICATION AND EVALUATION

There are **three types of jaundice**, referred to as **prehepatic, hepatic** and **post-hepatic** jaundice. **Biochemical evaluation of the three types of jaundice** can be done as shown in Table 35.4.

Table 35.4: Differential diagnosis of different types of jaundice based on various biochemical tests

Biochemical parameter	*Type of jaundice*		
	Pre-hepatic	*Hepatic*	*Post-hepatic*
Serum bilirubin	↑↑	↑↑	↑↑
Type of bilirubin	Unconjugated	Both	Conjugated
Urine urobilinogen	↑↑	N/↑	↓/ –
Urine bile pigments	– –	– –	↑
Stercobilinogen	↑	↓	↓/ –
SGPT/SGOT (mainly SGPT)	N	↑↑↑	↑
Serum alkaline phosphatase	N	↑	↑↑↑
Serum 5′-nucleotidase	N	↑	↑↑↑

- **Pre-hepatic jaundice:** Pre-hepatic jaundice, also called **hemolytic jaundice**, is **characterized by the excessive presence of unconjugated bilirubin**.

  Prehepatic jaundice may be a **result of increased production of unconjugated bilirubin** (such as in hemolysis), **decreased uptake of unconjugated bilirubin across the hepatocyte membrane** (as in Gilbert syndrome), or **decreased biotransformation** (such as in neonatal jaundice, Crigler-Najjar syndrome, etc.).

  - **Hemolysis:** In the **disorders which are associated with hemolysis** (hemolytic anemia), the **rate of bilirubin production is increased,** which, in turn, exceeds the amount that cannot be removed by the liver.
  - **Gilbert syndrome:** Gilbert syndrome is a **heterogeneous group** of disorders, inherited as **autosomal recessive trait.** Several defects include the **deficiency of bilirubin glucuronyl-transferase**, a **defect in hepatic uptake of bilirubin, or decrease in red cell survival**.
  - **Neonatal jaundice:** Neonatal jaundice is also called **physiological jaundice of the newborn. Every infant exhibits some transient unconjugated hyperbilirubinemia** (about 5 mg/dL) **between the second and the fifth day of life,** as at this stage hepatic glucuronyl-transferase activity is not fully developed. Activity of the enzyme increases **within 2 weeks after birth** when serum bilirubin level returns to normal.
    - Neonatal jaundice is **more pronounced in premature infants**.
    - Unconjugated bilirubin **levels above 18 mg/dL leads to deposition of bilirubin in the lipid-rich basal ganglia.** This is referred to as kernicterus.
  - **Crigler-Najjar syndrome:** This disorder is known to exist in two forms:
    - **Type I:** It is **clinically more severe** form of the disease, **due to complete absence of glucuronyl-transferase**.
    - **Type II:** It has **moderate clinical findings** and is **due to partial deficiency of the enzyme glucuronyl-transferase**.

    In both the conditions, unconjugated bilirubin is significantly raised.
- **Hepatic jaundice:** Hepatic jaundice is **due to some primary disease.** Plasma, usually, shows **elevated levels of both conjugated as well as unconjugated bilirubin,** e.g. in **viral hepatitis, liver cirrhosis,** etc. Besides bilirubin, there is **also an increase in SGOT and SGPT levels**.
  - Elevated levels of conjugated as well as unconjugated bilirubin along with the dark-brown pigmentation in the liver cells is also observed in **Dubin-Johnson syndrome (a benign, autosomal recessive condition)**.
  - **Inhalation, ingestion** or parenteral **administration of** several pharmacological and chemical agents, such as **carbon tetrachloride, acetaminophen, isoniazid or chlorpromazine** (which result in liver injury) also leads to hepatic jaundice.
- **Post-hepatic jaundice:** Post-hepatic jaundice, also referred to as **obstructive jaundice** or **post-hepatic cholestasis,** is **caused by obstruction of the bile duct** (may be due to gallstones, carcinoma of the head of pancreas or carcinoma of the bile duct). Serum of such a patient shows **excessive amount of conjugated bilirubin**. It is also characterized by the **presence of the excessive amount of** bilirubin **(bile pigments) in the urine**.

Some Important Questions

1. **Explain various liver function tests**
2. **What is jaundice? Describe various types of jaundice. How will you biochemically differentiate them?**
3. **Describe:**
   i. Liver function tests
   ii. Jaundice
   iii. Various functions of the liver

Chapter 36

Kidney Function Tests

Various metabolic processes occurring in the body produce a number of substances, many of which, such as CO_2, water, nitrogenous compounds and inorganic salts, are the waste products. If not regularly removed from the body, these toxic metabolites may severely affect normal health. **Kidneys excrete most of the water as well as organic and inorganic substances**, whereas CO_2 is expired through lungs.

FUNCTIONS OF THE KIDNEY

Kidney performs several functions (Table 36.1).

Table 36.1: Important functions of the kidney

- Filtration of blood and preparation of ultrafiltrate fluid as urine
- Reabsorption of useful substances such as glucose, amino acids, electrolytes, etc.
- Homeostasis of the extracellular volume
- Maintenance of the acid–base status, water and electrolytes
- Endocrine functions and activation of hormones such as synthesis of erythropoietin, activation of vitamin D, etc.

1. FILTRATION OF BLOOD AND EXCRETION OF WASTE PRODUCTS

Urine is an ultrafiltrate of plasma. Each kidney has nearly one million basic filtration units called **nephrons**.

- A nephron **consists of the glomerulus and the tubule**.
- The **glomerulus is a network of arteriolar afferent and efferent capillaries**, and is **surrounded by a double walled epithelial sac**, called **Bowman's capsule**.
- Bowman's capsule **leads to the tubule**, which is **divided into proximal convoluted tubule, loop of Henle** and **distal convoluted tubule**.
- Loop of Henle consists of the **descending limb**, a **thin segment** and the **ascending limb**.
- **Proximal convoluted tubule has its opening into the descending limb** of the loop of Henle, which continues into the thin segment, from where ascending limb arises.
- It **continues into the distal convoluted tubule**, which, finally, **opens into the collecting duct** (Fig. 36.1).

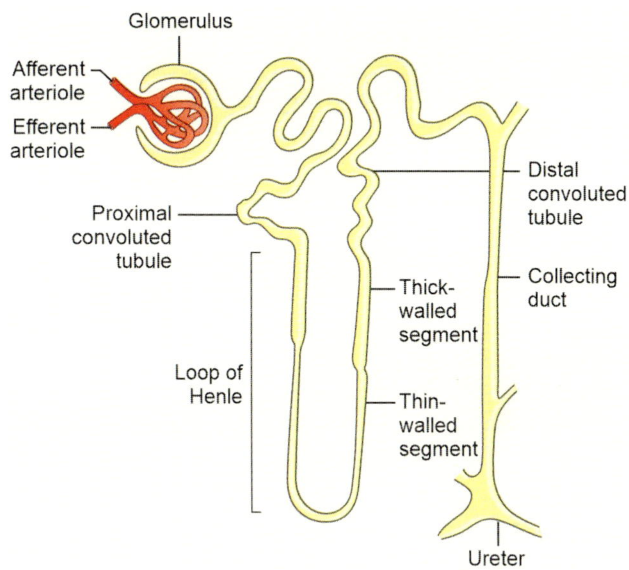

Fig. 36.1: Nephron

Filtration of Blood

- **Filtration of blood is carried out in the nephron through glomeruli** and as the blood passes through the glomeruli, **noncolloidal substances** (usually, of low molecular weight), **filter through capillaries, with the retention of protein** (not normally found in the urine).
- **Total amount of the filtrate formed per minute**, by all the nephrons of both the kidneys, **is known as glomerular filtration rate (GFR)**.
- Under **normal** physiological conditions, **GFR is 125 mL/min**.
- About **150–200 L of the ultrafiltrate passes through the glomeruli in 24 hours**.

Reabsorption of Useful Substances and Excretion of Waste Products

As mentioned above, nearly, **150–200 L of the plasma ultrafiltrate passes through the glomeruli in 24 hours.**

Its **volume is reduced to, nearly, 800–1500 mL per day, as urine**. This is due to the **reabsorption of water and useful solutes** in different regions of the tubule:

- **In the proximal tubule:**
  - Nearly, **60–80% of** water **(the ultrafiltrate) is absorbed in an obligatory fashion, along with the Na^+, Cl^-, HCO_3^-, Ca^{2+}, HPO_4^{2-},** and other ions in the proximal tubule.
  - **Glucose is also reabsorbed by a Na^+-dependent active transport process**, almost completely, in the proximal tubule.
  - **Uric acid is also reabsorbed here**.
  - When the blood level of creatinine increases above normal, **creatinine is secreted in this region**.
- **In the loop of Henle** Cl^- and more of the Na^+, but without water, are reabsorbed, **resulting in a diluted urine**.
- **In the distal tubule** and the **collecting duct, water reabsorption is regulated by** the antidiuretic hormone (**ADH** or vasopressin).
  - As secretion is the prominent activity in the distal tubule, so, **organic ions and K^+ are transported from the blood into the tubular fluid**.
  - This region **also secretes H^+** and **reabsorbs Na^+** and **HCO_3^-**.
  - At the same time, **certain solutes, such as hippuric acid and other organic waste products are added** to the fluid by an excretory function of the tubule.

Thus, Urine Carries off

- **Water and salts** in such amounts, so as **to maintain equilibrium between extracellular and intracellular fluids**,
- **Acids or bases, to maintain acid–base balance**,
- **Waste products,**
- **Toxic and detoxified substances,** and
- **Other substances, which may be present** in blood, **in excessive amounts.**

2. REGULATION OF WATER AND ELECTROLYTES

- **Regulation of water:** Kidney plays an important role in regulating water balance.
  - **If excessive amount of** water **(fluid)** is **ingested, kidney excretes** the same. On the other hand, **if intake is low**, kidney retain water and excretes more concentrated urine.
  - **Water regulation** (homeostasis) **is** intrinsically **linked to renal urea handling**. Only, about 40–50% of the filtered load of urea is reabsorbed.
  - Most of the glomerular filtrate is reabsorbed through tubule cells. Whereas, **about 90% of the water is reabsorbed as a result of the difference in pressure,** the remaining **10% is reabsorbed actively, by** tubular cells, as a result of **the action of ADH**.
  - **In the absence of ADH little water and urea are reabsorbed**, and a large amount of water is excreted. On the other hand, in the presence of ADH only 1.0–1.5 L of the filtrate is excreted as urine.
- **Regulation of electrolytes:** Kidney also plays an important role in the maintenance of electrolyte balance. **Depending upon the dietary intake and physiological needs, salts are either excreted or conserved,** by the kidney, by tubular reabsorption.
  - **Sodium and chloride ions** predominate in the glomerular filtrate. As the glomerular filtrate flows through the tubule, these electrolytes are absorbed into the blood.
    - **Reabsorption of Na^+ is required for the re-absorption of water, Cl^-, glucose, HCO_3^-, urea and amino acids.**
    - Approximately 80% of the Na^+, entering the tubular cells, is in exchange for H^+ secretion, which, in turn, leads to the entry of both Cl^- and HCO_3^-,– into the cells.
    - **Sodium transport is regulated by many factors, which include:**
      - Aldosterone
      - Na^+/K^+-ATPase
      - Na^+-H^+ exchanger
      - H^+-ATPase, etc.
  - **Calcium and phosphorus**
    - Approximately, **98% of the filtered Ca^{2+} is reabsorbed.** Out of which 65–75% in the proximal tubule, 20–25% in the thick ascending limb of the loop of Henle, 10% in the distal tubule and a small amount in the collecting duct.
    - Normally, **less than 20% of the filtered load of phosphorus is excreted in the urine.** Reabsorption of phosphorus, though dependent on Na^+ reabsorption, is regulated by many factors:
      - Protein kinase C-dependent phosphorylation
      - PTH
      - Active vitamin D
      - Calcitonin
      - Dopamine and serotonin

3. MAINTENANCE OF ACID–BASE BALANCE

Oxidation of various **metabolites** in the living organism **results in the formation of** a variety of **acids as well as bases.** For example:

- **Protons are generated from** ionization of various substances, such as organic acids (produced during metabolism of glucose, fatty acids and amino acids), **uric acid** (from purines), **sulfates** (from sulfur-containing amino acids) and **carbonic acid** (from CO_2).
- Similarly, **bases** arise **during catabolism of** various **metabolites,** such as **ammonia** (from amino acids), **bicarbonate, phosphates, acetate** and **citrates**.

- All **these acids and bases enter** the **blood plasma** and other extracellular fluids **for their disposal** from the body.
- **In spite of** the entry of **these acids and bases, pH of the blood** does not alter much and **remains within the normal limit of 7.35–7.45.**
- This is, **due to the presence of various defense mechanisms,** which include:
  - **Buffer systems** of the blood, tissue fluids and cells **(first line of defense)**
  - **Excretion or retention of CO_2** by the lungs **(respiratory response, the second line of defense)**
  - **Excretion of an acidic or alkaline urine** (**renal response,** the **third line of defense**)
  - Formation and excretion of ammonia as well as organic acids.

4. SYNTHESIS AND ACTIVATION OF HORMONES

- **Kidney synthesizes** some hormones (such as **erythropoietin, renin and prostaglandins**).
- **Kidney** is **also** the **site for the activation of vitamin D**.

KIDNEY FUNCTION TESTS

Various kidney function tests that are **useful in the assessment of a kidney disease include** routine laboratory tests (**physical and chemical,** i.e. **normal and abnormal constituents, examination of urine**), **estimation of blood urea, serum creatinine, electrolytes, uric acid** and **blood gas analysis** (**BGA or ABG;** Table 36.2).

Table 36.2: Commonly used biochemical tests for the assessment of the kidney functions

Routine laboratory tests	*Tests for glomerular functions*	*Tests for tubular functions*
Urine • Volume • pH • Normal constituents • Abnormal constituents	**Renal clearance test** • Inulin clearance • Urea clearance • Creatinine clearance **Renal plasma flow**	• Urine concentration test • Urine dilution test • Urine acidification test
Blood • Urea • Creatinine • pH, gases and electrolytes		

- **Routine laboratory tests:** Routine laboratory tests include:
  - **Physical examination of urine** such as **volume, color, general appearance and odor, specific gravity, pH,** and tests for **normal and abnormal constituents of urine**.
  - **Estimation of blood urea, serum creatinine, blood pH** and **gases, and serum electrolytes.**
    - **Blood urea: Normal blood urea level is between 15 and 45 mg/dL.**
      - Measurement of blood urea is **widely used as a test of renal function.**
      - **Increase in blood urea** concentration include acute or chronic **renal failure with reduction in glomerular filtration rate.** Estimation of plasma urea concentration, however, is a **less valuable test of renal function** than plasma creatinine concentration. This is **due to the reason that nearly 50% of the urea filtered at the glomerulus is passively reabsorbed through the tubules** and this fraction increases, if urine flow rate increases, such as in dehydration.
      - **Blood urea concentration is also affected by dietary protein intake.**
    - **Serum creatinine: Normal serum creatinine concentration varies between 0.8 and 1.5 mg/dL.**
      - Determination of serum creatinine is a **useful indicator of the degree of renal failure.** An **increased serum creatinine concentration** indicates a **fall in GFR.**
      - **Creatinine is freely filtered** at the glomerulus. Although it is **not reabsorbed by the renal tubules,** but a **small amount of it is secreted** and that its **secretion is increased with the increasing level of serum creatinine.**

Blood Urea and Serum Creatinine Levels in Renal Insufficiency

Renal insufficiency refers to some degree of renal failure, which, in turn reduces glomerular filtration rate (GFR), meaning thereby, that the kidneys may not be working as they should.

Generally, blood urea and serum creatinine, and GFR are estimated to assess functioning of the kidney. In renal insufficiency, since GFR is reduced, as a result of which both, blood urea and serum creatinine concentrations are increased.

- **Blood pH, gases and electrolytes: Diminished capacity of the kidney to excrete H^+ results in metabolic acidosis,** the severity of which may be **assessed by measuring arterial H^+, HCO_3^- and pCO_2** concentrations. Estimation of plasma **sodium, potassium, calcium and phosphorus** are also **of value in certain kidney conditions,** e.g. chronic renal failure or metabolic acidosis accompanied by hyponatremia, hyperkalemia, hypocalcemia and hyperphosphatemia.

- **Glomerular function tests:** Glomerular function tests include **renal clearance (urea, creatinine or inulin) and renal plasma flow.**

  Clearance is defined as the volume of plasma that is cleared-off a particular substance by the two kidneys in one minute.

- **Urea clearance:** Urea clearance is calculated in two different ways (depending upon the rate of flow of urine) as standard urea clearance and maximum urea clearance.
  - **Standard urea clearance** is calculated **when** the value of **urine volume is below 2 mL/min. Mean value** for standard urea clearance **is 54 mL/min.**
  - On the other hand, **maximum urea clearance** is calculated when **volume of urine excreted is 2 mL/min or more. Mean value** for maximum urea clearance **is 75 mL/ min.**
- **Creatinine clearance:** Creatinine clearance is **preferred as a measure of GFR. Normal value for creatinine clearance is 95–105 mL/min.**
- **Renal plasma flow:** Renal plasma flow is **determined with p-amino hippuric acid (PAH).** PAH clearance for normal adult male **is 700 ± 130 mL/min.**

- **Tubular function tests:** These include **urine concentration, dilution and acidification tests.**
  - **Urine concentration test:** Urine concentration test is done by measuring osmolality (number of solute particles per kg water) of the specimen of urine after water deprivation or administration of vasopressin (ADH).
  - **Urine dilution test:** Urine dilution test is done to assess ability of the kidney to eliminate excessive amount of water. The test is not advisable in patients with adrenal insufficiency.
  - **Urine acidification test**

Some Important Questions

1. **Describe various functions of the kidney.**
2. **Write notes on:**
   i. Kidney function tests.
   ii. Glomerular function tests
   iii. Tubular function tests

Chapter 37

Gastric Function Tests

The **stomach** functions as a temporary **storage** organ for food and secretes about **2–3 liters of gastric juice every day.** Most of this juice is **produced by exocrine glands** located **in the body and fundus of the stomach.**

FUNCTIONS OF THE STOMACH

These **exocrine secretory glands** contain **three types of secretory cells,** referred to as **the chief cells, the parietal cells** and **the mucous cells, each one of which has specific functions** (Table 37.1).

- **The chief cells:** The chief cells are located in the basal region of these glands and also in the glands of the antrum. These cells secrete pepsinogen (the inactive precursor of pepsin).
- **The parietal cells:**
  - Parietal cells secrete iso-osmotic solution of HCl, with a hydrogen ion concentration of about 150 mEq/L (pH near 0.9–1.0).

    HCl performs several functions:
    - HCl initiates conversion of pepsinogen to pepsin.
    - It also has some physical action on proteins and makes them more easily digestible.
    - HCl also converts the colloidal ferric hydroxide (which is found in the foodstuffs) to ferric ions that can be more readily reduced to ferrous ions by ascorbic acid, and cysteine and sulfhydryl groups of proteins of the food.
  - The parietal cells **also secrete intrinsic factor,** which is necessary for the intestinal absorption of vitamin B_{12} (required for the formation of RBCs).
  - **The mucous cells:** The mucous cells are **located at the neck of these glands, in the glands of the antrum** and scattered **throughout the gastric epithelial lining.**
    - Mucous cells **secrete alkaline mucous-containing fluid,** which **coats the gastric wall** and **protects** it against various forms of damage to the gastric mucosa.
    - Gastric mucin comprises mucoid, mucoprotease and glandulary mucoprotein.

Table 37.1: Biochemical functions of the various cells of the exocrine glands of the stomach

Cell type	*Functions*
Chief cells	Secretion of pepsinogen
Parietal cells	Secretion of HCl and intrinsic factor
Mucous cells	Secretion of mucous

    - Mucoprotein is the main carrier of the intrinsic factor that is necessary for the absorption of vitamin B_{12} (which is referred to as the extrinsic factor).

COMPOSITION OF GASTRIC JUICE

Gastric juice consists of water (99.4%), **HCl (hydrochloric acid), mucin** and several enzymes such as pepsin (as **pepsinogen**), carbonic anhydrase and lipase. Besides HCl, gastric residue contains **mucoproteins** and organic acids such as **lactic acid and butyric acid,** etc. which **contributes to the total acidity of the gastric juice.**

Residuum

The **content of the stomach after,** nearly, **12 hours of fast** is referred to as **gastric residue (residuum). For this purpose, fasting content of the stomach is aspirated and its volume is measured.** This is termed as the **basal acid output (BAO).**

- **In normal persons, the BAO ranges from 0 to 10 mEq/hour.**
- Complete **absence of gastric secretion** is referred to as **achylia gastrica.** This is observed in **advanced cases of gastric carcinoma.**
- **A large volume of BAO indicates obstruction of gastric outlet.**
- **A very high BAO suggests that the patient has Zollinger-Ellison syndrome.**

Stimulation of Gastric Secretion

Acid output after stimulation is termed as the **maximal acid output** (MAO). **Several compounds,** or processes, such as test meal, alcohol, caffeine, gastrin, pentagastrin or insulin **stimulate gastric secretion** and, in turn, the secretion of HCl.

- **Alcohol:** For stimulation of gastric stimulation, **50–100 mL of 7% ethyl alcohol** (3.5 mL ethanol in 50 mL of water) may be administered through the syringe that is attached to the tube, as a stimulant for HCl secretion.
- **Caffeine: Caffeine sodium benzoate, 500 mg in about 200 mL of water** may be administered into the stomach through a gastric tube, as a stimulant of gastric secretion.
- **Histamine:** Histamine is a powerful stimulant for the secretion of gastric juice. It causes secretion of an increased volume of highly acidic gastric juice with low pepsin content.

  Two types of histamine tests may be carried out:
  - **Standard histamine test:** In standard histamine test, subcutaneous injection of histamine **(0.01 mg/kg body weight)** is given and the gastric contents are removed.
  - **Augmented histamine test:** For this test, a large dose of histamine **(0.04 mg/kg body weight)** is given.

> *Note:* In pernicious anemia no free HCl is secreted, but in other forms of achlorhydria some amount of free HCl may be secreted, after augmented histamine stimulation test is performed.

Antihistaminics

Sometimes, high dose of histamine may cause a severe reaction mediated through H1-receptors. Under such a condition, an injection of antihistaminic may be given, intramuscularly. This does not interfere in gastric stimulation, because the gastric stimulation effect of histamine is mediated through H2-receptors.

- **Insulin:** Insulin **(0.1–0.2 U/kg body weight of soluble insulin, intravenously)** may also be given for the stimulation of gastric secretion. In this case, the gastric samples are withdrawn after every 15 min and this test is called **Hollander test**.

> *Note:* Insulin stimulation is helpful to ascertain the effectiveness of vagotomy in patients with duodenal ulcer. In these patients, concentration of free HCl may be as high as 1200 mEq/L. After successful vagotomy, since there is no response to insulin, gastric acidity remains at a low level of 15–20 mEq/L before as well as after insulin administration. As insulin may cause hypoglycemia the test is not preferred.

- **Gastrin and pentagastrin:**
  - **Gastrin** is the most powerful stimulus for gastric HCl secretion. It is administered in a single subcutaneous dose of **2 mg/kg body weight**.

Zollinger-Ellison Syndrome

Zollinger-Ellison syndrome is due to a **gastrin-secreting tumor** of the endocrine pancreas. **Excess gastrin overstimulates gastric acid secretion** resulting in **abdominal pain, mucosal ulceration and diarrhea**. It is suspected in patients of acid-peptic disease, who fail to respond to conventional treatment with H2 receptor blockers and proton pump inhibitors.

  - **Pentagastrin:** Pentagastrin is a **synthetic pentapeptide** with a physiologically active part of the gastrin molecule. It is administered subcutaneously (6 mg/kg body weight), and post-stimulation secretions are collected at 15 min intervals for the next one hour.

  This test is **useful in differentiating the diagnosis of achlorhydria and hyperchlorhydria**.

BIOCHEMICAL EVALUATION OF GASTRIC FUNCTIONS

Gastric functions are **assessed by performing physical and chemical examination of the gastric juice**, and **by estimating its free and total acidity**.

- **Physical examination of gastric residue:**
  - **Volume:** Total volume of the resting gastric residue, **normally**, varies from **20 to 50 mL**. An **increase** in the volume (>100 mL) **may be due to hypersecretion, retention or regurgitation** from duodenum and is considered abnormal. Various causes include **pyloric obstruction, duodenal ulcer or Zollinger-Ellison syndrome**.
  - **Consistency:** Resting gastric juice is **fluid in consistency**. It may be **viscous in the presence of mucus. Food particles may be present in carcinoma of the stomach**.
  - **Color:** The resting gastric content is, usually, **colorless**. It may be slightly **yellow or green due to regurgitation of bile**, or **red/brown due to the presence of blood**.
- **Chemical examination:**
  - **Bile:** Bile may be found in gastric residuum **as a result of intestinal obstruction or ileal stasis**.
  - **Mucus:** Small amount of mucus is found normally. **Increased amounts may be seen in gastritis and gastric carcinoma**.
  - **Blood: Accidental trauma** to the gastric mucous membrane during the passage of Ryle's tube may result in **traces of blood** in the gastric juice. **Increased amount** of blood may be present **due to gastric carcinoma, erosive gastritis or bleeding peptic ulcer**.
  - **Organic acids:** Organic acids, such as **lactic acid and butyric acid may be present in** large amounts in conditions of **hypoacidity, achlorhydria and carcinoma of the stomach. In the absence of free HCl, these organic acids are formed in increased**

amounts by bacterial fermentation of food, as food is retained in the stomach for longer period (usually more than 6 hours) at neutral or alkaline pH.

- **Estimation of free and total acidity of gastric juice:**
  - **Free acidity: HCl** present in the gastric juice **accounts for free acidity**. As mentioned above, it is secreted by the parietal cells at a concentration of about 150 mEq/L with pH <1.0.
    - Concentration of free acidity in gastric residue in normal individuals varies from **0 to 40 mEq/L**.
    - Free acidity concentration **above 50 mEq/L** may be suggestive of **hyperacidity**.
    - When free acidity is increased, the condition is called **hyperchlorhydria**. It occurs **in duodenal and gastric ulcers**, and in **diseases of the gall bladder**.
    - **Complete absence of HCl** is referred to as **achlorhydria**. It occurs **in pernicious anemia**.
    - In the absence of HCl, bacterial fermentation of food is increased, which leads to the formation of lactic acid. A small percentage of healthy individuals (about 4% of the young ones and 25% at age 60 years) may have no free HCl in the fasting stomach.
  - **Total acidity:** Total acidity in gastric residue **includes** hydrogen ions occurring as free **HCl, mucoproteins, acid salts and organic acids**. Total acidity is, generally, **up to 10 mEq/L more than free acidity**. Thus, total acidity in a normal state is, usually, **10–50 mEq/L**.

Some Important Questions

1. **Describe various biochemical functions of the stomach.**
2. **Describe various gastric function tests.**
3. **Write notes on:**
   i. Zollinger-Ellison syndrome
   ii. Antihistaminics
   iii. Stimulation of gastric secretion
   iv. Free and total acidity of gastric juice

Chapter

38

Acid–Base Regulation

Acid is a substance whose dissociation in water **releases hydrogen ions (H^+)**. The H^+ since does not contain any neutron and is essentially equivalent to a proton, an acid, therefore, is often referred to as a **proton donor**.

Addition of an acid to a solution increases concentration of free H^+ in the solution and results in a decrease in pH.

A strong acid such as HCl, completely dissociates in an aqueous solution. On the other hand, a weak acid gives up H^+ less rapidly and does not dissociate completely.

Most of the acids produced in living systems are weak acids.

BASE

A base releases hydroxyl ions (OH^-) in an aqueous solution and **decreases its H^+ concentration** by accepting or binding with the free H^+, resulting in an **increase in pH of the solution**. A strong base, such as sodium hydroxide (NaOH), dissociates completely. A weak base, such as bicarbonate (HCO_3^-), can also utilize H^+ and thus raises the pH of the solution.

pH

The pH is defined as the **negative logarithm to the base 10, of the molar concentration of hydrogen ions** (H^+) **in a solution, i.e.:**

$$pH = -\log[H^+], \text{ or}$$
$$= \log(1/[H^+])$$

Thus, pH of a solution is inversely related to free H^+ concentration $[H^+]$.

A **low pH indicates high H^+ concentration** while a **high pH indicates low H^+ concentration.**

The **scale of pH measurement** varies from **0 to 14.** If **pH of a solution is <7**, the solution is said to be **acidic**; if pH of the solution is **equal to 7**, it is referred to as **neutral**; and if pH is **>7**, the solution is said to be **alkaline** or basic in nature.

BUFFER

Buffer is a substance that tends to **resist a shock** and, thereby, **promotes relative stability**. A buffer **minimizes the change in pH** when either an acid or a base is added to a solution.

A **chemical buffer consists of a weak acid** (HA) **and its conjugate base** (A^-), or a **weak base and its conjugate acid**.

The effectiveness of a buffer, in minimizing changes in pH, depends upon two factors:

1. The **pKa of the buffer** in relation to the desired pH, e.g. pKa of the imidazole group of histidine in hemoglobin is close to 7.4 and, thus, it is an ideal buffer in the blood.
2. The **amount or concentration of the buffer**—Greater the concentration of a buffer, greater is its ability to bind or release H^+.

EFFECT OF DIET ON BLOOD pH

A diet results in a net production of acids, largely from the oxidation of protein. Food also contains basic anions, such as citrate, lactate and acetate. When these are oxidized to CO_2 and water, H^+ are consumed. A balance of acid-forming and acid-consuming metabolic reactions results in a net production of about 1 mEq H^+/kg body weight per day, in an adult person, on a mixed diet.

Generally, **vegetarians have less of a dietary acid burden** and a more alkaline urine pH than nonvegetarians, because most fruits and vegetables contain large amounts of organic anions that are metabolized to HCO_3^-.

MECHANISMS OF ACID–BASE REGULATION

As discussed above, acids are continuously produced in the body and threaten normal pH of the extracellular fluid (ECF) as well as intracellular fluid (ICF). However, despite constant threat to acid–base homeostasis, blood pH is maintained within the normal limit of 7.35 ±0.05, in a normal healthy person. This is due to three different lines of defense (Fig. 38.1).

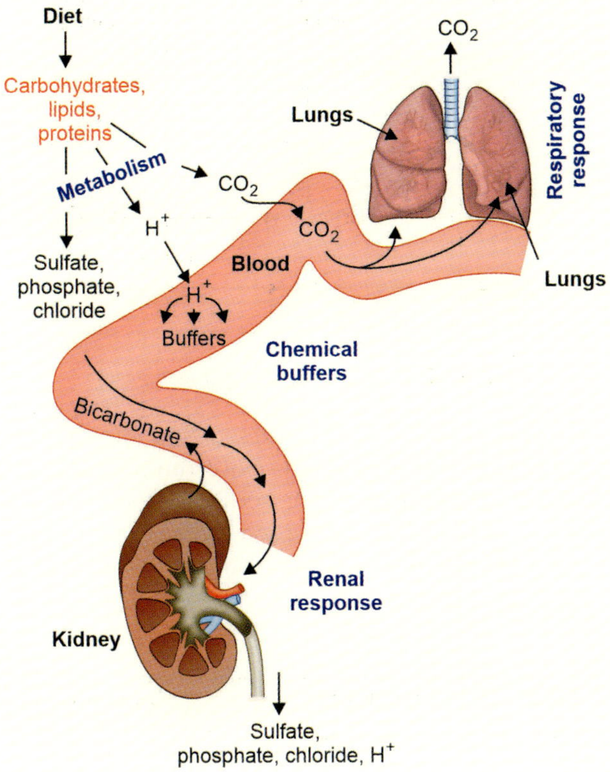

Fig. 38.1: Three lines of defence for regulation of acid–base balance

1. BODY BUFFERS

Chemical **buffers present in** the **extracellular and intracellular fluids** as well as in the bones are referred to as the **first line of defense** (Table 38.1).

Table 38.1: Major body buffers

Buffer	*Reaction*
Extracellular fluid	
Bicarbonate/CO_2	$CO_2 + H_2O \rightleftharpoons H_2CO_3 \rightleftharpoons H^+ + HCO_3^-$
Inorganic phosphate	$H_2PO_4^- \rightleftharpoons H^+ + HPO_4^{2-}$
Plasma proteins (HPr)	$HPr \rightleftharpoons H^+ + Pr^-$
Intracellular fluid	
Cell proteins, e.g. hemoglobin (HHb)	$HHb \rightleftharpoons H^+ + Hb^-$
Organic phosphates	Organic-$HPO_4 \rightleftharpoons H^+$ + organic-PO_4^{2-}
Bicarbonate/CO_2	$CO_2 + H_2O \rightleftharpoons H_2CO_3 \rightleftharpoons H^+ + HCO_3^-$
Bone	
Mineral phosphates	$H_2PO_4^- \rightleftharpoons H^+ + HPO_4^{2-}$
Mineral carbonates	$HCO_3^- \rightleftharpoons H^+ + CO_3^{2-}$

Bicarbonate/CO_2 Buffer

The HCO_3^-/CO_2 buffer pair is of **prime importance in acid–base regulation** due to several reasons:

- **High concentration of the two components:** The **concentration of HCO_3^- in plasma** or ECF, normally, averages **24 mmol/L** and that the **metabolic processes** in the body **generates unlimited supply of CO_2**.
- **Open system:** The HCO_3^-/CO_2 buffer system is more effective because it is open, i.e. **its both the components can be added to or removed from the body.**
- **Dual regulation:** It has dual regulation, i.e. it is **controlled,** both, **by the lungs and the kidneys.** Whereas, **lungs** (the respiratory system) **regulate the amount of CO_2** in the body by hyperventilation or hypoventilation. On the other hand, the **kidneys** regulate the amount of HCO_3^- in the ECF by forming new HCO_3^- (when excess acid has been added to the body) or by excreting HCO_3^- (when excess base has been added).

Phosphate Buffer

The pKa for the phosphate buffer is 6.8, which is comparatively closer to pH of blood (7.4). So, it is a good buffer.

In the ECF, phosphate is present as inorganic phosphate. Its concentration, however, is low. So, it plays a minor role in extracellular buffering. However, **phosphate is an important intracellular buffer for two reasons:**

- First, **cells contain large amount of phosphate** in various organic compounds, such as ATP, ADP and creatine phosphate. Though, these compounds, primarily, function in energy metabolism, they also act as pH buffers.
- Second, **intracellular pH is, generally, lower than the pH of ECF**, and is closer to the pKa of phosphate.

Protein Buffer

Protein is the largest buffering pool in the body and is the excellent buffer. Since proteins are amphoteric, they can function as, both, acids as well as bases. Proteins contain many ionizable groups, which can release or bind H^+. Plasma albumin and globulins are the major extracellular protein buffers. Cells also have large protein stores including hemoglobin in RBC.

2. RESPIRATORY RESPONSE

Respiratory response is also referred to as the second line of defense. It is due to the reason that, normally, CO_2 is expired at the same rate at which it is produced and, thus, pCO_2 is maintained. So,

- **If blood becomes acidic** by the addition of fixed acids, pulmonary ventilation is increased and **CO_2 is flushed out** at a rate greater than the rate at which it is produced. Consequently, **pCO_2 falls** and results in a **decrease in H^+ concentration of blood**. Hyperventilation, in turn, **lowers HCO_3^- concentration** and **reduces acidic shift in the blood.** Accordingly, the equilibrium reactions are pulled to the left (Fig. 38.2).

$$CO_2 + H_2O \rightleftharpoons H_2CO_3 \rightleftharpoons H^+ + HCO_3^-$$

Fig. 38.2: The equilibrium is pulled to the left during hyperventilation

- On the other hand, **if blood becomes more alkaline,** changes occur in the opposite direction. Accordingly, **hypoventilation takes place,** CO_2 is not removed at an adequate rate and the blood pCO_2 rises. Accordingly, the equilibrium reactions are pushed to the right (Fig. 38.3).

$$CO_2 + H_2O \rightleftharpoons H_2CO_3 \rightleftharpoons H^+ + HCO_3^-$$

Fig. 38.3: The equilibrium is pushed to the right during hypoventilation

Thus, hypoventilation results in a higher carbonic acid concentration in blood and a less alkaline shift in blood pH. This, however, is limited, because hypoventilation causes retention of CO_2, which further stimulates ventilation.

Buffering of acid–base disturbances by the respiratory response although is rapid, but is relatively coarse. It brings blood pH back, close to normal, but cannot eliminate a fixed acid or base from the body and so, it cannot restore pH to normal.

3. RENAL RESPONSE

It is also referred to as the third line of defense. Renal responses, in contrast to other two buffering mechanisms, are slow but more complete and that full renal compensation may take 1 to 3 days.

Kidneys regulate acid–base balance by controlling bicarbonate (HCO_3^-) reabsorption and secreting acid (H^+). In addition, kidneys also excrete anions, such as phosphate, chloride, sulfate, etc. which are liberated from the strong acids.

Carbonic anhydrase catalyzed reaction in the tubule cells generates bicarbonate (HCO_3^-) and hydrogen ions (H^+). The H^+ are actively secreted into the tubular fluid (lumen) in exchange for Na^+ (via Na^+/H^+-antiport system). Within the tubule cell, Na^+ combines with HCO_3^- and generates sodium bicarbonate ($Na^+ + HCO_3^-$), that is pumped out of the cell into the blood (interstitial fluid) and equilibrates with the plasma (Fig. 38.4).

The H^+ secreted into the tubular fluid result in acidification of urine by three mechanisms. These are associated with the addition of bicarbonate to the peritubular capillary blood by the kidney tubules.

i. **Reabsorption of the filtered bicarbonate:** HCO_3^- (bicarbonate) filtered by the glomeruli combines with H^+. This, in turn, results in the formation of carbonic acid, which is dissociated to CO_2 and water in the proximal convoluted tubule lumen, by carbonic anhydrase within the brush border membrane. CO_2 rapidly diffuses through the cell membrane where it combines with water and forms carbonic acid, which, in turn, gets dissociated into hydrogen and

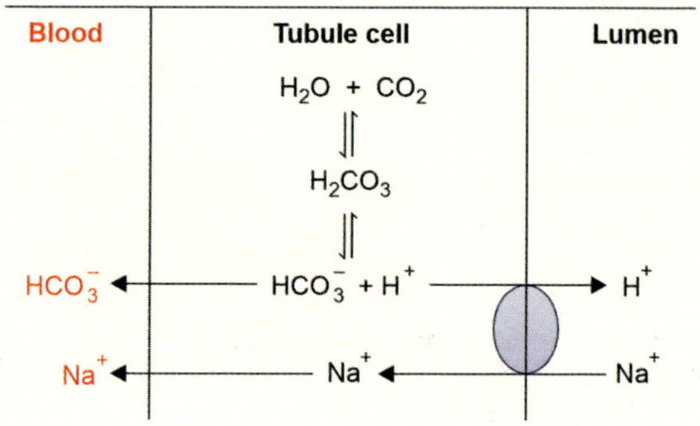

Fig. 38.4: Basic ion exchange mechanism

bicarbonate ions. The H^+ are secreted into the lumen while the bicarbonate ions exit from the basolateral membrane along with the sodium ions. The filtered HCO_3^-, thus, is not reabsorbed by direct transport out of the tubular urine, rather it is reabsorbed indirectly by the secretion of the hydrogen ions (Fig. 38.5).

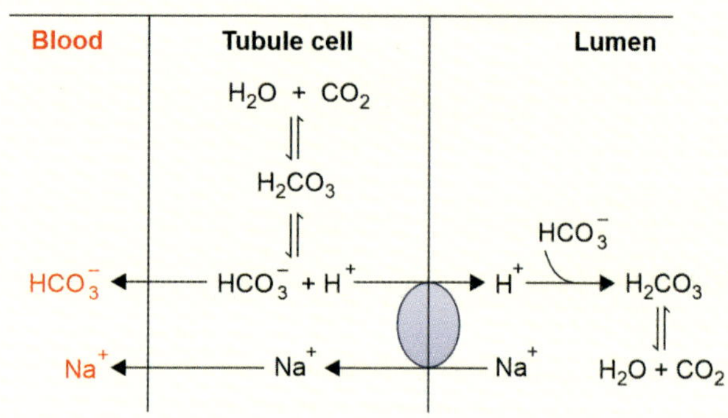

Fig. 38.5: Reabsorption of bicarbonate

ii. **Excretion of titratable acid:** As reabsorption of sodium bicarbonate proceeds, the tubular fluid becomes depleted of HCO_3^- and the pH drops. At this stage, H^+ are taken up by the phosphate buffer. As a result, the basic form of the phosphate (HPO_4^{2-}) is converted to its acidic form $H_2PO_4^-$. Thus, excretion of titratable acids not only eliminates H^+ from the body but also restores depleted plasma bicarbonate reserves, since for each mEq of H^+ excreted as titratable acid, a new HCO_3^- is added to the blood (Fig. 38.6).

iii. **Excretion of ammonia:** The third fate of H^+ in the tubular fluid is its neutralization by NH_3 which is mainly synthesized in the proximal tubule from amino acids (predominantly from glutamine). Ability of the kidney to synthesize NH_3 from glutamine is increased under conditions of excess acid in the body. Ammonia readily diffuses through the cell membrane and combines with the secreted H^+ and forms NH_4^+, which is, usually, accompanied by an anion, e.g. chloride, in the urine. For each H^+ excreted in the urine as NH_4^+, an equivalent quantity of HCO_3^- is added to the blood (Fig. 38.7).

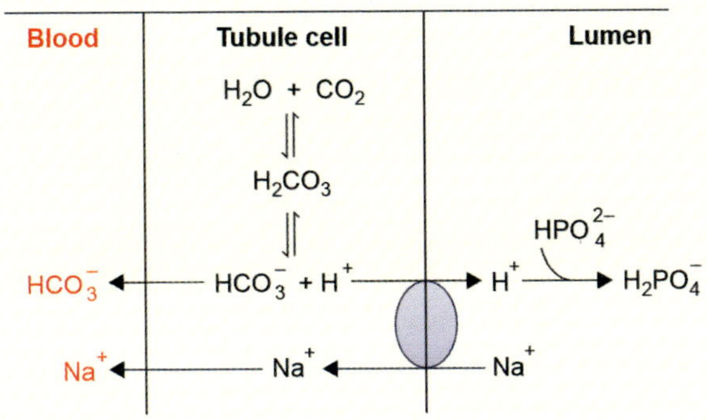

Fig. 38.6: Excretion of titratable acid

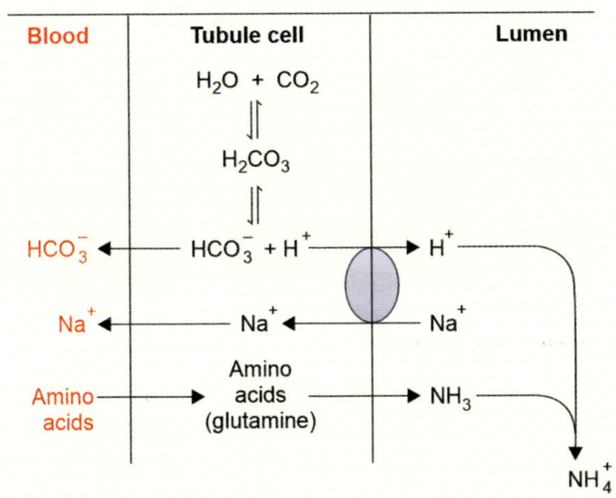

Fig. 38.7: Excretion of ammonia

ARTERIAL BLOOD GAS (ABG) ANALYSIS

Arterial blood gas **(ABG)** analysis is important in the assessment of acid–base imbalance. The disturbances of acid–base balance are accompanied by characteristic changes in blood **pH, pCO_2 and HCO_3^-**.

Normal values for which, **in the arterial blood, are** as follows:

pH	7.35–7.45
pCO_2	35–45 mm Hg
HCO_3^-	22–26 mmol/L

Besides the above measured parameters, the values for some of the calculated parameters is also useful. These include:

Base excess: Base excess is defined as the amount of acid required to titrate the blood to pH 7.4, at a pCO_2 of 40 mm Hg, at 37°C. The **normal value is in the range of –2.0 to +3.0 mmol/L.** If a blood sample is acidic, the base excess will be negative.

Anion gap: Anion gap is the difference between the sum of Na^+ plus K^+ (cations) from the sum of Cl^- plus HCO_3^- (anions).

$$\text{Anion gap} = (Na^+ + K^+) - (Cl^- + HCO_3^-)$$

Anion gap, thus, represents plasma anions other than Cl^- and HCO_3^-, which are not routinely measured, such as lactate, citrate, ketone bodies (acetoacetate and β-hydroxybutyrate), etc. **Normal value for anion gap is in the range of 12–16 mmol/L.**

ACID–BASE DISORDERS

Acidosis vs Alkalosis

Acidosis is an abnormal process that tends to produce **acidemia**, i.e. the **blood pH is below 7.35** (H^+ >45 nmol/L). On the other hand, **blood pH above 7.45** (H^+ <35 nmol/L) **is referred to as alkalosis (alkalemia).**

Respiratory Disorder vs Metabolic Disorder

The **disorder is of respiratory nature**, if there is a **disturbance in CO_2**, i.e. **too much or too little of CO_2**. On the other hand, **if the problem is too much or too little of HCO_3^-** then it is referred to as a **metabolic disorder** (non-respiratory disturbance).

Compensatory Mechanisms

In various acid–base disturbances, if the primary problem is a change in HCO_3^- or pCO_2, the pH can be brought closer to normal by changing the other member of the buffer pair in the same direction. For example, if pCO_2 is primarily decreased, a decrease in plasma HCO_3^- will minimize the change in pH. Under these situations, **lungs adjust the blood pCO_2** while **kidneys adjust the plasma HCO_3^- to reduce deviations of pH from normal. These adjustments are called compensations or compensatory mechanisms.**

Types of Acid–base Disorders

Four types of simple acid–base disorders are known to occur (Table 38.2).

- Respiratory acidosis
- Metabolic acidosis
- Respiratory alkalosis,
- Metabolic alkalosis

Table 38.2: Changes observed in major acid–base balance disorders

Acid–base disorder	*Arterial blood*			*Compensatory response*
	pCO_2	*pH*	*HCO_3^-*	
Respiratory acidosis	↑	↓	↑	Renal H^+ excretion increases plasma HCO_3^- concentration
Respiratory alkalosis	↓	↑	↓	Renal HCO_3^- excretion decreases plasma HCO_3^- concentration
Metabolic acidosis	↓	↓	↓	Hyperventilation decreases pCO_2
Metabolic alkalosis	↑	↑	↑	Hypoventilation increases pCO_2

Respiratory Acidosis

Respiratory acidosis is most often due to inadequate ventilation **(hypoventilation)** of the alveoli, **resulting in retention of CO_2** and **fall in blood pH**.

- **Alveolar hypoventilation** occurs when the **depth or rate of respiration is diminished**, such as in airway obstruction or a pulmonary disease.
- This, in turn, will result in a **rise in pCO_2**.
- As pCO_2 rises, plasma pH drops and **HCO_3^- concentration rises.**
- **Kidneys compensate** for respiratory acidosis **by increasing the output of H^+ in urine.**
- Accordingly, the **filtered HCO_3^- is reabsorbed** and the **increased amounts of H^+ combine with the urinary buffers** and are **excreted in urine**.
- Thus, **by excreting H^+ in urine, kidneys increase plasma HCO_3^-** concentration.

Respiratory Alkalosis

Respiratory alkalosis is produced by **hyperventilation,** which results in the **excessive removal of CO_2 from the blood**. This, in turn, causes a **fall in arterial blood pCO_2,** a **fall in plasma H^+ concentration**, i.e. a **rise in pH** and a **fall in plasma** HCO_3^- concentration.

- Hyperventilation may be **caused by anxiety, central nervous system injury involving the respiratory center, salicylate poisoning or fever**.
- At **high altitude** also, due to decrease in total atmospheric pressure, alveolar pCO_2 falls and results in chronic respiratory alkalosis.
- **Kidneys compensate** for the respiratory alkalosis **by excreting HCO_3^- in the urine**.
- Low pCO_2 leads to **decreased H^+ secretion** by the tubular epithelium.
- This, in turn, **reduces reabsorption of the filtered** HCO_3^- and **increases HCO_3^- excretion in urine**.
- This results in further **decrease in plasma HCO_3^-** and **plasma pH towards normal.**

Metabolic Acidosis

- Metabolic acidosis is characterized by the **accumulation of nonvolatile acids** (gain of fixed acids other than H_2CO_3), or **loss of HCO_3^-**. This **gain of metabolically produced acid may be due to** several reasons, such as:
- **Uncontrolled diabetes mellitus** leading to the **production of large quantities of ketone bodies.**
  - **Acidemia stimulates pulmonary ventilation** resulting in a **compensatory lowering of alveolar and arterial blood pCO_2 (respiratory compensation).**
  - The consequent **reduction in blood H_2CO_3 moves blood pH back toward normal.**
  - **Kidneys also reabsorb filtered HCO_3^- (Renal compensation).**
  - Kidneys also **increase excretion of titratable acid,** part of which is composed of ketone bodies.
  - Increased renal synthesis and excretion of ammonia.
- **Diarrhea or abnormal excretion of HCO_3^- in urine** results in a decrease in plasma **HCO_3^-** concentration. Two compensatory mechanisms are usually available to deal with the excess acid:
  - Due to the acidic pH, **respiratory system is stimulated to hyperventilate**. This, in turn, **lowers pCO_2** and hence, carbonic acid concentration in blood.
  - The other mechanism which begins almost instantly, is the **renal compensation. Kidneys increase H^+ excretion**.

Metabolic Alkalosis

Metabolic alkalosis is characterized by the intake of excess of alkali, i.e. by the **gain of strong base or HCO_3^-,** or **abnormal loss of acid other than HCO_3^-.** For example, **ingestion of excess sodium bicarbonate used in treating gastric** ulcer while a **common cause of abnormal loss of acid** causing metabolic alkalosis **is prolonged vomiting or gastric lavage** since loss of stomach contents **results in net addition of HCO_3^- to the blood**.

- Characteristic arterial blood changes include a **primary increase in plasma HCO_3^-** concentration, a **rise in pH**, and a **compensatory rise in pCO_2**.
- As the primary defect is an increase in plasma HCO_3^- concentration, **immediate physiological compensation is hypoventilation, followed by increased renal excretion of HCO_3^-.**
- Ventilation is inhibited by the alkaline blood pH, resulting in a **rise in pCO_2** (Respiratory compensation).
- **Renal compensation is enhanced excretion of HCO_3^-.**

Some Important Questions

1. **Define buffer. Name important buffers present in the body. Explain the role of various body buffers in acid–base regulation.**
2. **Explain:**
   i. Role of kidney in the acid–base regulation
   ii. Mechanisms of H^+ secretion
   iii. Disturbances of acid–base balance
   iv. Biochemical measures of acid–base gas analysis
   v. Role of lungs in the acid–base regulation
3. **Write notes on:**
   i. pH
   ii. Chemical buffers in the body
   iv. Respiratory acidosis
   v. Respiratory alkalosis
   vi. Metabolic acidosis
   vii. Metabolic alkalosis
   viii. Base excess
   ix. Anion gap

Chapter 39

Electrolyte Balance

An electrolyte is **a substance that ionizes, when dissolved in suitable ionizing solvents** such as water. This includes most soluble salts, acids and bases. Chemically, electrolytes are substances that become ions in solution and acquire the capacity to conduct electricity.

Electrolytes are present in the human body and the **balance of the electrolytes in our body is essential for normal function of cells and organs.**

Osmolality: Concentration of the dissolved particles, such as sodium and potassium, etc. is referred to as osmolality. **High osmolality suggests increased concentration of electrolytes in the serum.**

Common electrolytes that are measured in blood include **sodium and potassium**. Their important biological functions are described in Table 39.1.

SODIUM

An **adult human body contains, nearly, 100 g of sodium,** as sodium ions (Na^+). Sodium is the **major cation in** the ECF (extracellular fluid).

- Sodium **exists in the body in association with several anions,** such as chloride, bicarbonate, phosphate, lactate and proteinate.
- **High concentration of Na^+** (along with low K^+) **in the ECF is maintained by** Na^+/K^+-ATPase **(Na^+/K^+ pump).**
- It is **completely absorbed by the gastrointestinal tract.**
- Sodium is **freely filtered by the glomerulus.** About 70% of the filtered sodium is reabsorbed by the proximal tubules, 15% by the loop of Henle, 5% by the distal convoluted tubules and about 10% by the collecting ducts.
- It is, mainly, **excreted by the kidneys.** Under normal physiological conditions, its daily urinary excretion is equal to its intake.
- **Sodium homeostasis is influenced by several general factors,** including aldosterone, renin-angiotensin system and natriuretic factor (ANF).
- Only, **less than 2% of the ingested sodium is eliminated in the feces.**
- **Active reabsorption of Na^+** in the proximal tubule results in the **passive reabsorption of Cl^- and HCO_3^-** along **with water**. This helps to **maintain electrical neutrality of the** ECF while **reabsorption of water ensures normal osmotic pressure.**

Sources of Sodium

Most important source of sodium is the **common table salt,** i.e. sodium chloride. Besides, meat, seafoods, milk, cheese and bread are also good sources of sodium. Plant sources are, usually, low in sodium.

RDA of Sodium

ICMR-NIN (2020) has recommended daily intake of sodium as **2000 mg/day**.

Table 39.1: Biological functions of sodium and potassium in the body

Sodium	*Potassium*
1. Regulation of osmotic pressure of extracellular fluid	1. Regulation of intracellular osmotic pressure
2. Regulation of acid–base balance of extracellular fluid	2. Regulation of intracellular acid–base balance
3. GI and renal absorption of monosaccharides and amino acids	3. GI secretions
4. Maintenance of neuromuscular irritability and excitability	4. Maintenance of neuromuscular irritability and excitability
5. Maintenance of blood viscosity	5. Storage of proteins and glycogen
6. Cofactor for Na^+/K^+-ATPase	6. Cofactor for enzymes, e.g. Na^+/K^+-ATPase, pyruvate kinase, etc.

POTASSIUM

Potassium is the **chief cation in the ICF** (intracellular fluid). Its functions are described along with sodium in Table 39.1.

Potassium is completely **absorbed from the gastrointestinal tract**. It is freely **filtered at the glomerulus** and is **excreted,** almost, entirely **by the kidneys.**

Sources of Potassium

Potassium is **widely distributed in plants as well as animals,** as the chloride, phosphate and carbonate salts of inorganic acids, organic acids and proteins. The good sources of potassium are coffee, cocoa, dried beans, wheat bran, most of the vegetables such as potato, tomato, dairy products, fish, eggs, meat and fruits like banana, peach and oranges.

RDA for Potassium

ICMR-NIN (2020) has recommended daily intake of potassium as **3500 mg/day**.

DISTRIBUTION OF ELECTROLYTES IN BODY FLUIDS

Electrolytes are **distributed unevenly between the** intracellular fluid **(ICF)** and the extracellular fluid **(ECF)**, two major compartments of the water in the body.

- **ICF is composed of the fluid within the trillions of cells in our body.** On the other hand, **ECF is composed of fluid outside the cells.**
- In a young adult man, **two-thirds of the body water is in the ICF** while the remaining **one-third is in the ECF.**
- **ECF** can be further **subdivided into** two sub-compartments, which are separated from each other by the endothelium of blood vessels, as **plasma**, and the **interstitial fluid and lymph**.
- Differences in chemical composition between ICF and plasma are shown in Table 39.2.

Table 39.2: Electrolyte distribution in various fluid compartments

Electrolyte	*Concentration (mmol/L)*	
	Intracellular fluid	*Plasma*
Total anions	205	154
Cl^-	2	103
HPO_4^{2-}	148	4
Others	55	47
Total cations	205	154
Na^+	10	142
K^+	160	4
Others	35	8

ELECTROLYTE BALANCE

Adequate hydration (water) and normal levels of electrolytes are important for proper functioning of the body. Various mechanisms which maintain a normal electrolyte balance in body fluids are shown in Fig. 39.1.

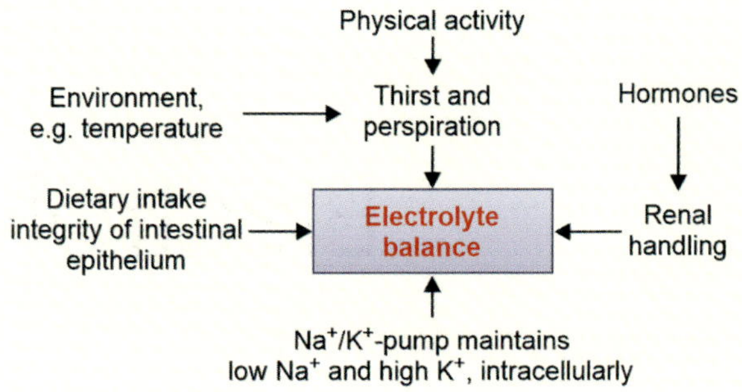

Fig. 39.1: Electrolyte balance. (Aldosterone secreted by the adrenal cortex, facilitates the retention of Na^+ and excretion of K^+ by the kidneys. Hypofunctioning of the adrenal cortex as in Addison's disease results in hyponatremia with hyperkalemia while hyperfunctioning of the adrenal cortex such as in Cushing's syndrome results in hypernatremia with hypokalemia)

Among the **hormones,** the **most important** one is **aldosterone** and that the **main driving force for the secretion of aldosterone** in the adrenal zona glomerulosa **is angiotensin II,** which is **generated via renin-angiotensin system (under the influence of low plasma Na^+,** or low blood volume or pressure).

Renin-angiotensin System

Renin-angiotensin system, also referred to as **renin-angiotensin-aldosterone system** or **RAAS,** is an important system that participates in various homeostatic mechanisms, such as water balance, electrolyte balance and maintenance of blood pressure.

- **Renin**, a proteolytic enzyme **produced and stored in the granules of the juxtaglomerular cells of the afferent arterioles in the kidneys,** is **induced by hypovolemia** (low blood volume) **and hyponatremia** (low blood sodium concentration).
- Renin **acts on angiotensinogen** (a plasma α_2-globulin, which is synthesized in the liver) and **cleaves it to angiotensin I** (a decapeptide).
- Thereafter, **angiotensin-converting enzyme (ACE) converts** angiotensin I **to angiotensin II (an octapeptide)**, which counteracts a decrease in mean arterial pressure by several mechanisms, such as arteriolar vasoconstriction, increased Na^+ reabsorption by the proximal tubules, release of aldosterone (which promotes Na^+ reabsorption in the distal tubules) and release of vasopressin (a vasoconstrictor).
- **By** the action of an **aminopeptidase, angiotensin II** is further **degraded to angiotensin III** amongst the renal handling by the hormones, the most important factor is the renin-angiotensin system (a heptapeptide; Fig. 39.2).
- Both, **angiotensin II and angiotensin III bind to angiotensin receptors** and **activate phosphatidylinositol system** to **generate IP_3 and DAG.**

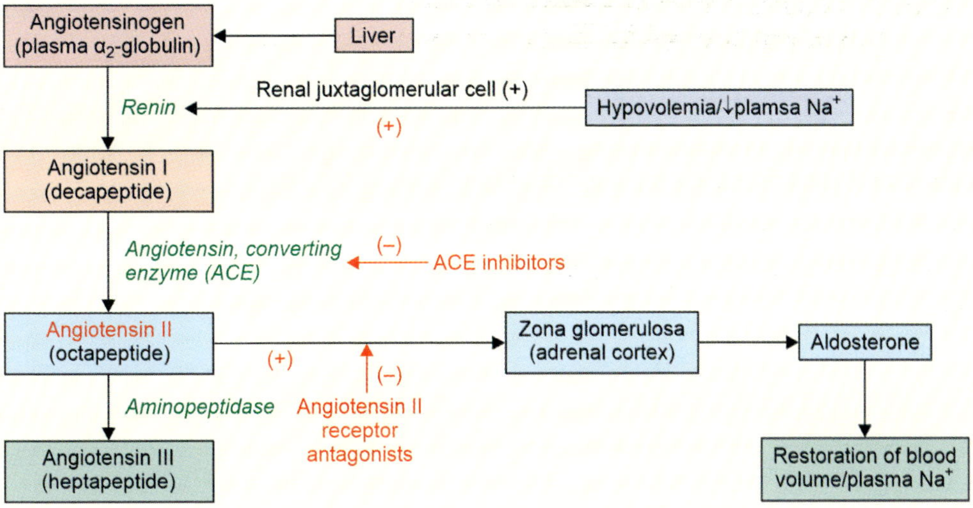

Fig. 39.2: Renin-angiotensin-aldosterone system (RAAS)

- **IP_3 stimulates release of Ca^{2+} from** the **intracellular calcium storage vesicles.**
- **Increased cytosolic Ca^{2+} along with** the **DAG stimulates protein kinase C,** which, in turn, leads to the **phosphorylation of proteins,** which **stimulate rate-limiting steps of aldosterone biosynthesis.**
- **Increased level of aldosterone** is **secreted** into the blood and **enters the distal cells in the kidney,** where it **binds to its receptors.**
- This, in turn, **stimulates expression of proteins,** which **increase transport of Na^+ from the glomerular filtrate** to the blood.

ELECTROLYTE IMBALANCE

Electrolyte imbalance may result in **hyper or hyponatremia,** or **hyper or hypokalemia.**

- **Hyponatremia:** Hyponatremia is defined as **plasma Na^+ concentration <135 mEq/L.** It is the **most common disorder of body fluid and electrolyte imbalance.** General **symptoms include muscle cramps, lethargy, fatigue, disorientation, headache, anorexia, nausea, agitation, hypothermia, seizures and coma.** These symptoms, mainly **neurological,** are a consequence of swelling of the brain cells, as plasma osmolality falls. Excessive brain swelling may be fatal, or may cause permanent damage.
- **Hypernatremia:** Hypernatremia is defined as **plasma Na^+ concentration >150 mEq/L.** It is always **hyperosmolar** and is **characterized by edema, azotemia and anemia.** Accumulation of Na^+ in the body has been shown to result in a concomitant rise in blood pressure, referred to as **essential hypertension. Symptoms are** primarily **neurological,** which include **tremors, irritability, confusion and coma.**
- **Hypokalemia:** Hypokalemia is defined as **serum potassium concentration <3.5 mEq/L.** It is seen **in individuals taking potassium losing diuretics** (carbonic anhydrase inhibitors, loop diuretics or thiazides), those with **severe liver disease, gastrointestinal losses,** and metabolic alkalosis.

  Hypokalemia can also be a result of hyperaldosteronism, which, in turn, causes increased excretion of potassium accompanied by increased retention of Na^+ both of these leads to depletion of plasma K^+. Hypokalemia, affects both, **cardiac and skeletal muscles**. Deficiency symptoms include **muscular weakness, mental apathy, cardiac arrhythmias** (irregular heartbeat), **tachycardia** (heartbeat more rapid than usual), **hypotension, paralysis, bone fragility,** etc. It **can be corrected by** oral **KCl supplements** and, if necessary, by suitable intravenous electrolytes.
- **Hyperkalemia:** Hyperkalemia is defined as **serum potassium concentration >5.5 mEq/L.** It arises when **K^+ excretion by the kidney is depressed** such as in acute renal failure. **Acidosis** and **potassium-sparing diuretics may lead to hyperkalemia. Hyperkalemia,** in turn, **may lead to CNS depression, mental confusion, numbness or tingling of extremities and weakness of the respiratory muscles,** resulting in difficulty in breathing and speech. High concentration of potassium is also **toxic to muscles and may cause paralysis.**

BIOCHEMICAL EVALUATION OF WATER AND ELECTROLYTE IMBALANCE

The following estimations are performed for the biochemical evaluation of water and electrolyte imbalance:

1. Serum electrolyte concentration, i.e. **sodium, potassium, chloride and bicarbonate.**
2. **Serum creatinine and urea concentration**

3. **Serum osmolality**
4. **Urine volume, osmolality and sodium concentration.**

Some Important Questions

1. **What are electrolytes? Describe their physiological functions in the body.**
2. **Discuss various factors responsible for the regulation of electrolytes.**
3. **Describe physiological functions of electrolytes.**
4. **Write note on:**
   i. Hyponatremia
   ii. Hypernatremia
   iii. Hypokalemia
   iv. Hyperkalemia

Unit X

Practicals

Chapter 40

Practical Exercises

I. QUALITATIVE TESTS FOR CARBOHYDRATES

Several tests are done for the detection of a carbohydrate. The unspecific tests include Molisch test, which is based on the formation of furfural or its derivative in the presence of concentrate acid. Other tests, e.g. Fehling's test, Benedict's test, etc. are based on their reducing properties. Complex formation, such as the formation of phenylhydrazone crystals, is used as a specific test for some of the carbohydrates. For testing polysaccharides, iodine is commonly used.

MOLISCH TEST

Take about 2 ml of a carbohydrate solution in a test tube. Add a drop of the Molisch reagent and mix cautiously. Continuously pour down about 1 ml of concentrate H_2SO_4 so that two distinct layers are formed (the bottom layer being that of the acid). A reddish-violet zone appears at the junction of the two layers.

Molisch reagent is 10% solution of α-naphthol in ethanol.

This reaction is due to the formation of the furfural or its derivative (Fig. 40.1)

Furfural and furfural derivatives are highly reactive substances. They react with a number of compounds to produce complex-colored products.

It is not a specific test for carbohydrate. It is, however, an indication of the presence of a carbohydrate.

TESTS FOR REDUCING SUGARS

Due to the presence of a free aldehyde or ketone group, carbohydrates are readily oxidized and behave as reducing agents. Only the reducing sugar, therefore, will give a positive reaction. Non-reducing sugar like sucrose will respond to these reactions after its hydrolysis to glucose and fructose.

The following tests are based on the reducing properties of a sugar.

Fehling's Test

Add 1 ml of a sugar solution (a few drops at a time) to 4 ml of warm Fehling's solution and heat the mixture.

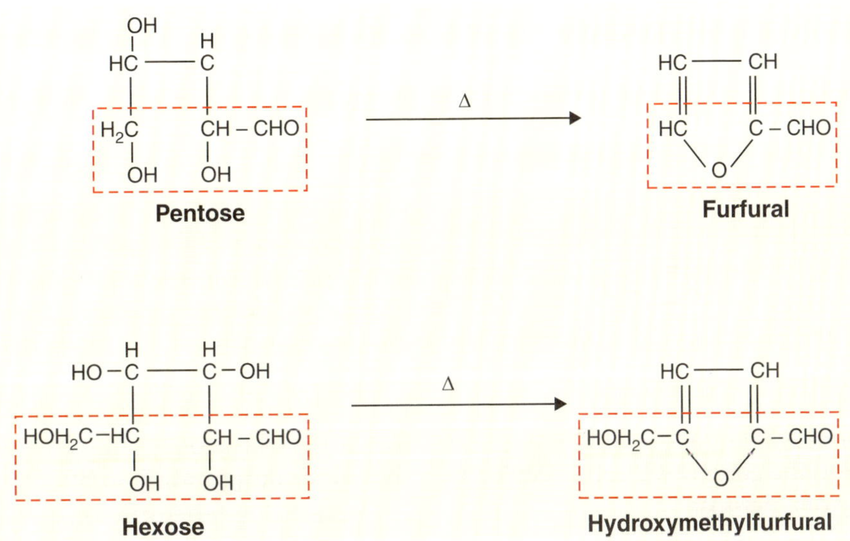

Fig. 40.1: Formation of furfural or its derivatives

Red precipitate indicates the presence of a reducing sugar.

Fehling's solution is a mixture of copper sulfate (1) and sodium-potassium tartarate (2). The two solutions are mixed afresh in equal volumes, immediately before use. This test is positive due to the reduction of copper sulfate ($CuSO_4$) to cuprous oxide (Cu_2O) in an alkaline medium.

Benedict's Test

Add 5 ml of the Benedict reagent (qualitative Benedict reagent) to 0.5 ml of a sugar solution in a test tube. Mix and heat the contents. In case of a reducing sugar, there is the appearance of a red precipitate.

Benedict qualitative solution is prepared by dissolving sodium citrate and sodium carbonate in water. Copper sulfate solution is slowly added with constant stirring to the above citrate-carbonate mixture. In the presence of a reducing sugar, a red precipitate is observed.

This test is routinely used in the examination of urine for the detection of a reducing sugar.

Benedict's test is more specific for a reducing sugar than the Fehling's test. In the Fehling's test, reduction of $CuSO_4$ takes place in a strong alkaline medium where even a small quantity of a reducing substance will give red precipitate while in the Benedict's test reduction occurs in a weak alkaline medium. Hence, Fehling's test is more sensitive but less specific whereas Benedict's test is less sensitive but more specific.

Barfoed Test

Mix 5 ml of the Barfoed reagent with 0.5 ml of the carbohydrate solution in a test tube and heat in a boiling water bath for 5 min. Appearance of the red precipitate within 5 min indicates the presence of a monosaccharide. If red precipitate is seen after 5 min, it confirms the presence of a reducing disaccharide (lactose or maltose).

Barfoed reagent is prepared by dissolving neutral copper acetate in water, thereafter glacial acetic acid is added to it. Barfoed test is also a copper reduction test. It, however, differs from the Fehling's or the Benedict tests. In Barfoed test, reduction of copper sulfate occurs in acidic medium, instead of the alkaline medium in the other two tests.

When a sugar solution is boiled for a long time with the Barfoed reagent, a disaccharide is hydrolyzed, by the acetic acid present in the reagent, and the monosaccharides give a positive test. Hence, monosaccharides respond quickly than a disaccharide.

Test for Pentoses

Take 3 ml of the orcinol reagent and add 0.5 ml of the sugar solution to it. Boil the contents. Deep-green color indicates the presence of a pentose.

Orcinol reagent contains orcinol and ferric chloride in concentrate HCl.

Pentoses react with HCl to form furfural, which then reacts with a phenol compound such as orcinol, and forms a deep-green colored complex.

Test for Galactose

Take 2 ml of the sugar solution in a test tube. To it, add 2 ml of concentrate HCl and 1 ml of fluoroglucinol solution. Boil slowly. A red color confirms the presence of galactose. This test is referred to as ***Tollen test***.

Galactose forms a red-colored complex with fluoroglucinol in concentrate HCl.

Lactose, after hydrolysis in hot acid reagent also gives the positive test due to the presence of galactose.

Test for Keto Sugars

To 0.5 ml of the sugar solution, add 5 ml of the Saliwanoff reagent. A blank (containing water) is prepared without the sugar solution, to judge for the color. Place the test tube in a boiling water bath for 1 min. Red color indicates the presence of a keto sugar such as fructose. This test is called ***Saliwanoff test***.

Saliwanoff reagent is resorcinol in concentrate HCl.

A ketose gives a fiery-red color. Aldoses, such as glucose, may also give the weak test. If boiling is prolonged, the positive test may be obtained even with glucose, due to its partial conversion to fructose.

This test may also be given by sucrose, which is hydrolyzed during the course of the test, yielding fructose as one of the products. However, the test will be positive after 1 min.

Osazone Test

Take about 200–300 mg (nearly 2–3 spoon) of phenylhydrazine mixture in a test tube. Add few drops of glacial acetic acid and about 5 ml of the sugar solution. Shake well and heat the contents in a boiling water bath for 15–30 min. Remove the test tube and allow it to cool, slowly. Yellow crystals of phenylhydrazine, called osazone crystals, appear. This test is called ***phenylhydrazine test or osazone test***.

Crystals of the maltose and the lactose appear only on cooling and not in the hot solution while that of glucose appear even when the tube is in the water bath.

Collect some of the crystals by a pipette, transfer them to a glass slide and examine under microscope.

Fine needle-shape yellow crystals are characteristic of a monosaccharide. Glucose, mannose and fructose give identical osazones. This is due to the reason that except first two carbons (which are identically involved in the formation of osazones); the remaining four carbons have the same configuration in the three sugars.

Sucrose does not form osazone because of not having a free reducing group available for its reaction with phenylhydrazine.

Crystals of lactose are puff-shaped while that of maltose are petal-shaped.

Phenylhydrazine mixture is prepared by mixing equal quantities of the phenylhydrazine hydrochloride with anhydrous sodium acetate.

TEST FOR POLYSACCHARIDES

Take 5 ml of starch solution in a test tube. Add a drop of dilute iodine solution and note the presence of blue color. This test is called ***iodine test***.

Heat the test tube. The blue color disappears but reappears on cooling. Blue colored substance is an adsorption complex between the starch and the iodine. Since this complex dissociates on heating, therefore, the color disappears when heated.

The complex is formed under neutral or acidic conditions. Under alkaline conditions I_2 reacts with NaOH so blue color disappears. If alkali is neutralized with acid, I_2 is released and blue color reappears. Color formed by iodine test depends upon the chain length of the polysaccharide.

Amylose gives deep-blue color; **amylopectin** (branched-chain compound) gives a purple color while **glycogen** (highly branched structure) gives a reddish brown color. **Erythrodextrin,** that is formed by the partial degradation of the starch, gives brownish-red color, as the linear chain length becomes smaller. On extensive degradation of the starch, the **achrodextrin** is formed, which may not give any color.

SCHEME FOR THE IDENTIFICATION OF AN UNKNOWN CARBOHYDRATE

The presence of a particular carbohydrate can be identified in an unknown solution by the **Molisch test.**

Thereafter, **Fehling's and Benedict tests** confirm the presence of a reducing sugar. A reducing sugar may be a monosaccharide or a disaccharide.

Barfoed test confirms the presence of a disaccharide, which can be further identified by the phenylhydrazine test.

Orcinol test, Tollen test and Saliwanoff test confirm the presence of pentose, galactose and fructose, respectively

The non-reducing sugar may be a polysaccharide or sucrose. **Iodine test** confirms the presence of a polysaccharide. If iodine test is negative, the non-reducing sugar is sucrose (Fig. 40.2).

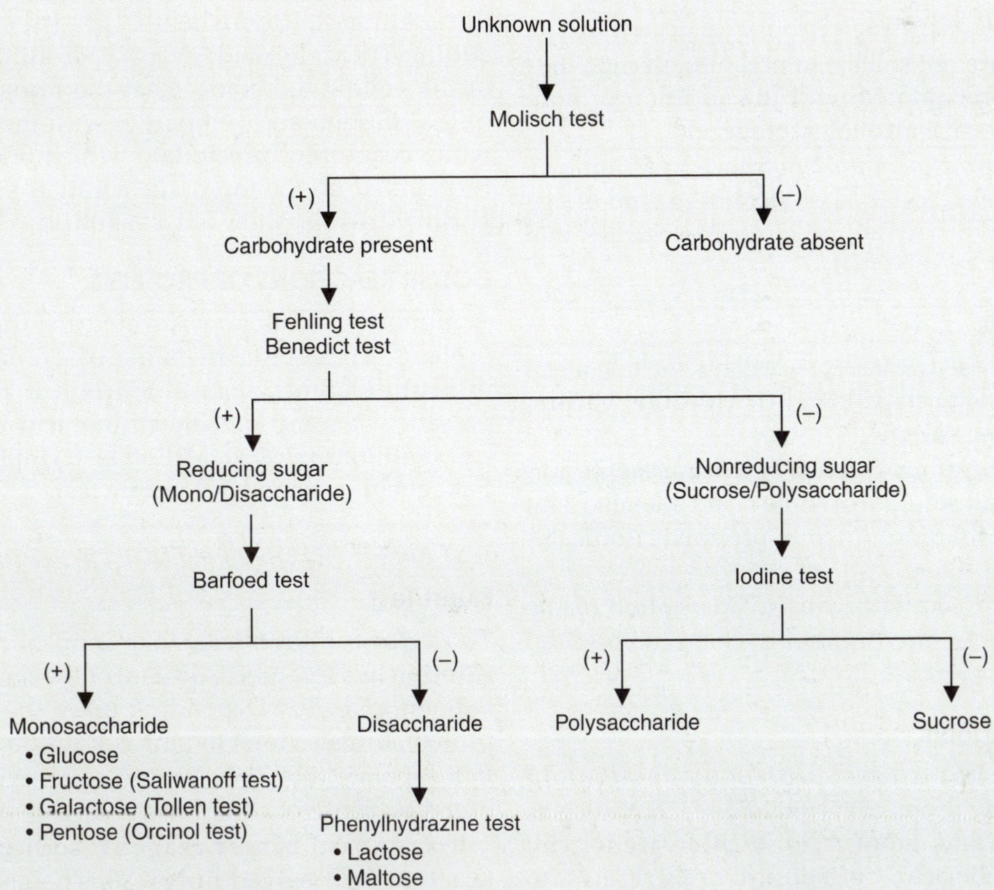

Fig. 40.2: Scheme for the identification of an unknown carbohydrate

II. QUALITATIVE TESTS FOR PROTEINS AND AMINO ACIDS

PRECIPITATION OF PROTEINS

By Salts

Proteins are the large molecular weight substances that can be easily precipitated by the addition of a salt solution. This process is known as **salting out**. Highly soluble salts, like NaCl and $(NH_4)_2SO_4$, are used for this purpose.

For the ***precipitation of globulins*** from egg white, add **equal** volume of saturated solution of **ammonium sulfate** to **egg white** solution. Mix and wait for 10–15 minutes. Filter the precipitate. Residue on the filter paper contains **globulins**.

For the ***precipitation of albumin***, add ammonium sulfate powder to the filtrate to **saturate it completely. Albumin** is precipitated.

This shows that albumin is more soluble in water than globulin, since, at full saturation albumin precipitates whereas at half saturation only globulins precipitate.

Precipitation of protein by a salt solution is, apparently, due to the neutralization of charges as well as dehydration of the molecule. Protein, which has been precipitated by a salt solution, remains native and usually gets redissolved when again put in the solvent.

By Non-aqueous Solvents

Since proteins are not soluble in organic solvents, they can be easily precipitated with the addition of non-aqueous solvents like **alcohol, acetone**, etc.

For the ***precipitation of protein*** from egg albumin ***by an organic solvent***, add 5 ml of **alcohol** to 3 ml of egg albumin solution. A white precipitate indicates that protein has been precipitated.

By Heavy Metals

Most commonly used protein precipitants, include metal salts such as **lead acetate, mercuric chloride, barium chloride and zinc sulfate**.

For the ***precipitation of protein by a heavy metal***, add few drops of a salt solution of some heavy metal to 2 ml of egg albumin solution. A white precipitate indicates precipitation of protein.

Protein gets precipitated due to adsorption of the metallic cations by the negatively charged colloidal particles of the protein.

By Alkaloid Reagents

To see the ***precipitation of protein by an alkaloid solution***, add few drops of an alkaloid reagent, such as **sulphosalicylic acid, tannic acid, trichloroacetic acid, phosphomolybdic acid,** tungstic acid or picric acid, to a tube containing 2 ml of egg albumin. A precipitate indicates the presence of protein.

Precipitation by an alkaloid reagent is due to the formation of an insoluble salt between the anions of the reagent and the positively-charged protein particles. This test is used for the detection of protein in urine.

PROTEIN DENATURATION

Usually, proteins are soluble in water due to their organized structure. On **heating** or adding a **strong acid**, protein looses its native structure and gets precipitated. This is referred to as **denaturation**. Usually, on denaturation protein **looses** its **biological activity**.

To **demonstrate the process of denaturation** of protein, take 3 ml of concentrate HNO_3 in a test tube and pour some protein solution from the side of the tube in a way that two solutions do not mix. A white precipitate, due to the precipitation of protein, appears at the junction of two fluids.

This test is used for the detection of protein (albumin) in urine and is referred to as **Heller test**.

PROTEIN COAGULATION

On heating protein gets coagulated. Coagulation is the maximum at pI.

To ***demonstrate the process of heat coagulation***, fill nearly 2/3rd of the test tube with egg albumin solution. Add a drop of chorophenol red and adjust the pH of the solution to approximately 5.4 (pI of albumin) by adding 1% acetic acid, drop by drop, till appearance of the yellow-red color. Heat the upper-half portion of the solution and compare it with the lower-half. A white coagulum (precipitate, which floats at the top) is observed on the top of the solution while the lower portion does not show any coagulum.

COLOR REACTIONS OF PROTEINS

A number of tests is performed for the detection of proteins. These tests are either based on the presence of **peptide bonds**, such as **biuret test**, or indicate the presence of some **specific amino acid** in the protein, e.g. **xanthoproteic test, Millon test, Hopkins-Cole test, Sakaguchi test and lead acetate test**.

TEST BASED ON THE PRESENCE OF PEPTIDE BONDS

Biuret Test

To perform biuret test, take 2 ml of some **protein solution** in a test tube, add 2 ml of the qualitative biuret reagent and mix. Depending upon the nature of the protein, **bluish-violet** to pink color is obtained.

In a separate tube, mix 2 ml of water with 2 ml of the biuret reagent, for comparison.

To prepare **biuret reagent**, sodium-potassium tartarate is dissolved in NaOH. Thereafter, $CuSO_4$ is added and the contents are mixed, until dissolved. Then add potassium iodide to it.

Principle of the Biuret Test: Peptide bonds (–CO–NH–), which are present in the protein, are responsible for the biuret test. A minimum of two consecutive peptide linkages give a positive test, i.e. minimum of a tripeptide (having two peptide linkages) is essential for the test. This test is called biuret test because biuret, which is formed on heating urea, also gives the positive test (Fig. 40.3).

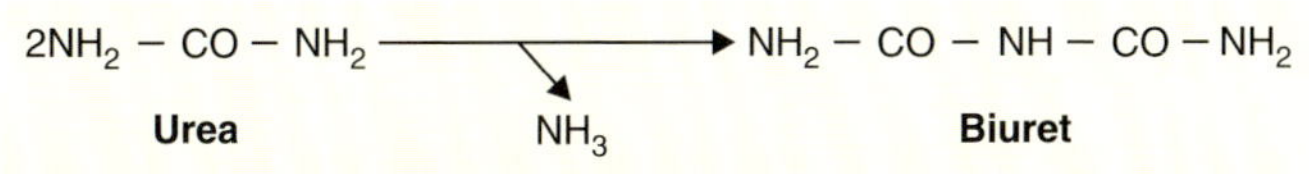

Fig. 40.3: Formation of biuret

TESTS BASED ON THE PRESENCE OF SPECIFICAMINO ACIDS

Xanthoproteic Test for Aromatic Amino Acids

To perform xanthoproteic test, heat 2 ml of a protein solution with 1 ml of concentrate nitric acid. Cool and add few drops of 10% NaOH. Orange color is obtained, which indicates the presence of aromatic amino acids.

This reaction is due to the presence of benzene ring that gets nitrated in the presence of concentrate nitric acid and forms nitrobenzene derivatives, which are yellow in color.

Among the 20 amino acids, which occur in most of the proteins, only 3 have a benzene ring. They are tyrosine, phenylalanine and tryptophan. These amino acids are referred to as **aromatic amino acids**.

Millon Test for Tyrosine (Phenol group)

To perform Millon test, take 3 ml of some protein solution in a test tube and add 3 to 4 drops of Millon reagent. Mix and heat the contents of the tube over a flame, so as to bring the solution to boil. Usually, protein is precipitated under this condition (at high temperature, in the presence of a strong acid). A white precipitate is obtained, which slowly turns to red, on continuous heating. This indicates the presence of tyrosine.

Millon reagent is prepared by dissolving Hg metal in fuming HNO_3, with gentle heating. Thereafter, 2 parts of water are added to it.

Tyrosine, due to the presence of the phenolic group, gives positive test with Millon reagent.

Hopkins-Cole Test for Tryptophan (Indole group)

To perform Hopkins-Cole test, take 3 ml of some protein solution, add 2 ml of the Hopkins-Cole reagent and mix. Then, cautiously pour down about 1 ml of concentrate H_2SO_4, so that the two layers do not mix together. A violet ring is formed at the junction of the two fluids, indicating the presence of tryptophan.

Hopkins-Cole reagent is an aqueous solution of glyoxylic acid. It is prepared by mixing magnesium powder with water. The mixture is shaken, cooled and, thereafter, cold saturated oxalic acid is added to it. The mixture is then thoroughly shaken and filtered.

Indole derivatives, such as **tryptophan**, give colored condensation products when treated with an aldehyde, like glyoxylic acid, in the presence of H_2SO_4 or HCl.

Sakaguchi Test for Arginine (Guanidino group)

To perform Sakaguchi test, take 3 ml of some protein solution and add 1 ml of 5% of NaOH, 2 drops of 1% alcoholic solution of α-naphthol and 1 drop of 10% sodium hypochlorite solution to it. Mix well. A bright-red color is observed due to the presence of arginine, an amino acid containing a guanidino group.

Lead Acetate Test for Sulfur-containing Amino Acids

To perform lead acetate test, heat 1 ml of some protein solution with 1 ml of 40% NaOH. Thereafter, add few drops of 10% lead acetate solution and again heat. A black precipitate is observed due to the formation of PbS, indicating the presence of sulfur-containing amino acids.

III. BIOCHEMICAL EVALUATION OF SALIVA

Saliva is a **mixture of secretions from salivary glands**. Salivary glands are three pairs of bilateral glands, referred to as the parotid, **the submandibular and the sublingual glands**. They are located along the jaw, from the base of the ear to the chin.

Secretion of one set of glands differs from that of the other. Secretion from the **parotid gland** is a serous fluid and contains an enzyme, referred to as **amylase. Sublingual glands** secrete a mucoid type of fluid, which contains mucous while secretion of the **submandibular gland is seromucous.**

COMPOSITION

Saliva, a mixture of three different secretions, is a colorless, slightly opalescent and viscous fluid with a specific gravity of 1.002–1.008. Its pH may vary from 6.4–7.3. Whereas, the resting saliva is slightly acidic (pH 6.4–6.9), saliva secreted under the influence of a stimulus is neutral to slightly alkaline (pH 7.0–7.3).

On an average, saliva contains nearly 99.4% water and 0.6% solids. Primary secretion is isotonic with plasma and contains both **organic** and **inorganic substances.** Nearly 65% of the total solids are organic substances while the remaining are inorganic salts (Fig. 40.4).

Organic Constituents

Organic constituents of saliva include various **enzymes, albumin, globulins, mucin, uric acid and urea.** Amino acids and glucose are also present in very small amounts.

High protein diet increases the level of urea in the salvia. Urea in turn acts as a buffer for the neutralization of acids, which are formed by bacterial fermentation.

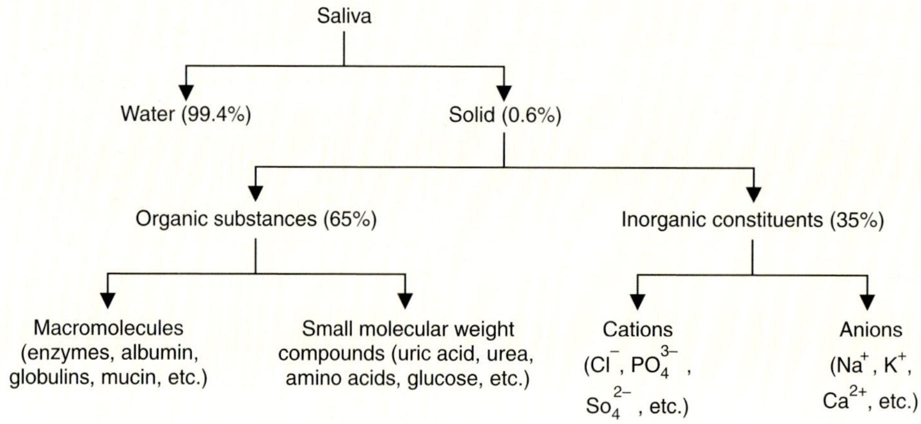

Fig. 40.4: Composition of saliva

Enzymes

Principal enzyme of the human saliva **is amylase**. Lipase, lysozyme, maltase, catalase, urease and proteases are also present in traces.

Salivary Amylase: Salivary amylase (the S-type enzyme) is a most important enzyme present in saliva. It is secreted chiefly, by the parotid glands. It is also referred to as **ptyalin.**

Salivary amylase is an **α-amylase**. It has important role in the **digestion of polysaccharides**. It hydrolyses polysaccharides, **like starch, glycogen, and dextrin into glucose, maltose, maltotriose** and a mixture of branched oligosaccharide and dextrins. Action of salivary amylase occurs mainly, in the mouth for a short period only (5–6 min, i.e. till the food enters the stomach and mixes with the gastric juice). **Salivary amylase is α-1,4-glycosidase** because of its specific hydrolytic action on **α-1,4-glycosidic** bonds. **Optimal pH** for the enzyme **is 6.8.**

Lesions in salivary glands, such as caused by infections, irradiation, obstruction, surgery or tumor, produce **hyperamylasemia**. Mumps and maxillary surgery may cause two-fold elevation while salivary gland irradiation can produce 9–10 fold elevation of serum amylase. Increased levels of salivary amylase also occur in biliary tract diseases, such as in cholecystitis, intra-abdominal events, e.g. ruptured ectopic pregnancy, peritonitis and acute appendicitis.

Lingual Lipase: The lingual serous glands secrete lingual lipase. It is of particular importance in neonates where it hydrolyses dietary fat.

Lysozyme: Lysozyme is a polysaccharidase, which hydrolyses complex polysaccharides that are present in the bacterial cell wall. Its activity in saliva, is nearly equal to that of the blood and is only about 1% of that present in tears.

Mucin

Mucin is a **mucoprotein, secreted** chiefly **by the sublingual and submandibular pairs.** It is mainly responsible for giving viscosity to saliva. It acts as a lubricant and **facilitates swallowing of food.**

Inorganic Constituents

Chief inorganic ions present in the saliva are **K^+, PO_4^{3-} and Cl^- with small amounts of Na^+, Ca^{2+} and SO_4^{2-}.** Of these, Ca^{2+} helps to stabilize salivary amylase while Cl^- acts as an activator for it.

Ionic concentration of saliva varies with its rate of flow. Under resting conditions, concentrations of Na^+ and Cl^- are lower than that of the plasma while those of K^+ and HCO_3^- are higher than the plasma.

Some of these inorganic ions may combine and form insoluble precipitates, such as $Ca_3(PO_4)_2$ or $CaCO_3$. This, in turn, may lead to the formation of **salivary calculi.**

REGULATION OF SECRETION OF SALIVA

Total flow of saliva in an adult man is nearly **1.0–1.5 L/day.** It may vary widely, depending upon the intake of water and food, character of food and the process of chewing. Under resting conditions, about **0.5 ml** of the saliva is secreted per min. The presence of food in the mouth may increase the rate of secretion of saliva, up to 8 ml/min. Rate of secretion of saliva is entirely under the control of the nervous system.

A variety of **stimuli**, by reflex stimulation, cause **increased rate of flow**. These include:

1. **Psychic stimuli**, such as **sight, smell or thought of the palatable food** increase salivary secretion by conditioned reflex mechanism.
2. **Mechanical stimulation**, such as **chewing of food**, and
3. **Chemical stimulation**, e.g. **contact of sugar, salt, acid or spices on the taste buds.**

Stimulation of certain taste receptors, e.g. sour food, causes more profused secretion than other types of taste receptors.

Aging causes atrophy of the cells in the salivary glands, resulting in decreased salivary flow and changes its composition.

Decreased salivary flow leads to **dryness of mouth** called **xerostomia**. Lack of saliva causes dryness of the oral mucosa, and makes chewing and swallowing more difficult. It **also increases the incidence of dental caries**. Chewing stimulates salivary flow and helps in prevention of xerostomia.

PHYSIOLOGICAL FUNCTIONS OF SALIVA

Various physiological functions of saliva are shown in Table 40.1.

Table 40.1: Important physiological functions of saliva
• Formation of food bolus • Hydrolysis of starch • Bactericidal action • Protection of teeth and gums against decay • Excretion of toxic substances • Perception of taste • Speech • Helps in absorption of vitamin B_{12}

1. During mastication, saliva gets mixed with the **food** and **changes** it **into a semisolid form** called **food bolus**, which can be easily swallowed.
2. Due to the presence of α-amylase, **digestion of starch** starts in the mouth. This role of salivary amylase, however, is limited, since as the food bolus reaches stomach and mixes with the gastric juice, acidic pH stops this action.
3. Saliva **contains** buffering substances, e.g. **bicarbonate, phosphates and mucin**. It, thus, keeps the mouth at neutral pH and **protects teeth from decalcification.** Saliva also contains several proteolytic enzymes and antibodies that have **bactericidal action.** Saliva thus, has a **protective effect on** the development of **dental caries**.
4. Normally, tooth enamel is continuously bathed in saliva. As there is exchange of nutrients, particularly minerals, between the enamel and the saliva, it contributes to the **resistance to tooth decay.** Adequate saliva production is, therefore, essential to maintain integrity of teeth as well as other oral structures.
5. Saliva also has **excretory functions**. It acts as a channel for **excretion of toxic substances**, such as lead and mercury, which enters mouth along with the food material.

   Some of the **waste products of metabolism**, such as urea, uric acid, ammonia and other detoxified

DIAGNOSTIC SIGNIFICANCE OF SALIVA

Estimation and/or isolation of the various substances from saliva is helpful in clinical evaluation of certain diseases (Table 40.2):

1. Most of the **steroids** of clinical interest can be measured in saliva. For some of the steroids, such as cortisol, estriol and progesterone, measurement of **their salivary level is a reliable indicator of free concentrations in plasma.**
2. Measurement of cortisol in saliva is a more practical and convenient approach for assessing the concentration of free hormone. Salivary cortisol measurement reflects concentration of nonprotein-bound cortisol in blood, which is independent of salivary flow rate.
3. Morning salivary cortisol concentration is decreased in adrenal insufficiency (Addison's disease) while evening values are increased in hyperactivity of the adrenal gland (Cushing's syndrome).
4. Salivary **testosterone concentration** also correlates well with the free testosterone level in plasma. It has been suggested as an indicator of the androgen status.
5. Saliva is tested for **secretary IgA** in infantile hypogammaglobulinemia and β-macroglobulinemia, in Sjögren's syndrome.
6. Measurement of a drug in the saliva can be used as an estimate of free and pharmacologically active **concentration of the drug** in the serum.
7. Saliva can also be used for the **isolation of viruses**, such as mumps virus, rabies virus, Epstein-Barr virus or herpes simplex virus.
8. Saliva can also be used for identifying a suspect in a **forensic** laboratory.

Table 40.2: Diagnostic significance of saliva
• Estimation of steroids • Estimation of proteins, including antibodies in a disease condition • Estimation of drugs • Isolation of viruses • Forensic applications

products, e.g. thiocyanate, are also partially, excreted in the saliva.

Iodine, which is produced as a result of deiodination of thyroxine in the parotid and submaxillary glands, is also excreted via saliva.

Some of the **drugs**, such as morphine and alcohol, may also be excreted through saliva.

6. Saliva also **serves as a solvent** for the transport of molecules so that they reach taste receptors, in the taste buds.
7. Saliva also **helps in speech** by keeping the mouth, lips and tongue moist.
8. Saliva also helps in **absorption of vitamin B_{12}**. At low pH of stomach, most of the cobalamin is temporarily bound to a salivary protein, called R-protein (R refers to rapid electrophoretic mobility). This complex reaches duodenum where R-protein is degraded by the pancreatic proteases so that vitamin B_{12} can bind to the intrinsic factor (IF). IF-B_{12} complex is resistant to proteolysis and directly passes into the distal ileum, which is the site of vitamin B_{12} absorption.

COLLECTION OF SALIVA

Take about 15–20 ml of water in mouth and chew it for about 2–3 minutes. Collect the secretion in a beaker.

PRACTICAL EXERCISES WITH SALIVARY AMYLASE

To Demonstrate the Effect of Salivary Amylase on Hydrolysis of Starch

Salivary amylase catalyses the hydrolysis of α-1,4-glycosidic linkages present in amylose and amylopectin (two components of starch), and glycogen, randomly.

Hydrolysis of starch by salivary amylase yields polysaccharides of gradually diminishing molecular size, i.e amylodextrin, erythrodextrin and achrodextrin (Fig. 40.5).

Starch (Blue)
↓
Amylodextrin (Violet)
↓
Erythrodextrin (Red)
↓
Achrodextrin + Maltose (No color)

Fig. 40.5: Hydrolysis of starch by salivary amylase

Time taken by the enzyme to hydrolyze starch, to the stage of achrodextrin, i.e. when it fails to change the color of iodine, is referred to as **achromic point**. Normally, it is 8–10 minutes.

To demonstrate the effect of salivary amylase on the hydrolysis of starch and to find out the achromic point, saliva is collected, as above. It is mixed with the reaction mixture containing starch, NaCl, and buffer. The mixture is thereafter, periodically added to iodine and the change in color of iodine is observed.

Procedure: Take 5 ml of starch **in a test tube. Add 2** ml of phosphate buffer **(pH 6.8)** and 1 ml of NaCl **solution (5%) to it. Incubate this** reaction mixture **at 37°C for 4–5 min.**

Take 0.5 ml of iodine solution in 10–12 tubes and place them in a rack, at room temperature.

Thereafter, add 2 ml of the salivary amylase (collected salivary secretion) to the tube containing the above reaction mixture, which was kept in a water bath at 37°C. Mix the contents and take a drop from the mixture. Add it to the first tube containing iodine. Starch gives blue color. Thereafter, repeat the same, after every one minute by adding a drop of the reaction mixture, each time to a new tube containing iodine, and continue up to 10–15 minutes. Decrease in blue color gives the idea of starch hydrolyzed by the enzyme. Note the time required for achieving the **achromic point**.

As we know, several factors are known to affect salivary amylase activity. These include pH, temperature, etc.

Effect of pH on Salivary Amylase

Amylase has optimum pH of 6.8–7.0. Its activity is reduced with change in pH.

Procedure: To demonstrate the effect of pH on salivary amylase, take 2 test tubes. Mark them as control and test, and add various solutions as shown in Table 40.3.

Table 40.3: Procedure to demonstrate the effect of pH on salivary amylase

Solution	*Control*	*Test*
Starch solution	5 ml	5 ml
Buffer	2 ml (pH 6.8)	2 ml (pH 5.0)
NaCl solution	1 ml	1 ml
Mix and incubate at 37°C for 3–4 min.		
Saliva (enzyme)	2 ml	2 ml

Mix the contents and incubate at 37°C. Take one drop from each of the above two tubes, containing reaction mixtures, after every one min. and add to two separate tubes containing iodine solution.

Note the achromic point for each tube. Compared to the control tube (pH 6.8), achromic point is prolonged in the tube containing buffer of pH 5.0 (test).

It demonstrates that low pH reduces enzyme activity.

Effect of Temperature on Salivary Amylase

Optimum temperature for salivary amylase is between 37–40°C. When temperature is increased beyond 50°C, its activity is reduced. On boiling, enzyme gets denatured and its activity is lost.

Procedure: To demonstrate that enzyme is destroyed on boiling, take 2 ml of saliva (enzyme) in a tube, boil it over the flame (to denature the enzyme) and cool it.

Take 2 test tubes and mark them as control and test. Add various solutions to them as shown in Table 40.4.

Table 40.4: Procedure to demonstrate the effect of temperature on salivary amylase

Solution	*Control*	*Test*
Starch solution	5 ml	5 ml
Buffer (pH 6.8)	2 ml	2 ml
NaCl solution	1 ml	1 ml
Mix and incubate at 37°C for 3–4 min.		
Saliva (enzyme)	2 ml (normal enzyme)	2 ml (boiled enzyme)

Mix the contents and incubate at 37°C. Add a drop from each of the two tubes containing reaction mixtures, to two separate tubes containing iodine solution. Repeat after every one minute. Note the achromic point for the control tube.

Continue with the other tube labelled as test for about 10 more minutes. Achromic point is not observed in this tube as the enzyme has been denatured on boiling and lost its activity.

Effect of Activator (chloride ions, Cl^-) on Salivary Amylase

Chloride ions (Cl^-) act as activator for salivary amylase whereas fluoride, oxalate, citrate and EDTA act as inhibitors for the enzyme.

Procedure: To demonstrate the effect of (Cl^-) as activator for salivary amylase, take 2 test tubes and label them as control and test. Add various solutions to these tubes, as shown in Table 40.5.

Table 40.5: Procedure to demonstrate the effect of Cl^- as activator on salivary amylase

Solution	*Control*	*Test*
Starch solution	5 ml	5 ml
Buffer (pH 6.8)	2 ml	2 ml
NaCl solution	1 ml	—
Distilled water	—	1 ml
Mix and incubate at 37°C for 3–4 min.		
Saliva (enzyme)	2 ml	2 ml

Mix the contents and incubate at 37°C. Add a drop of the reaction mixture from each of the above two tubes, to two separate tubes containing iodine solution. Repeat after every one minute till achromic point is reached.

Achromic point is prolonged in the tube which contains distilled water instead of NaCl. It demonstrates that Cl^- ions are required as activator for salivary amylase.

IV. BIOCHEMICAL ANALYSIS OF MILK

During recent years although dried milk foods are being used extensively for feeding infants, human milk is still regarded as the ideal food for feeding infants during the early months of life, universally.

Colostrum: Milk secreted during the first few days after delivery is known as colostrum. It is comparatively more yellowish and contains more proteins. There is a steady fall in protein content of milk with the advancement of lactation.

Modification of the Animal Milk for Infant Feeding

Milk from animal source can be modified for infant feeding by adjustment of some of the nutrients by dilution, boiling and adding sugar. This is also referred to as **humanization of the animal milk**.

Dilution and boiling: Dilution with water is essential to reduce its protein and mineral contents. Animal milk is generally diluted with equal amount of water, for feeding infants (1–2 months of age). As an infant grows, proportion of water is gradually reduced.

Boiling also brings physicochemical changes in milk and improves it digestibility.

Adjustment of fat: Animal milk, particularly from buffalo, should be partially skimmed, to reduce its fat to about 3.5%.

Addition of sugar: Sugar is added to bring its level to about 5% after dilution.

CHEMICAL ANALYSIS OF MILK

Milk contains large amount of casein which is first precipitated at its isoelectric point (pH 5.4) and thereafter removed by filtration. The precipitate and the filtrate are thereafter tested separately, as follows:

1. Precipitate for fat and protein (casein). Since casein is a phosphoprotein, test for phosphorus will also be positive with the precipitate.
2. Filtrate for lactose, proteins (lactalbumin and lactoglobulin), Ca^{2+} and phosphorus.

PRECIPITATION OF CASEIN

Take 1 test tube full of milk and transfer it to a beaker. Thereafter, add 1 test tube of water and 1 test tube of 1% acetic acid. Keep for 5 min and centrifuge/filter.

TESTS WITH THE PRECIPITATE

Test for Fat

Take a small amount of the precipitate in a test tube and add 2 ml of alcohol. Heat the contents to solubilize lipids.

COMPOSITION OF MILK

In general, milk contains **80–90% water**. Amongst the various nutrients, **lactose, fat,** and **proteins** are the major constituents of milk.

Milk contains **three types of proteins,** called **casein**, albumin and globulins, also referred to as **lactalbumin** and **lactoglobulins**.

Casein is a phosphoprotein and has high biological value. It can be precipitated at pH 5.4, by the addition of acid. After the precipitation of casein, lactalbumin and lactoglobulin remain in the filtrate. **Lactoglobulin provides immunity** to the child.

Milk fat contains **triglycerides, short and medium chain fatty acids, phospholipids** (particularly lecithin) and small amount of **cholesterol**. In addition, milk also contains large amounts of **calcium, phosphorus, vitamin A and riboflavin.** Thiamin, vitamin C, vitamin D, and iron are present in small amounts.

Milk from different species differs in the relative amounts of protein, fat, lactose, minerals, and vitamins. They also differ in digestibility. For example, human milk contains more lactose compared to cow's milk while cow's milk contains more protein, calcium, and phosphorus.

Data regarding chemical composition of human milk as compared with those from some other species are shown in Table 40.6.

Table 40.6: Composition of milk from different sources (values are per 100 ml of milk)

Nutrients	*Human milk*	*Cow milk*	*Buffalo milk*	*Goat milk*
Calories (kcal)	71	69	100	76
Protein (g)	1.2	3.3	3.8	3.3
Fat (g)	3.8	3.7	7.5	4.1
Lactose (g)	7.0	4.8	4.4	4.7
Calcium (mg)	33	125	210	130
Phosphorus (mg)	15	96	130	106
Vitamin A (mg)	48	47	60	36
Riboflavin (μg)	40	180	100	120

Add few drops of water. Fat droplet appears. Shake and put a drop on a paper. A greasy-spot is observed on the paper.

Tests for Proteins

To confirm the presence of casein, biuret test for protein and color reactions for various amino acids are done with the precipitate, after its suspension in water.

Biuret test: Take a small amount of the precipitate in a test tube and suspend it in 2 ml of water. Add 3 ml of qualitative biuret reagent. Purple color indicates the presence of protein.

Ninhydrin test: Heat the suspension of casein with 2–3 drops of ninhydrin. Deep-blue color is observed due to the presence of free α-amino groups of amino acids in the protein.

Xanthoproteic test: To 2 ml of suspension of casein in a test tube, add 1 ml of concentrate nitric acid. Boil and add 2–3 drops of NaOH solution. Orange color is observed due to the presence of aromatic amino acids in the protein.

Millon's test: To 2 ml suspension of casein in water, add 1–2 drops of Millon's reagent. Boil and cool the contents, and add 1 ml of sodium nitrite. Red color confirms the presence of tyrosine in the protein.

Hopkins-Cole test: To 2 ml water suspension of casein in a test tube, add 2–3 drops of Millon's reagent and 2–3 drops of formalin. Mix and add concentrate H_2SO_4 along the side of the test tube. Violet colored ring indicates the presence of tryptophan in the protein.

Sakaguchi test: Take 2 ml of water suspension of casein in a test tube. Add 1 ml of 10% NaOH and 2–3 drops of alcoholic solution of α-naphthol. Mix and add 2–3 drops of sodium hypobromide solution. Red color confirms the presence of arginine in the protein.

Lead acetate test: Take 2 ml water suspension of casein in a test tube. Add 1 ml of 40% NaOH and 2–3 drops of lead acetate solution. Heat the contents. Black precipitate is seen due to the presence of sulfur-containing amino acids in the protein.

TESTS WITH THE FILTRATE

Tests for Reducing Sugar (Lactose)

Lactose may be determined either by Benedict, Barfoed's or KOH reduction test.

Benedict's test: Take 5 ml of the qualitative Benedict's reagent in a test tube. Add 0.5 ml of the filtrate to it and boil. Red precipitate appears due to the presence of a reducing sugar.

Barfoed's test: Take 5 ml of Barfoed's reagent in a test tube. Add 0.5 ml of the filtrate to it. Mix and place the tube in a boiling water bath. Appearance of the red precipitate after 5 min confirms the presence of a reducing disaccharide.

KOH reduction test: Take 5 ml of the filtrate in a test tube. Add 2 ml of ammonium hydroxide and few drops of 15% KOH solution. Mix and place the tube in boiling water bath. Orange color indicates the presence of lactose.

Tests for Lactalbumin

Heat coagulation test: As the isoelectric pH for albumin is 4.6, hence it does not get precipitated at the isoelectric pH of casein (5.4) and appears in the filtrate.

Take a test tube nearly 2/3 filled with the filtrate. Add a drop of chlorophenol red. Yellow color is observed. Add 1% acetic acid drop by drop to lower the pH from 5.4 to 4.6 (isoelectric pH for albumin), till the solution turns pink. Heat upper half of the solution, a white coagulum appears due to coagulation of lactalbumin at its pI.

Color reactions for the presence of various amino acids: Perform following tests with the filtrate:

- Biuret test
- Ninhydrin test
- Xanthoproteic test
- Millon's test
- Hopkins-Cole test
- Sakaguchi test, and
- Lead acetate test

All the tests will be positive.

Test for Calcium

Take 2 ml of filtrate in a test tube and add 2–3 drops of potassium oxalate solution to it. White precipitate of calcium oxalate is observed, due to the presence of Ca^{2+} in the filtrate.

Test for Phosphorus

Take 2 ml of filtrate in a test tube. Add 2 ml of concentrate sulfuric acid and 2–3 drops of concentrate nitric acid. Heat the contents and add 2–3 drops of ammonium molybdate reagent. Yellow precipitate of phosphomolybdate indicates the presence of phosphorus.

This is referred to as **Neumann's test.**

V. ANALYSIS OF GASTRIC JUICE

COLLECTION OF SAMPLE

The gastric fluid is obtained by aspiration through a gastric tube (such as Ryle's tube).

The patient is asked to sit with the head tilted slightly forward. Place the tip of the tube on the tongue, hold well and push it towards the throat or introduce the tube along the floor of the nose, until it is felt that the top turns down into the pharynx. Thereafter, the patient is asked to swallow it slowly until it is passed to the desired length.

EXAMINATION OF THE GASTRIC RESIDUE

The content of the stomach after nearly 12 hours of fast is referred to as **gastric residue (residuum).** It is examined for physical characteristics, chemical constituents and free and total acidity.

Physical Examination

Color: Resting gastric content is usually colorless. It may be slightly yellow or green due to the regurgitation of bile. It may be dark-red or brown due to the presence of blood.

Volume: Total volume of the resting gastric residue normally varies between 20 and 50 ml. Volume above 100–200 ml may be considered abnormal. It may be due to hypersecretion, retention or regurgitation from the duodenum. Other causes include pyloric obstruction, duodenal ulcer or Zollinger-Ellison syndrome.

Consistency: Resting gastric juice is a fluid of low specific gravity. It may be viscous due to the presence of mucus. Food particles may be present in carcinoma of the stomach.

Chemical Examination

Bile: A small amount of bile may regurgitate into the stomach during intubation. Increased amount may be a result of intestinal obstruction or ileal stasis.

Mucus: Small amount of mucus is normally found. Excessive amount may be due to excessive amount of saliva in the gastric juice. Increased amount may also be seen in gastritis and gastric carcinoma.

Blood: Normally, blood is not present in the gastric juice. Accidental trauma to the gastric mucous membrane, during the passage of the tube, may result in traces of blood. Increased amount of blood may be present due to lesion, such as gastric carcinoma or gastric ulcer.

Organic acids: Lactic acid and butyric acid may be present in large amounts in hyperacidity, achlorhydria and carcinoma of the stomach.

In the absence of free HCl, organic acids are formed in increased amounts by bacterial fermentation of food, as food is retained in the stomach for longer period.

Pepsin: Absence of pepsin is seen in a condition called **achylia gastrica**.

Decreased levels of pepsin are seen in diseases, such as atrophic gastritis and gastric carcinoma.

Increased pepsin activity may be observed in diseases associated with increased gastric output or in patients with gastrinomas, Zollinger-Ellison syndrome, duodenal ulcer and gastritis as well as after omeprazole administration.

FREE AND TOTAL ACIDITY

Free Acidity

HCl is the main acid in the gastric juice, which is a strong mineral acid and accounts for free acidity. It is secreted by the parietal cells, at a concentration of about 155 mmol/L (mEq/L) and has pH less than 1.0. As parietal secretion gets mixed with other gastric constituents, concentration of hydrogen ions usually reaches less than 40 mEq/L, with pH between 1.5 and 2.5.

Free acidity concentration in the gastric residue, in a normal individual, varies from 0–40 mEq/L.

Increase in free acidity (more than 45 mEq/L) is referred to as **hyperchlorhydria.** It occurs in duodenal and gastric ulcers, Zollinger-Ellison syndrome, etc.

Decreased secretion of HCl is called **hypochlorhydria.** It is observed in gastric carcinoma, chronic gastritis, constipation and anemia.

Complete absence of HCl in the gastric juice is called **achlorhydria**. It occurs in pernicious anemia. Achlorhydria may also be seen in tuberculosis, gastric carcinoma and atrophic gastritis.

In the absence of HCl bacterial fermentation of food is increased, which in turn, leads to the formation of lactic acid.

Total Acidity

Total acidity in the gastric residue is due to hydrogen ions occurring as free HCl, mucoproteins and organic acids, such as lactic acid and butyric acid. Total acid concentration in a normal state is usually between 10–50 mEq/L.

STIMULATION OF GASTRIC SECRETION

Many compounds or processes such as test meal, alcohol, caffeine, gastrin, pentagastrin or insulin stimulate gastric secretion and thus secretion of HCl.

By alcohol: Fifty to hundred ml of 7% ethyl alcohol (3.5 ml of ethanol in 50 ml of water) is administered through Ryle's tube.

By caffeine: Caffeine sodium benzoate (500 mg in about 200 ml of water) can also be administered into the stomach through the Ryle's tube.

By histamine: Histamine is a powerful stimulant for the secretion of gastric juice. It causes secretion of increased volume of highly acidic gastric juice with low pepsin content.

Two types of histamine tests are carried out:

Standard histamine test: Subcutaneous injection of histamine (0.01 mg/kg body weight) is given and gastric contents are removed. Absence of free HCl in gastric secretion after giving histamine indicates **achylia gastrica**.

Augmented histamine test: A large dose of histamine (0.04 mg/kg body weight) is given. In pernicious anemia no free HCl is secreted but in other forms of achlorhydria some amount of free HCl may be secreted after augmented histamine test.

Sometimes high dose of histamine may cause a severe reaction. Under such conditions, injection of some antihistamine (100 mg) may be given, intramuscularly. Administration of antihistamine does not interfere in gastric stimulation.

By insulin: Intravenous injection of insulin (0.1–0.2 U/kg body weight) may be given for the stimulation of gastric secretion and samples are withdrawn after every 15 min. This is called **Hollander's Test**.

Insulin stimulation is helpful to ascertain the effectiveness of vagotomy in patients with duodenal ulcer where concentration of free HCl may be as high as 100 mEq/L. After successful vagotomy since there is no response to insulin, gastric acidity remains at a low level of 15–20 mEq/L before as well as after insulin administration.

This test is not preferred as insulin may result in hypoglycemia.

By gastrin/pentagastrin: Gastrin is a powerful stimulus for HCl secretion. It is administered in a single subcutaneous dose of 2 mg/kg body weight.

Pentagastrin is a synthetic pentapeptide with physiologically active part of gastrin. It is also a potent stimulus for HCl secretion and is commonly used now-a-days.

Fasting content of stomach is aspirated. Secretions are collected at 15 minute intervals, up to 1 hour, pooled and volume is measured. This is termed as **basal acid output (BAO)**.

After the aspiration of the fasting sample, pentagastrin is given (6 mg/kg body weight), subcutaneously and post-stimulation secretions are collected at 15 min intervals, up to next one hour. This is termed as **maximal acid output** (MAO).

This test is useful in differentiating the diagnosis of achlorhydria and hyperchlorhydria.

ESTIMATION OF FREE AND TOTAL ACIDITY

Principle: Acids present in the gastric juice are titrated with a strong alkali. During titration with alkali (0.1 N NaOH) HCl is completely neutralized at about pH 3.5 whereas weak acids are neutralized in the alkaline range (at about pH 8.0). Thus, titration is done by using

Topfer's reagent as indicator during titration for free acidity while phenolphthalein is used for titrating total acidity.

Topfer's reagent has a pH range of 2.9 (red) to 4.0 (yellow). On the other hand, phenolphthalein works in the pH range of 8.2 (colorless) to 10.0 (pink).

Procedure: Fill 0.1 N NaOH solution in the burette. Take 10 ml gastric juice in a conical flask or china dish and add a drop of Topfer's reagent to it.

On adding the indicator if yellow color is seen, this indicates the absence of free acid (HCl). If red color appears, titrate with 0.1N NaOH till salmon pink color appears. Note the volume of NaOH used. This gives the value of free acidity.

Add a drop of phenolphthalein and again titrate with 0.1N NaOH. Note the change in color from salmon pink to colorless. Note the volume of NaOH used. This gives the value for total acidity.

Calculation:

$$\textbf{Free acidity (mEq/L)} = \frac{\text{ml of 0.1 N NaOH required to titrate 10 ml of gastric juice with Topfer's reagent (A)}}{} \times \frac{100}{10}$$

or $= A \times 10$

$$\textbf{Total acidity (mEq/L)} = \text{ml of 0.1 N NaOH required to titrate 10 ml of gastric juice with phenolphthalein (B)} \times \frac{100}{10}$$

or $= B \times 10$

The result may also be expressed in terms of **clinical units**.

One clinical unit is defined as the **amount of 0.1 N NaOH required to neutralize** the amount of acid present in **100 ml of gastric juice**.

Normally, free HCl is 0–30 mEq/L. Concentration above 50 mEq/L may be suggestive of hyperacidity.

Total acidity includes free HCl and combined acidity.

Combined acidity refers to the amount of organic acids (mainly lactic acid) and H^+ bound with proteins. Total acidity is up to 10 mEq/L more than free acidity.

VI. ESTIMATION OF BLOOD GLUCOSE

There are several photometric oxidation-reduction methods besides the enzymatic method to measure blood glucose concentration. Some of these are relatively nonspecific and result in false increased values.

SAMPLE COLLECTION

In methods for self-monitoring of glucose though whole blood can be used, in most of the clinical chemistry laboratories plasma or serum is used for glucose determination.

Fasting whole blood glucose concentration is nearly 10–15% lower than plasma. This is due to lower water content with in red blood cells.

During fasting, capillary blood glucose concentration is nearly 3–5 mg/dL higher than the venous blood.

In a normal blood sample, serum glucose concentration is decreased by 5–7% in 1 hour, at room temperature. In separated non-hemolysed sterile serum, glucose concentration is generally stable for nearly 8 hours at 25°C and up to 72 hours at 4°C.

Glycolysis in the red blood cells reduces blood glucose value by nearly 5% each hour, at room temperature. To prevent this loss, most commonly, the sample is collected in a vial containing a mixture of sodium fluoride (2 mg/dL) and potassium oxalate (2 mg/dL). Alternatively, either the sample should be analyzed within 30 min of its collection or an inhibitor of glycolysis, such as sodium fluoride, should be added. Sodium fluoride (NaF) prevents glycolysis by inhibiting enolase.

METHODS OF ESTIMATION OF BLOOD GLUCOSE

OXIDATION-REDUCTION METHODS

Many procedures for measuring glucose are based on its property of acting as a reducing agent in a hot alkaline solution.

The principle of these methods is that in a hot alkaline solution aldehyde group of glucose readily reduces cupric ions (Cu^{2+}) to cuprous ions (Cu^+), which, in turn, form cuprous oxide (Cu_2O).

Standard solution is also analyzed in the same manner as protein free filtrate. It is due to the reason that this reaction is dependent on the alkalinity, the time and temperature of heating, and the concentration of reagents.

Thereafter, phosphomolybdic or arsenomolybdic acid is added, which in turn is reduced by the cuprous ions and forms molybdenum blue (the compound with lower oxidation state of molybdenum and is blue in color). The intensity of the color is measured colorimetrically.

Most commonly used oxidation-reduction methods include Folin-Wu method and Somogyi-Nelson method.

Folin-Wu Method

As in some of the laboratories it is still being used, its details are given below.

This is based on the reducing property of glucose and may over estimate blood glucose value by 15–20%. This is due to the presence of other reducing substances, such as glutathione, vitamin C, other sugars, etc. in the blood.

Principle: In Folin-Wu method, proteins are precipitated with tungstic acid and the protein-free filtrate is used in the reaction with cupric ions. Re-oxidation of cuprous ions by oxygen, from the air, is prevented by using a specially designed constricted tube, referred to as the Folin-Wu tube. The cuprous oxide, so formed, is treated with phosphomolybdic acid solution. Blue color is formed whose intensity is compared with the standard.

Preparation of protein-free filtrate: Take 3 test tubes and label them as blank (B), Standard (S) and test (T). Add distilled water, standard, blood and other solutions, as shown in Table 40.7.

Table 40.7: Preparation of protein-free filtrate for the estimation of blood glucose by Folin-Wu method

Contents	*B*	*S*	*T*
Distilled water	3.4 ml	3.2 ml	3.2 ml
Standard (0.1 mg/ml)	—	0.2 ml	—
Blood	—	—	0.2 ml
10% Sodium tungstate	0.3 ml	0.3 ml	0.3 ml
2/3 N H_2SO_4	0.3 ml	0.3 ml	0.3 ml

Mix the contents and centrifuge/filter after 5 min to obtain a protein-free filtrate.

Procedure: Take 3 Folin-Wu tubes and label them as blank (B), standard (S) and test (T). To each Folin-Wu tube, add 2 ml of filtrate/supernatant from the above respective tubes. Thereafter, add 2 ml of alkaline copper reagent to each tube. Mix and keep the tubes in a boiling water bath for 6 min. Cool and add 2 ml of phosphomolybdic acid solution to each tube.

Mix and dilute the contents of each tube to 25 ml mark with distilled water. Mix and read optical density at 420 nm against water.

Calculation:

$$\begin{matrix}\text{Blood sugar}\\ \text{(mg/dl)}\end{matrix} = \frac{OD_{T-B}}{OD_{S-B}} \times \begin{matrix}\text{Concentration}\\ \text{of standard}\end{matrix}$$

$$= \frac{OD_{T-B}}{OD_{S-B}} \times 100$$

Reference value of blood sugar, for fasting venous blood, by this method is 80–120 mg/dL. Out of this, reducing substances, other than glucose, constitute nearly 20–30 mg/dL of whole blood.

Somogyi-Nelson Method

In Somogyi-Nelson method, proteins are precipitated by the addition of barium hydroxide [$Ba(OH)_2$] and zinc sulfate ($ZnSO_4$). In this method, besides proteins, sulfhydryl compounds, such as glutathione, are removed as zinc salts while other reducing substances like uric acid and creatinine, etc. are precipitated and adsorbed on barium sulfate ($BaSO_4$). The resultant filtrate is, thus, free of non-sugar reducing substances.

O-Toluidine Method

Principle: An aldohexose, such as glucose, when heated with O-toluidine in acidic medium forms a condensation product called glycosylamine and subsequently, a Schiff's base, which has blue-green color.

O-Toluidine reagent: O-Toluidine reagent contains O-toluidine, glacial acetic acid and thiourea.

Preparation of protein-free filtrate: Take 0.2 ml of blood/serum in a test tube. Add 1.8 ml of 4% trichloracetic acid, mix and centrifuge/filter after 10 min.

Procedure: Take 3 test tubes and mark them as blank (B), standard (S) and test (T). Add distilled water, standard, protein-free filtrate and O-toluidine reagent, as shown in Table 40.8.

Table 40.8: Procedure for the estimation of blood glucose by O-toluidine method

Contents	*B*	*S*	*T*
Distilled water	0.5 ml	—	—
Standard (0.1 mg/ml)	—	0.5 ml	—
Protein-free filtrate	—	—	0.5 ml
O-Toluidine reagent	2.5 ml	2.5 ml	2.5 ml

Mix and keep in a boiling water bath for 10 min. Cool under tap water and read the optical density at 630 nm, against blank.

Calculation:

$$\begin{matrix}\text{Blood glucose}\\ \text{(mg/dL)}\end{matrix} = \frac{OD_T}{OD_S} \times \begin{matrix}\text{Concentration}\\ \text{of standard}\end{matrix}$$

or

$$= \frac{OD_T}{OD_S} \times 100$$

GLUCOSE OXIDASE METHOD

It is based on the principle that glucose is oxidized by glucose oxidase. This in turns leads to the formation of H_2O_2 and gluconic acid. With the addition of the second enzyme, i.e. peroxidase, and a chromogenic oxygen acceptor, such as O-dianisidine or 4-aminophenazone, a colored compound is formed, intensity of which is directly proportional to the concentration of glucose.

This is also referred to as glucose oxidase-peroxidase (GOD/POD) method.

NORMAL VALUES

Normal value for glucose, by methods other than Folin-Wu, varies between 60 and 90 mg/dL of whole blood or 70–100 mg/dL of serum or plasma, in adults.

In neonates, blood glucose concentration varies between 30 and 60 mg/dL of serum/plasma, which is still lower in premature neonates.

GLUCOSE TOLERANCE TEST

Glucose tolerance test (GTT) determines the ability of an individual to tolerate an extra load of glucose.

Oral GTT is helpful in patients who have fasting blood glucose concentration in the upper normal limit, those with transient or sustained glycosuria without the symptoms of diabetes or those with family history of the disease, etc.

Procedure: For GTT, fasting venous blood sample (after 12–16 hours of fast) is drawn, in a fluoride-oxalate bottle. Thereafter, 75 g of glucose (about 1 g/kg body weight) is given, in nearly 200–300 ml of water, to drink. Blood samples are again drawn after every 30 minutes, till 2 to 2½ hours.

Urine specimens are also collected, simultaneously.

Each sample is analyzed and glucose tolerance curve is plotted.

Interpretation: Fasting blood glucose, maximum value of glucose, rate at which it returns to the fasting value and glycosuria give idea about the disease.

For a normal individual, fasting blood glucose value is within the normal limit. It is increased by more than two-fold within 60 min and thereafter returns to normal after about two hours of the ingestion of glucose. Moreover, glycosuria is not observed in any of the sample (Fig. 40.6).

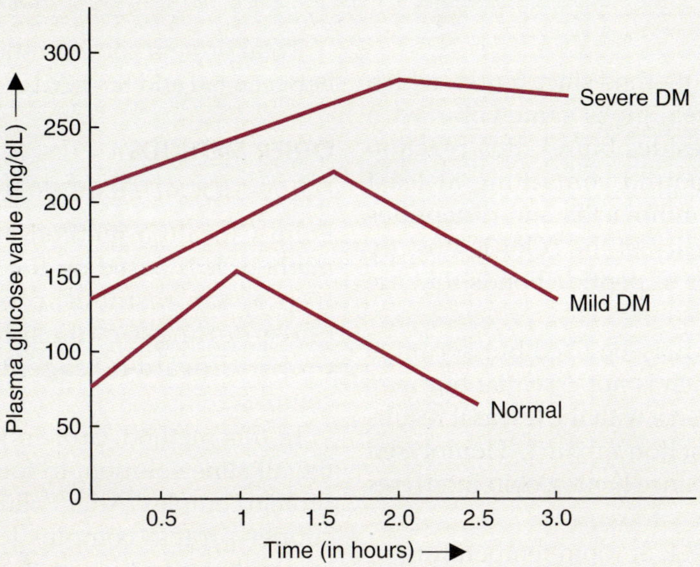

Fig. 40.6: Glucose tolerance curves

Any deviation from the above is referred to as abnormal glucose tolerance curve. In a patient with diabetes mellitus fasting blood glucose level is above the normal and/or curve is raised as well as prolonged. This is also accompanied with glycosuria.

In a patient of renal glycosuria, glucose tolerance curve is normal but there is glycosuria.

Recently, International Committee of Diabetologists has recommended simplifying the glucose tolerance test to require only an overnight fasting measurement and 2 hours sample after 75 g of oral glucose load.

An oral glucose tolerance test is normal if the fasting venous plasma glucose value is less than 100 mg/dL and the 2-hours value falls below 140 mg/dL.

A fasting value of 126 mg/dL or higher or 2 hour's value of greater than 200 mg/dl is diagnostic of diabetes mellitus.

Values between the upper limits of normal and those diagnostic of diabetes (fasting between 100 and 125 mg/dL and 2-hour value between 140 and 200 mg/dL) refer to impaired glucose tolerance (Table 40.9).

Table 40.9: Criteria for evaluating the glucose tolerance test

GTT	*Fasting Plasma Glucose (mg/dL)*	*Two hours after 75 g of glucose (mg/dL)*
Normal	<100	<140
Impaired GT	100–125	>140–199
Diabetes mellitus	>126	>200

Blood glucose concentration increases with age by about 2–3 mg/dL, per decade.

Glucose concentration in the cerebrospinal fluid (CSF) is nearly 60–65% of the serum/plasma level.

Hypoglycemia (plasma glucose concentration below 40 mg/dL) is a common and potentially dangerous complication of insulin treatment, particularly in tightly controlled diabetes. Insulinoma (benign adenoma of pancreatic islets) can also cause hypoglycemia. Estimating plasma insulin concentration, which is raised during fasting, confirms its diagnosis.

VII. ESTIMATION OF SERUM PROTEINS

Routinely, total protein estimation in serum is done by the biuret method.

BIURET METHOD

It is referred to as the biuret method since biuret, which is obtained on heating urea, gives same color with cupric ions as proteins. Besides biuret, this reaction can occur with any compound containing at least two peptide bonds. Free amino acids and dipeptides do not give this test. Intensity of the color is directly proportional to the number of peptide bonds that are present in the protein.

Either serum or plasma may be used but serum is preferred. A fasting specimen is not essential but may be preferred. Lipemia interferes with the test as it results in turbidity in the final reaction mixture. Hemolysed sample should not be used since hemoglobin interferes in this reaction.

Sample is stable for 1 week at room temperature or for 1 month at 2–4°C, if stored in a tightly stoppered bottle.

Biuret reagent: Biuret reagent which is used for the quantitative estimation of protein in serum is referred to as quantitative biuret reagent. It has copper sulfate, sodium potassium tartarate, potassium iodide and sodium hydroxide.

Principle of biuret method: Proteins and peptides (containing at least two adjacent peptide bonds) react with cupric ions (Cu^{2+}) in an alkaline solution and form violet colored complex, which has absorption maxima at 540 nm.

The complex is formed between the Cu^{2+}, and the carbonyl oxygen and amide nitrogen of the peptide bond.

Procedure: Take 3 test tubes and label them as blank (B), standard (S), and test (T).

Add distilled water, standard solution of albumin, serum and biuret reagent, as shown in Table 40.10.

Mix the contents and place the tubes for 10 min at 37°C or for 15 minutes at room temperature (if below 37°C). Read the optical density at 540 nm.

Table 40.10: Procedure for the estimation of serum protein by biuret method

Contents	*B*	*S*	*T*
Distilled water	2.5 ml	—	2.4 ml
Standard protein solution (2.8 mg/ml)	—	2.5 ml	–
Serum	—	—	0.1 ml
Biuret reagent	3.5 ml	3.5 ml	3.5 ml

Calculation:

$$\text{Serum protein (g/dL)} = \frac{OD_T}{OD_S} \times \text{Conecentration of the standard}$$

$$= \frac{OD_T}{OD_S} \times 7$$

Total protein concentration in a normal serum varies between 6.0 and 8.3 g/dL.

OTHER METHODS

FOLIN-CIOCALTEU METHOD

Folin-Ciocalteu method is also referred as Lowry's method. It is based on the principle that tyrosine and tryptophan residues, present in a protein, reduce phosphotungstic-phosphomolybdic acid reagent (Folin-Ciocalteu reagent) and form blue colored complex.

In this method, protein first reacts with the Cu^{2+} in the alkaline solution, to form a copper-peptide bound protein complex. After Folin-Ciocalteu reagent is added, copper-protein complex joins with the tyrosine and tryptophan residues, in the reduction process. Most of the color produced depends upon the Cu^{2+} complex, absorbency of which can be measured between 650–700 nm.

Detection limit of this method is 100 times lower than the biuret reaction. Thus, it is more suitable for the estimation of very low concentration of protein in a sample.

It is widely used in research to measure tissue protein and enzyme concentrations, in the purified preparations. This is, however, not satisfactory for measuring total protein concentration in urine or CSF because reagent reacts nonspecifically with the non-protein compounds.

KJELDAHL METHOD

It is based on the principle that acid digestion of a protein (after heating a protein in the presence of a strong mineral acid) converts protein nitrogen to ammonium ions (NH_4^+), concentration of which is evaluated by titration or nesslerisation. This value of ammonia nitrogen is multiplied with 6.25 (considering the average nitrogen content of the protein as 16%) to get the concentration of protein in the sample.

It is a very accurate method but time consuming and inconvenient in practice. So, it is not used routinely. It is, however, used for the standardization of the reference material for the biuret method.

REFRACTOMETERY

It is a quick alternative to chemical analysis for serum total protein when a rapid estimation is required. Refractometery is based on the principle that refractive index of water at 20°C is 1.33. When a solute is added to water, the refractive index value of the solution is increased linearly, proportionately to the concentration of the solute.

> **ALBUMIN: GLOBULIN RATIO**
>
> **Albumin:** Globulins ratio (A : G ratio) can be calculated by estimating albumin and then subtracting its value from the value of the total serum protein.
>
> Globulins = Total serum protein – albumin
>
> $$\text{A : G ratio} = \frac{\text{Concentration of albumin (g / dl)}}{\text{Concentration of globulins (g / dl)}}$$
>
> Normal value for A : G ratio varies from 1.5 : 1 to 2.5 : 1.

Clinical refractometers are pre-calibrated for total solids and the concentration of protein in the sample is directly expressed in g/dL.

Large positive errors occur with azotemia and hyperglycemia. At protein concentration less than 3.5 g/dL, results are not very accurate.

SERUM ALBUMIN

Serum albumin is estimated by dye binding method.

Dyes, such as bromocresol green (BCG), bind very specifically to albumin. On addition of alkali, color of BCG is changed from green to blue, intensity of which is proportional to the amount of albumin present in the serum.

SEPARATION OF PLASMA PROTEINS BY ELECTROPHORESIS

Electrophoresis is a technique for the separation of the charged particles by means of electric current. A charged particle, when placed in an electric field, migrates either towards the anode or the cathode, depending upon the net charge carried by the particles.

Different molecules migrate at different speeds depending upon their charge, particle size and shape. Their movement occurs in a liquid medium (a buffer), supported on an inert material, like filter paper, cellulose acetate strip, agar gel, starch gel or polyacrylamide gel.

Paper Electrophoresis

In paper electrophoresis, a strip of filter paper is dipped in a buffered solution (barbitone buffer, pH 8.6) and is laid on a platform. Two ends of the strip are dipped in the buffer. Entire apparatus is covered with a sheet to minimize evaporation. Two electrodes are also dipped in two compartments containing buffer. Current is supplied through a power supply which either supplies constant current and/or voltage. Current is carried by the charged particles and depending upon the charge, protein migrates towards either anode or cathode.

Procedure: About 10 ml of serum is applied along a thin line near the cathode. Since at pH 8.6, all the proteins carry a net negative charge and tend to migrate towards the anode, thus, on passing a constant current (about 1–2 mA per strip), different proteins migrate at different rates. At the end, their positions are revealed by some dye, such as bromophenol blue, which stains proteins. Different proteins form separate bands on the paper strip.

In the normal serum five bands are observed. Since albumin carries largest number of the negative charges, it moves fastest while γ-globulin has less negative charges and moves the least. Starting from anode, these bands are designated as albumin, α_1-globulin, α_2-globulin, β-globulin and γ-globulin.

Pattern of serum protein on electrophoresis may be used in the diagnosis of a disease, e.g. multiple myeloma (*see* Chapter 26).

ALTERATIONS IN SERUM PROTEINS

Alterations in serum proteins may be observed due to a change either in plasma water or concentration of a specific plasma protein (albumin or globulin).

Hypoproteinemia

Decrease in total protein concentration in serum below normal is referred to as hypoproteinemia.

Increase in plasma volume (hemodilution) is reflected as relative hypoproteinemia. Hemodilution may occur with water intoxication or salt retention, during massive intravenous infusion or physiologically when a recumbent position is assumed. The latter, in turn, decreases total protein concentration by 0.3 to 0.5 g/dL.

Hypoproteinemia is consistently related to low concentration of albumin (hypoalbuminemia) which may be a result of:

1. Decreased protein intake such as in kwashiorkor,
2. Decreased synthesis of albumin, e.g. in a chronic liver disease (hepatitis, cirrhosis, etc.),
3. Increased loss of albumin from body, e.g. in protein losing enteropathy or a renal disease, such as nephrotic syndrome, or
4. In a protein catabolic state, like high grade fever or acute infections, such as tuberculosis.

Hyperproteinemia

Increase in total protein concentration in serum, above normal, is referred to as hyperproteinemia.

It may be a result of:

1. **Hemoconcentration:** Hemoconcentration (decrease in volume of plasma water) is reflected as relative hyperproteinemia, e.g. in burns (above 20%). It may also be observed in dehydration due to either inadequate intake of water or excessive water loss, such as severe vomiting, diarrhea, Addison disease, diabetic acidosis, etc.
2. **Hyperglobulinemia:** High levels of the monoclonal immunoglobulins produced in multiple myeloma and other malignant paraproteinemia may cause marked hyperproteinemia.

VIII. ESTIMATION OF SERUM CREATININE

The amount of creatinine, which is produced daily, is related to muscle mass and does not vary greatly. Thus, its level in the blood remains fairly constant.

Free creatinine is a waste product of creatine. It is present in all body fluids and secretions. Creatinine is freely filtered by the glomerulus. Although, it is not reabsorbed, a small amount of it is secreted by renal tubules. Hence, its clearance is measured as an indicator of GFR.

Principle: Estimation of creatinine is based on the reaction with alkaline picrate, first described by **Jaffe**. In this reaction, creatinine reacts with picrate ions, in alkaline medium to yield an orange-red complex.

For the estimation of creatinine in serum, a protein-free filtrate is prepared.

Preparation of protein-free filtrate: Take 1 ml of serum in a test tube. Add 1 ml each of distilled water, sodium tungstate and sulfuric acid (2/3 N). Mix the contents and filter/centrifuge after 10 min to obtain protein-free filtrate.

Procedure: Take 3 test tubes and mark them as blank (B), standard (S) and test (T).

Add distilled water, standard, protein-free filtrate and other reagents, as shown in Table 40.11.

Mix the contents and read optical density at 520 nm, after 15 min.

Table 40.11: Procedure for the estimation of serum creatinine

Contents	*B*	*S*	*T*
Distilled water	4 ml	3 ml	2 ml
Standard creatinine solution (0.01 mg/ml)	—	1 ml	—
Protein-free filtrate	—	—	2 ml
NaOH	1 ml	1 ml	1 ml
Picric acid	1 ml	1 ml	1 ml

Calculation:

$$\text{S. creatinine (mg/dL)} = \frac{OD_T}{OD_S} \times \text{Concentration of standard}$$

Or

$$= \frac{OD_T}{OD_S} \times 2$$

Normal value for serum (plasma) creatinine is 0.8–1.5 mg/dl.

Value is slightly increased in elderly individuals due to its decreased excretion. Serum level is lower in women than in men. Serum creatinine is increased in renal failure and obstruction to urine outflow.

IX. NORMAL AND ABNORMAL COSTITUENTS OF URINE

NORMAL COSTITUENTS OF URINE

INORGANIC SUBSTANCES

Chloride

To demonstrate the presence of chloride in urine, take 5 ml of urine in a test tube. Add few drops of concentrate nitric acid and 2–3 drops of silver nitrate solution. A white precipitate, due to the formation of silver chloride, is observed indicating the presence of chloride in urine.

Nitric acid is added to prevent precipitation of phosphates, urates and other organic radicals, which may be present in the urine.

Phosphates

To demonstrate the presence of phosphates, take 3 ml of urine in a test tube and add few drops of concentrate nitric acid. Then add 3 ml of 5% ammonium molybdate solution to it. A yellow precipitate of ammonium phosphomolybdate is seen, which indicates the presence of phosphates in urine.

Sulfates

To demonstrate the presence of sulfates, take 5 ml of urine in a test tube and add 2–3 drops of concentrate hydrochloric acid. Add few drops of barium chloride solution. A white precipitate of barium sulfate is observed, indicating the presence of sulfates in urine.

Hydrochloric acid is added to prevent precipitation of phosphates and other salts of barium.

Ammonia

To demonstrate the presence of ammonia, take 5 ml of urine in a test tube. Cautiously, add dilute sodium hydroxide until the mixture is faint pink. Dip a glass rod in the solution of phenolphthalein. Boil the contents of the tube and hold the glass rod on the top of it. Phenolphthalein turns pink due to vapors of ammonia.

NONPROTEIN NITROGENOUS SUBSTANCES

Urea

Presence of urea in the urine can be shown by the alkaline hypobromite test where urea is decomposed under the influence of sodium hypobromite and liberates CO_2 and N_2. CO_2 is absorbed by sodium hydroxide and the effervescences are observed due to evolution of nitrogen.

To demonstrate the presence of urea in urine, take 5 ml of urine in a test tube and add 3–4 drops of the hypobromite reagent. Effervescences are observed due to the evolution of N_2 which is liberated from urea, thereby showing the presence of urea in urine.

Hypobromite reagent is prepared by mixing equal volume of concentrate sodium hydroxide solution with bromine water.

Uric Acid

Using Benedict's uric acid reagent (alkaline phosphotungstic acid solution), uric acid can be detected qualitatively. Uric acid reduces this reagent and leads to formation of tungsten blue, producing blue color.

To demonstrate the presence of uric acid in urine, take 2 ml of urine in a test tube. Make it alkaline by adding a pinch of sodium carbonate. Add few drops of uric acid reagent and mix the contents. Deep blue color is observed, confirming the presence of uric acid in urine.

Creatinine

Creatinine is detected by alkaline picric acid solution. This is known as Jaffe's reaction.

To demonstrate the presence of creatinine in urine, take 5 ml of urine in a test tube and add 1 ml of saturated picric acid solution. Make this mixture alkaline with the addition of 1 ml of 10% sodium hydroxide solution. A reddish-orange color, due to the formation of creatinine picrate, is observed indicating the presence of creatinine in urine.

ABNORMAL CONSTITUENTS OF URINE

Sugar

Presence of sugar in the urine can be detected by **Benedict test.**

Take 5 ml of qualitative Benedict's reagent in a test tube and add 0.5 ml (8–10 drops) of the urine sample. Contents of the tube are boiled for 1–2 min and allowed to cool, thereafter. In the presence of a reducing sugar, red colored precipitate of cuprous oxide is seen.

Depending upon the quantity of sugar in the sample, contents of the tube may be seen as green, yellow, orange or red. This intensity of the precipitate can also be indicated by arbitrary signs as 1+, 2+, 3+ or 4+. This test not only indicates the presence of sugar in the urine but also its approximate concentration indicating that it is a semiquantitative test (Table 40.12).

Table 40.12: Qualitative Benedict test

Color of the solution (with precipitate)	*Arbitrary sign (unit)*	*Approximate concentration of sugar in urine (g/dL)*
Green	1+	Up to 0.5
Yellow	2+	About 1.0
Orange	3+	About 1.5
Red	4+	2.0 or above

Ketone Bodies

Ketone bodies may be detected by **Rothera test**, using sodium nitroprusside.

Take 5 ml of urine in a test tube and saturate it with ammonium sulfate powder, by shaking. Add 2–3 drops of 5% sodium nitroprusside solution. Mix and add few drops of liquid ammonia (ammonium hydroxide) from the side of the tube. Development of purple/violet color indicates the presence of ketone bodies.

Proteins

Presence of protein in the urine can be confirmed by various tests such as **sulphosalicylic acid test, heat coagulation test or nitric acid test**.

Sulphosalicylic acid test: To 2 ml of urine, add few drops of 20% sulphosalicylic acid solution. White precipitate (turbidity), due to denaturation of albumin by sulphosalicylic acid, indicates the presence of protein in urine.

Heat coagulation test: Fill two-thirds of test tube with the urine and adjust its pH to 4.6 (the isoelectric pH of albumin). It may be done by adding a drop of chlorophenol red, followed by few drops of either dilute acetic acid (until the red color is discharged) or dilute sodium carbonate (till pink color appears). Gently heat the upper part of the fluid to boiling. Turbidity indicates the presence of protein or phosphates.

Add few drops of dilute acetic acid. Phosphates are dissolved. If turbidity persists, it is due to coagulation of albumin.

Nitric acid test: Take 5 ml concentrate nitric acid in a test tube. Slowly add urine along the side of tube so that it forms a separate layer, above the acid. A white ring, due to precipitation of protein by nitric acid, is observed. This is referred to as **Heller test**.

Test for Bence-Jones Proteins: Take 5 ml urine in a test tube. Heat it carefully by immersing in a beaker of warm water. Urine becomes turbid at 40°C and shows a precipitate, up to 60°C. On increasing the temperature above 60°C precipitate disappears. It again reappears on cooling.

Blood

Benzidine test or O-toluidine test can show presence of blood (hemoglobin) in the urine.

Take 3 ml of benzidine/O-toluidine reagent (saturated solution of benzidine or O-toluidine in glacial acetic acid) in a clean and dry test tube. Add 3 ml of hydrogen peroxide, mix and pour one-half of it to another tube. To one of the tubes, add few drops of water (to serve as control). To the other tube add few drops of urine. Fluid rapidly acquires a deep-blue color, due to the presence of hemoglobin.

The principle of the test is that hemoglobin acts as pseudoperoxidase and decomposes hydrogen peroxide. Oxygen is liberated, which, in turn, oxidizes benzidine/O-toluidine and forms blue-colored complex. On exposure to air, blue color rapidly changes to brown within few minutes.

Bile

Bile salts: Bile salts are surface-active agents. They form a layer on the surface of water and lower its surface tension.

This principle is used to detect the presence of bile salts in the urine and is referred to as **Hay's sulfur test**.

Fill the test tube with urine and sprinkle powdered sulfur on the top of it. Sulfur powder sinks.

When similar test is repeated with water, sulfur does not sink.

Due to surface tension (unbalanced force at the surface) sulfur powder floats on the surface. When bile salts are present, they lower surface tension and sulfur goes down.

Bile pigments: Bile pigments are the degradation products of heme. On oxidation, heme forms a series of colored compounds, such as biliverdin (green) and bilirubin (yellow).

Following tests are commonly performed to show to presence of bile pigments in the urine:

Gmelin test: Take 3 ml of fuming HNO_3 in a test tube and add 3 ml of urine (without disturbing the HNO_3 layer). Gently rotate the tube. At the junction of the two fluids, multicolored rings are formed due to the oxidation of bilirubin by HNO_3. Starting from the acid layer to the bile layer, the color is yellow, red, violet, blue and green.

Fouchet test: Take 5 ml urine in a test tube and acidify it by adding 1–2 drops of acetic acid. Add 5 ml of 10% barium chloride solution and 2–3 drops of the saturated solution of ammonium sulfate. Mix, allow to stand for 5 min and filter. Collect the precipitate.

Bilirubin is adsorbed on the precipitate of barium sulfate, giving it a yellow color. Unfold the filter paper, allow extra water to drain (by laying on dry filter papers) and carefully add 1 drop of Fouchet reagent on the precipitate. Blue-green color indicates the presence of bile pigments.

Fouchet reagent consists of trichloroacetic acid and ferric chloride.

Ammonium sulfate and $BaCl_2$ react to form the precipitate of BaSO4 which adsorbs bile pigments. They are released by trichloroacetic acid and react with $FeCl_3$, which oxidizes bilirubin (blue) to biliverdin and gives green color.

Urobilinogen

Presence of urobilinogen can be tested by **Ehrlich test**.

One ml of Ehrlich's reagent is added to 10 ml of urine in a test tube. A deep-red color is seen. Color remains light red with the normal sample. Rapidity and intensity of the color gives the idea about the quantity of urobilinogen in urine.

Ehrlich's reagent is prepared by dissolving *p*-dimethylaminobenzaldehyde in hydrochloric acid.

X. SAMPLE COLLECTION AND REFERENCE VALUES

SAMPLE COLLECTION

COLLECTION OF BLOOD

Biochemical tests are performed on any kind of body fluid but mostly on **blood, plasma** or **serum**. The type of test required dictates what type of sample is to be used? Proper sample collection and handling is an integral part of obtaining a valid and timely laboratory test result. Specimens must be obtained using proper phlebotomy techniques, collected in the proper container, correctly labelled (in the presence of the patient) and promptly transported to the laboratory.

Timing of Collection

Blood composition is significantly altered after consuming food, which consequently alters many clinical chemistry tests.

- In routine, the basal state, i.e. the **early morning** (approximately 12 hours after the last ingestion of food) is recommended for determining concentration of the various body constituents, such as glucose, lipoproteins, cholesterol, triglycerides, electrolytes and proteins.
- However, for glucose alone, fasting of four hours is sufficient.
- When the primary lipids of interest are serum total cholesterol and high density lipoprotein cholesterol, blood can be taken at any time of the day, i.e. with the subject even nonfasting.
- It is necessary to provide the patient, in advance, with appropriate collection instructions and information on fasting, diet and medication restrictions, when necessary.

Position of the Subject

Position of the subject can influence results of some of the analytes thus, standardization of the position is necessary. It is, generally, recommended that all blood

DRY CHEMISTRY

In clinical practice presence of an abnormal constituent can also be detected in the urine by the use of strips, called dipsticks. A dipstick is a thin strip of plastic with one or more cellulose pads fixed on it. Each pad is saturated with buffer and certain chemicals, which are present on the pad in the dry form. Hence, this technique is called **dry chemistry**.

Dipsticks are also referred to as **uristicks (uristixs)** since they are used for the analysis of urine.

Principle: Various chemicals, fixed on the pad, get activated when they soak water (from the urine sample). These reagents then react with the test component of the urine and change the color. Presence of an abnormal constituent in the urine can thus be detected and its approximate concentration can be found by comparing the color with the chart provided by the manufacturer.

Table 35.13 lists basic principle of each test with the use of dipsticks.

Table 40.13: Basic principle of urine analysis with dipsticks

Test	*Principle*	*Reagent used*
pH	Double indicator	Methyl red and bromothymol blue
Protein	Protein error of indicators	Citrate buffer (pH 3.0), bromophenol blue, and protein absorbent
Glucose	Double sequential enzyme reaction	Glucose oxidase-peroxidase and buffer
Ketone bodies	Sodium nitroprusside	Sodium nitroprusside and glycine buffer
Blood	Pseudoperoxidase activity of hemoglobin	O-toluidine, H_2O_2, and buffer
Bile pigments (bilirubin)	Diazo reaction	Diazo reagent
Urobilinogen	Ehrlich reaction	Buffered *p*-dimethylaminobenzaldehyde

Various types of dipsticks are commercially available. Some of these are specific for a particular test and have a single pad whereas others have two or more pads and are used for various test combinations.

Precautions: There are a number of precautions, which should be observed for the successful use of these dipsticks:

1. As reagents (most of them enzymes) have a fixed shelf life, dipsticks should not be used after the date of expiry.
2. Dipsticks should be properly stored in an area free from moisture, as moisture may inactivate the chemicals.
3. Test area of the strip (pad) should not be physically touched.
4. The test strip should be immersed in the sample only for a very short period (2-seconds) and should be tapped thereafter to remove the excess of water. Immersion for longer time may dissolve chemicals and wash the pad.
5. Allowable time, before color comparison, as per manufacturer, should be strictly complied with.

samples should be drawn in a sitting position and that the participant remain in sitting position for 15 minutes prior to blood collection. This waiting period will allow equilibration of the concentration of blood components.

Venipuncture

Venipuncture, venopuncture or venepuncture, in medicine, is the process of obtaining intravenous access for blood sampling of **venous blood**. This procedure is performed by medical laboratory technologist, medical practitioner, phlebotomist nursing staff. It is one of the most routinely performed invasive procedures carried out to obtain blood for diagnostic purposes as well as to monitor levels of blood components.

There are many ways in which blood can be drawn from a vein. The best method varies with the age of the patient, equipment available and tests required:

- Venipuncture, **using a needle and tube**, is the most common method for the collection of blood.
- Blood collection can also be done with an evacuated tube system called **vacutainer**, which consists of a plastic hub, a hypodermic needle and a vacuum tube.
- On some occasions, blood may be collected by puncturing the skin with a retractable **lancet** device.

Use of tourniquet: Prolonged venous occlusion can cause changes in the concentration of blood constituents. Therefore, use of a tourniquet should be minimized. If a tourniquet is used, **it should be released before withdrawal of blood begins**. In any case, the use of a tourniquet should be limited to less than one minute.

Site of venipuncture: Preferably, blood should not be collected from the arm that is used for blood pressure measurement, i.e. blood should usually be drawn from **the left arm**.

- Blood samples should be taken from the vein in the antecubital fossa.
- Before blood collection, the subject should remove tight clothes that might constrict the upper arm.
- During blood collection, the arm should rest on some supportive prop.
- Though larger median cubital and cephalic veins are the usual choice but the basilic vein on the dorsum of the arm or dorsal hand veins are also acceptable.
- Foot veins are a last resort because of the higher probability of complications.

Venipuncture procedure: The venipuncture procedure is complex, requiring both, knowledge and skill, to perform. Several essential steps are required for every successful collection procedure:

1. The first step to the collection is to positively **identify the patient** by two forms of identification, i.e. ask the patient to state and spell his/her name and give you his/her age. Check these against the requisition form.
2. **Check the requisition form** for requested tests, patient information and any special requirement.
3. **Gather the tubes** and supplies that one will need for the drawl of blood.
4. **Position the patient** in a chair, or sitting or lying on a bed.
5. **Wash your hands.**
6. **Select a suitable site for venipuncture** by placing the tourniquet 3 to 4 inches above the selected puncture site on the patient. Do not put the tourniquet too tightly or leave it on the patient for longer than 1 minute.
7. **Put on** non-latex **gloves** and **palpate for a vein**.
8. When a vein is selected, **clean the area** in a circular motion, beginning at the site and working outward. Allow the area to air dry. After the area is cleansed, it should not be touched or palpated again. If you find it necessary to re-evaluate the site by palpation, the area needs to be re-cleaned before the venipuncture is performed.
9. **Grasp the patient's arm** firmly, using your thumb to draw the skin taut and anchor the vein.
10. **Swiftly insert the needle** through the skin into the lumen of the vein. The needle should form a 15–30 degree angle with the arm surface (Fig. 40.7).
11. **Avoid excess probing**.
12. When the last tube is filling, **remove the tourniquet**.
13. **Remove the needle** from the patient's arm using a swift backward motion.
14. **Place gauze immediately on the puncture site.** Apply and hold adequate pressure to avoid formation of hematoma. After holding pressure for 1–2 minutes, tape a fresh piece of gauze to the puncture site.
15. **Dispose of the contaminated materials**/supplies in designated containers.

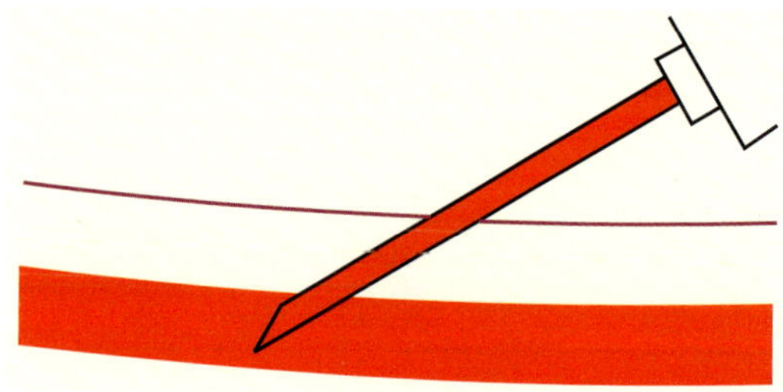

Fig. 40.7: Collection of blood sample

Disposal of the Syringe, Needle and other Material

Needle disposal boxes should be available for all personnel, drawing blood samples.

- Needles should be released from adapters directly to the needle disposal box.
- Needles should never be re-sheathed after use.
- The disposal box should not be allowed to become overfull to avoid potential hazard.

Whole Blood, Serum or Plasma?

It is imperative that the *in vivo* state of a constituent remains unchanged after withdrawal from the body fluid of a patient, to obtain a valid medical laboratory result. Historically, serum is the preferred assay material for determining extracellular concentrations of the constituents in blood. These days even plasma is preferred for many, but not all, laboratory investigations.

Whole blood: Blood is a bodily fluid that delivers necessary substances, such as nutrients and oxygen to the cell, and transport metabolic waste products away from the cells.

- Whole blood is **composed of cells suspended in blood plasma.** The blood cells are mainly red blood cells (also called RBCs or erythrocytes) and white blood cells, including leukocytes and platelets.
- In a venous, arterial or capillary blood sample, concentrations and properties of cellular and extracellular constituents remain relatively unaltered when compared with their *in vivo* state.

- Anticoagulation, *in vitro*, stabilizes the constituents in a whole blood sample for a certain period of time.

Serum: Serum is the **undiluted, yellow watery part of blood that is left after blood** has been allowed to clot and all blood cells have been removed. This is most easily done by centrifugation which packs the denser blood cells and platelets to the bottom of the centrifuge tube, leaving the liquid serum fraction, resting above the packed cells. Serum is used for many tests. For this purpose:

- Blood is collected into a tube **without any anticoagulant** and allowed to clot.
- **Leave** the container at room temperature, for at least **30 minutes**, to separate serum from blood cells. This period is shorter when coagulation has been activated.

Plasma: Plasma is the **cell-free supernatant of blood containing anticoagulant**, obtained after centrifugation. It constitutes about 55% of the blood fluid. It is mostly water (92% by volume) and contains dissipated proteins, glucose, mineral ions, hormones and carbon dioxide. It is obtained by centrifugation, before clotting of blood occurs.

- Plasma samples can be centrifuged directly after sample collection, unlike serum in which coagulation is completed after 30 minutes.
- Nearly 15 to 20% more volume can be obtained than serum, from the same volume of blood.
- Blood collected in additive tubes (anticoagulant tubes) must be mixed by gently inverting the tube several times, to ensure even distribution of the additive in the specimen. For this purpose, tilt the tube repeatedly (do not shake and avoid foaming), immediately after filling, to mix the sample thoroughly with the anticoagulant.
- Only the recommended quantity of the anticoagulant should be added to avoid errors in results.

Use of Anticoagulants

Anticoagulants are the additives that inhibit blood from clotting, ensuring that the constituent to be measured is not significantly changed. Anticoagulation occurs by binding calcium ions, such as by EDTA or citrate, or by inhibiting thrombin activity, e.g. by heparin. Commonly used anticoagulants that are mixed with blood, immediately after sample collection, include:

EDTA: Dipotassium (K_2), tripotassium (K_3) or disodium (Na2) salt of EDTA (ethylene diamine tetra-acetic acid) is used in a concentration of 1.2 to 2.0 mg/mL of blood, in a powdered form. It strongly and irreversibly chelates calcium ion to prevent blood from clotting.

Some of tests are interfered with the addition of EDTA especially potassium while using K_2 EDTA. In such a case heparin should be used, as an alternative. Tubes with liquid EDTA reduce the risk of hemolysis that sometimes may occur with the tubes using EDTA in the powder form.

Citrate: Trisodium citrate (3–4%) or citric acid, as buffered-citrate (pH 5.5 to 5.6), is used in the liquid form, in the tubes for coagulation tests as well as in blood transfusion bags. A mixture of one part of citrate with nine parts of blood is recommended for coagulation tests while one part of citrate is mixed with four parts of blood to determine the erythrocyte sedimentation rate (ESR).

Citrate binds calcium ions but not as strongly as EDTA. Correct proportion of the anticoagulant solution is important to avoid excessive dilution of the blood.

Oxalate: Oxalate acts by the mechanism similar to that of citrate. It is an anticoagulant used in fluoride-oxalate tubes for glucose and lactate determinations.

Heparin: About 12 to 30 IU/mL of unfractionated sodium, lithium or ammonium salt of heparin is recommended, to obtain heparinized plasma. Calcium-titrated heparin at a concentration of 8 to 12 IU/mL of blood is recommended for the determination of ionized calcium.

Fluoride: Fluoride tubes are used for blood glucose determination.

Hemolytic, Icteric or Lipemic Sample?

Laboratory tests are affected by several endogenous and exogenous factors in the sample matrix. The relevant observation should be mentioned for each sample, e.g. **hemolytic, icteric, opalescent** and **turbid** or **lipemic**, if a relevant color or turbidity is seen.

Hemolytic sample: Hemolysis is defined as release of the intracellular components of erythrocytes and other blood cells into the extracellular fluid of blood. After separation of the blood cells, hemolysis may be visible by the red color of serum or plasma. Cell constituents, particularly those with an intracellular concentration of 10 times higher than the extracellular concentration, will increase in plasma/serum during hemolysis, e.g. potassium, lactate dehydrogenase, aspartate aminotransferase, etc. Sample associated with greater degree of hemolysis may also interfere with other laboratory tests.

Icteric sample: Bilirubin occurs in plasma as a free molecule as well as covalently bound to albumin. In addition, water soluble bilirubin conjugates also exist as mono- and di-glucuronides. Conjugated bilirubin also appears in urine when present at increased concentration in blood. In patients with proteinuria, bilirubin bound to albumin can also appear in urine.

Bilirubin interferes in oxidase/peroxidase based test systems. Proportionally to its concentration, bilirubin reacts with H_2O_2 which is formed in the test system. This in turn causes systematically lower

Table 40.14: Sequence of filling the tubes for various biochemical tests

Type of analysis	*Specimen type*	*Volume required and type of tube*
Lipids	Serum	10 ml, plain tube
Glucose	Plasma	4 ml, tube filled with glycolytic inhibitors, i.e. potassium oxalate and sodium fluoride
Glycated-hemoglobin	Whole blood	3 ml, tube with anticoagulant K2•EDTA

results in enzymatic procedures that are used for the measurement of glucose, cholesterol, triglycerides, uric acid and creatinine.

Bilirubin also competitively interferes with dyes, which bind to albumin.

Lipemic sample: Lipemia is a turbidity of serum or plasma which is caused by the elevated lipoprotein concentration and is visible by the eye. A sufficiently transparent sample container must be used to detect lipemia. Post-centrifugal coagulation of serum samples of heparinized patients can also be the cause of turbidity.

Most often, lipemia results from increased triglycerides concentration in plasma/serum. This can be due to food intake, altered lipid metabolism or infusion of lipids. After intestinal absorption, triglycerides are present in plasma, as chylomicrons, for 6 to 12 hours. Lipemia in plasma or serum is visually observed at triglycerides concentration above 300 mg/dL. In whole blood, triglycerides concentration above 1000 mg/dL cause turbidity that can be detected by visual inspection. Centrifugation for 10 minutes at 1000 g is effective, when chylomicrons are present and turbidity is seen.

Sequence of Filling the Tubes for Various biochemical tests

The order, in which various tubes are filled, is determined by the risk of contamination and coagulation. The following sequence for filling tubes with blood from a patient is recommended to avoid contamination, i.e. serum, citrate, heparin and EDTA-containing tubes. So, EDTA samples should be drawn last and plain tubes first.

The recommended order is:

1. Blood for blood culture
2. Tubes for serum (avoid serum as first tube when electrolytes shall be measured)
3. Citrate-filled tubes
4. Heparin-filled tubes
5. EDTA-containing tubes, and
6. Tubes containing additional stabilizers (e.g. fluoride as glycolytic inhibitor).

Another consideration that might affect the order of tube filling is the priority of the assay for which the tubes are needed.

If there are any problems with blood flow during its withdrawl, e.g. collapsing vein, the procedure should be discontinued and an attempt should be made on the other arm.

Depending on the scheduled analyses, tubes should be filled in the following order, as shown in Table 40.14.

Before the subject leaves the examination site and the rack is moved, all the tubes should be labelled with the subject identification code.

Storage and Transport of the Sample

Non-centrifuged samples should not be stored at room temperature for longer time. Do not freeze whole blood samples before or after centrifugation. Samples may be refrigerated to 4°C.

For transport, samples should be properly marked and transfer list should be kept, in order to check for any possible loss of the sample.

COLLECTION OF URINE

For the quantitation of creatinine, protein, 17-ketosteroids or VMA in urine, 24 hours sample is collected in 2 litres bottle with few crystals of thymol.

For calcium 10 ml of 6 N HCl is added in the bottle.

First morning and midstream urine sample (about 25–30 ml) is collected for Bence Jones protein as well as urobilinogen.

REFERENCE RANGES OF SOME IMPORTANT CONSTITUENTS OF URINE, CSF, GASTRIC JUICE AND BLOOD

The range of reference values of some important constituents of blood, urine, CSF and gastric juice are shown for male adults, in the fasting state, in conventional units, in Tables 40.15–40.18.

Table 40.15: Reference values for some of the constituents in urine

Constituent	*Normal range*
D-xylose	1–2 g/5 hr
Total nitrogen	10–20 g/24 hr
Creatinine	1.0–2.0 g/24 hr
Calcium	0.1–0.7 g/24 hr
Chloride	110–250 meq/24 hr
Sodium	40–220 meq/24 hr
Potassium	25–125 meq/24 hr
Phosphorus	0.6–1.5 g/24 hr
Urea	20–35 g/24 hr

Table 40.16: Reference values of some of the constituents in CSF

Constituent	*Normal range*
Total protein	15–40 mg/dL
Glucose	50–75 mg/dL
Chloride (as NaCl)	700–750 mg/dL 118–132 mmol/L

Table 40.17: Reference values for some of the parameters in gastric juice

Parameter	*Normal range*
Volume	2–3 L/24 hr
pH	1.6–1.8
Titrable acidity (fasting sample)	15–35 mEq/L
Basal Acid Output	
Males	1.0–5.0 mEq/hr
Females	0.2–3.8 mEq/hr
Maximal Acid Output (After Histamine/Pentagastrin)	
Males	18–28 mEq/hr
Females	11–21 mEq/hr

Table 40.18: Reference values of some of the constituents of blood

Constituent	*Normal range*
Common Constituents	
Bilirubin (total)	0.2–0.8 mg/dL
Calcium (total)	9–11 mg/dL
Cholesterol (total)	140–220 mg/dL
Creatinine	0.8–1.3 mg/dL
Glucose (fasting)	60–100 mg/dL
Phosphorus (inorganic)	3.0–4.5 mg/dL
Urea	15–40 mg/dL
Uric acid	3–7 mg/dL

Contd...

Table 40.18: Reference values of some of the constituents of blood (*Contd...)*

Constituent	*Normal range*
Proteins	
Total serum proteins	6.0–8.3 g/dL
Serum albumin	3.7–5.3 g/dL
Serum globulins	1.8–3.7 g/dL
A/G ratio	1.2–2.0
Lipid Profile	
Serum triglycerides	50–160 mg/dL
Total cholesterol	140–220 mg/dL
HDL-cholesterol	30–60 mg/dL
LDL-cholesterol	60–160 mg/dL
VLDL-cholesterol	up to 32 mg/dL
Electrolytes	
Sodium	136–145 mEq/L
Potassium	3.5–5.0 mEq/L
Chloride	98–107 mEq/L
Enzymes	
Acid phosphatase	1–3.5 KA units/L
Alkaline phosphatase	3–13 KA units/L
Amylase	60–180 Somogyi U/L
LDH	100–190 U/L
SGOT	up to 40 U/L
SGPT	up to 40 U/L
CPK (Total)	20–90 U/L
Hormones	
Cortisol	5–25 mg/dL (8 AM)
T_3	70–200 ng/dL
T_4	5–12 ng/dL
TSH	0–5 mU/ml
Acid–Base Analysis and Blood Gases	
pH	7.35–7.45
Total CO_2	22–28 mmol/L
Bicarbonate (actual)	22–26 mmol/L
pCO_2	31–45 mm of Hg
pO_2	85–95 mm of Hg
Oxygen saturation	96–100%
Anion gap $[(Na^+ + K^+) - (Cl^- + HCO_3^-)]$	12–16 mmol/L
Base excess	–2 to +3 mmol/L

Index